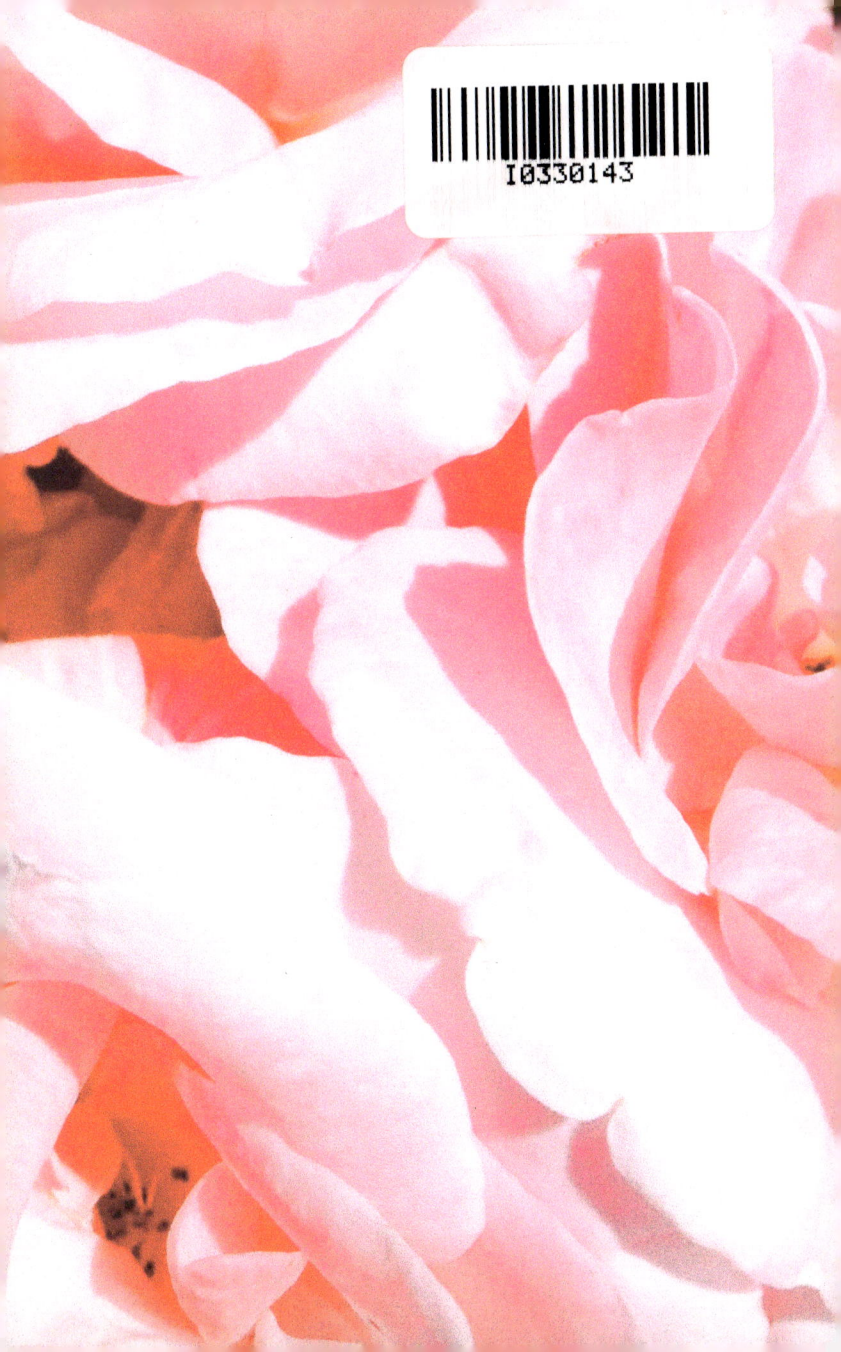

365 days of happiness

A Lifetime of Joy

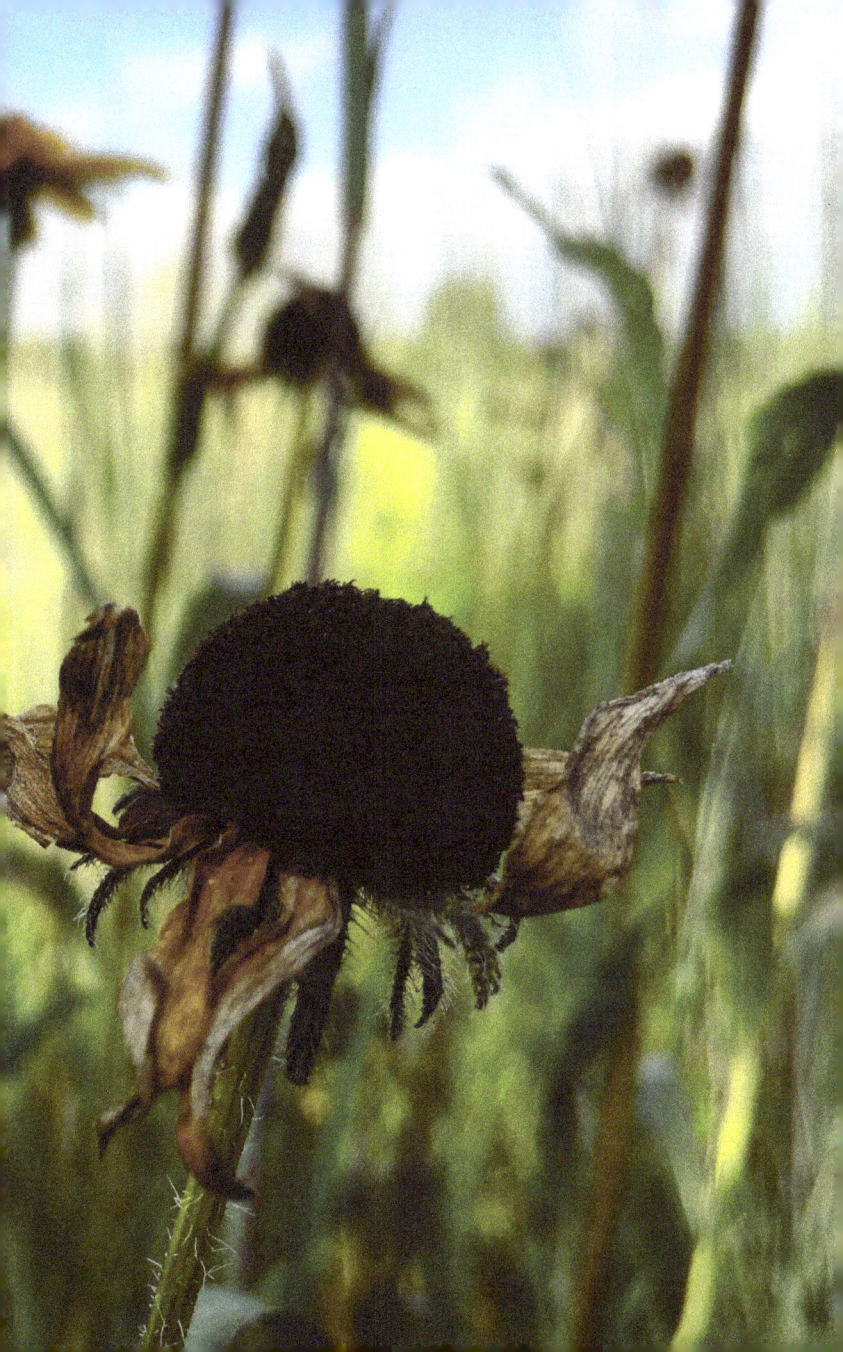

Copyright © 2016 Laura Paulisich
Photographs copyright © 2016 Laura Paulisich
www.laurapaulisich.com

All rights reserved.
First Printing, 2016
ISBN 978-0-9981899-1-8

Design by Laura Paulisich

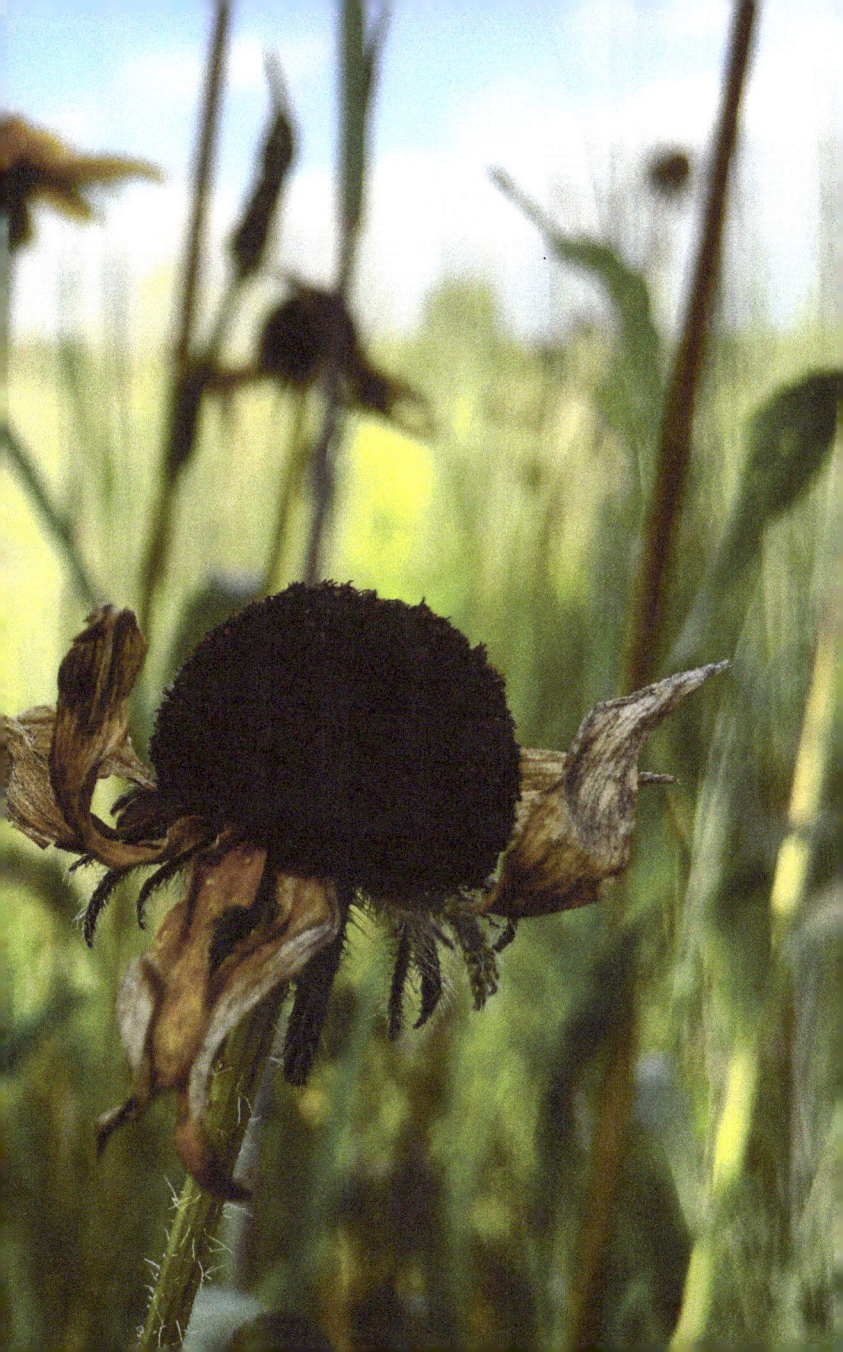

FOREWORD

In this short book of daily meditations Laura compiled the great wisdoms of current and past wise sages, wisdoms gleaned through woken heart, hard work, and hopeful journeys harvested through a soul centered in the deep wells of the sacred! It's a treasure chest full of incredibly satiating, healing, and healthy marrow for the heart, the mind, and the whole Being!!

Kifah A. Abdi

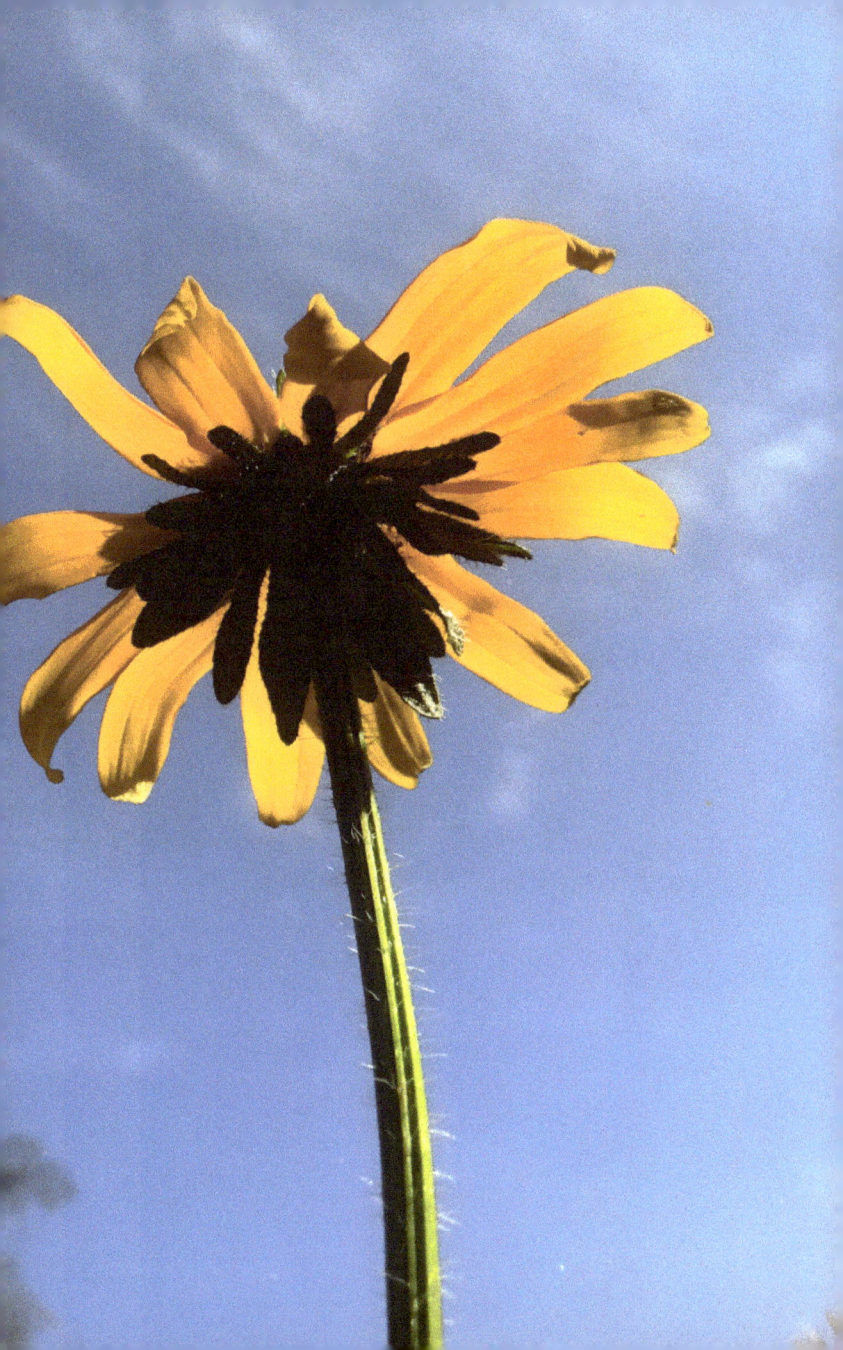

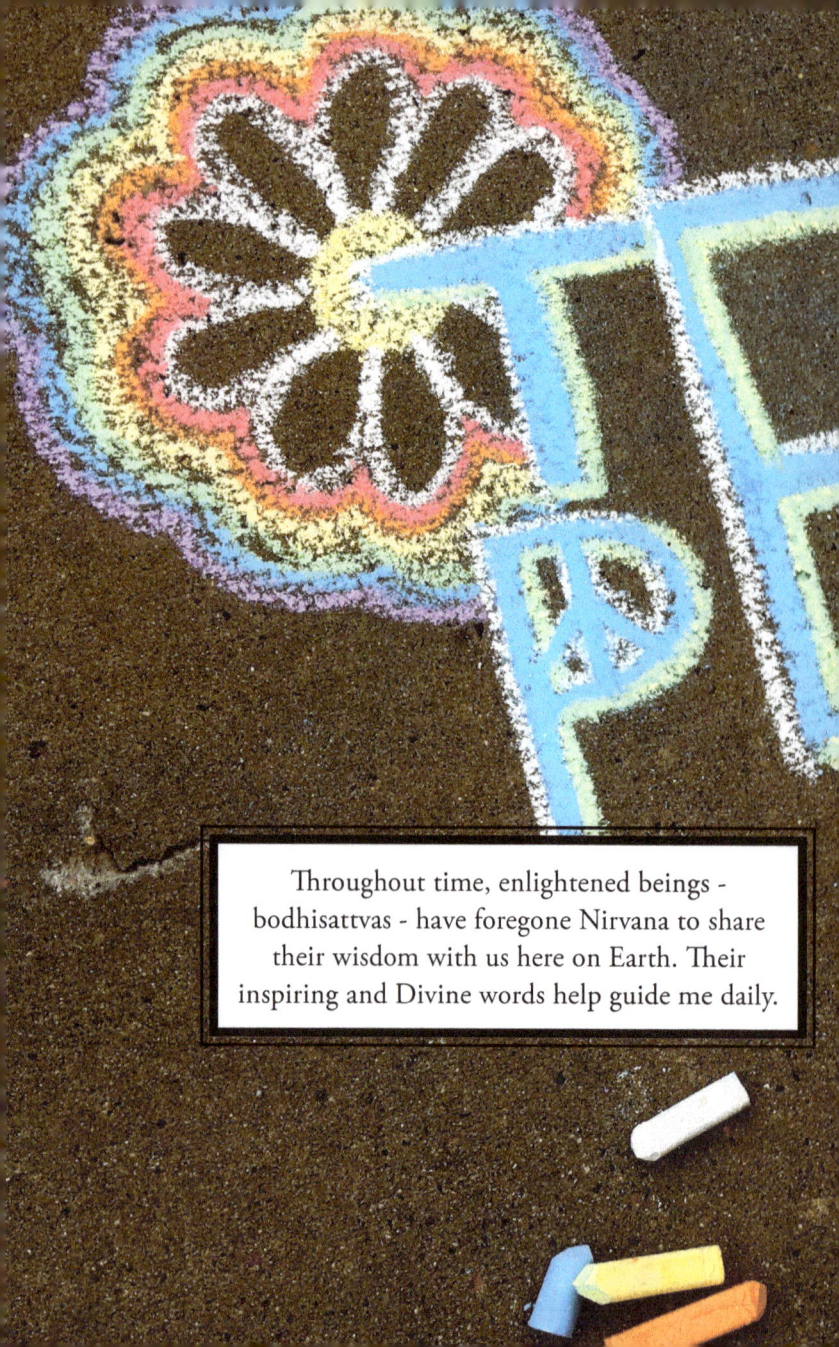

Throughout time, enlightened beings - bodhisattvas - have foregone Nirvana to share their wisdom with us here on Earth. Their inspiring and Divine words help guide me daily.

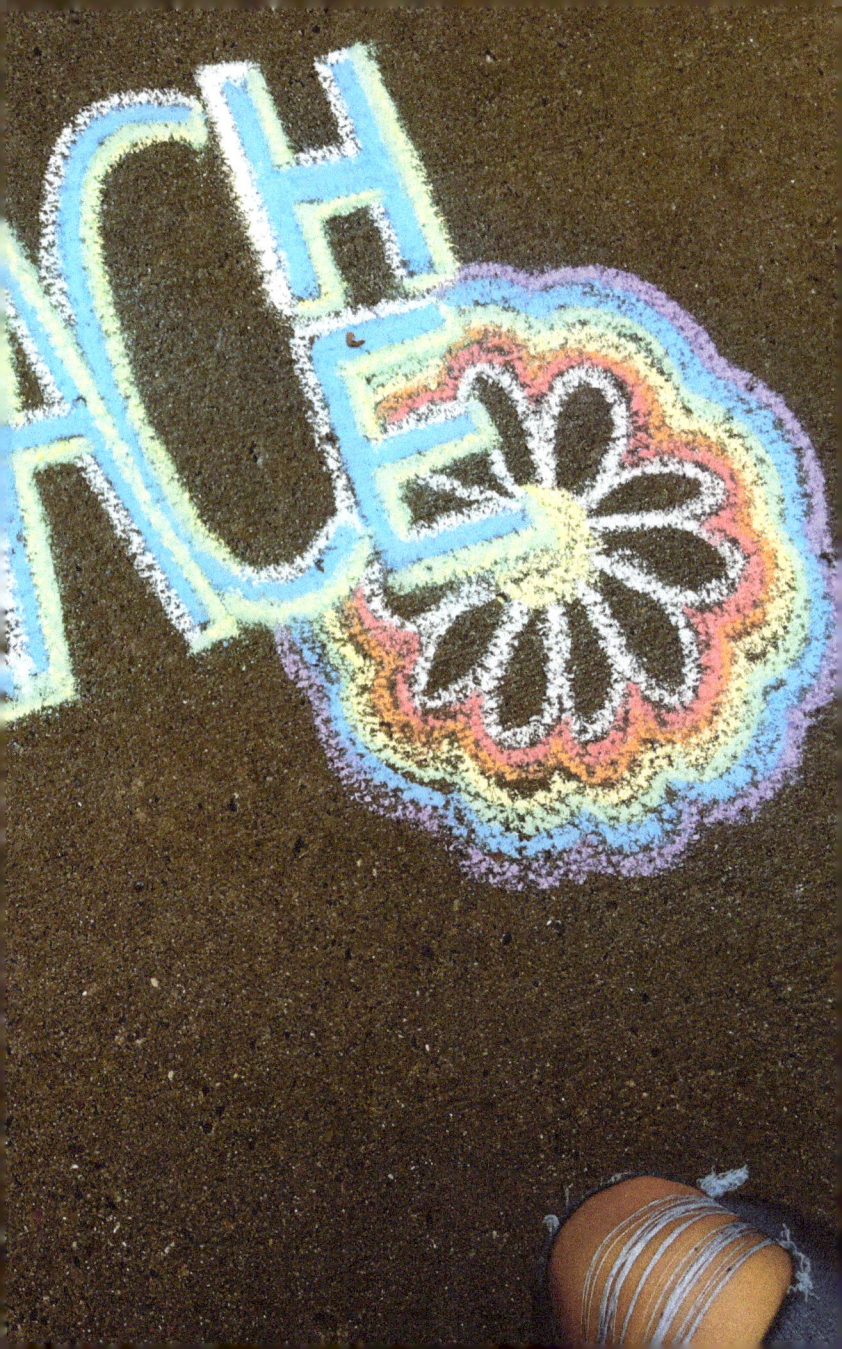

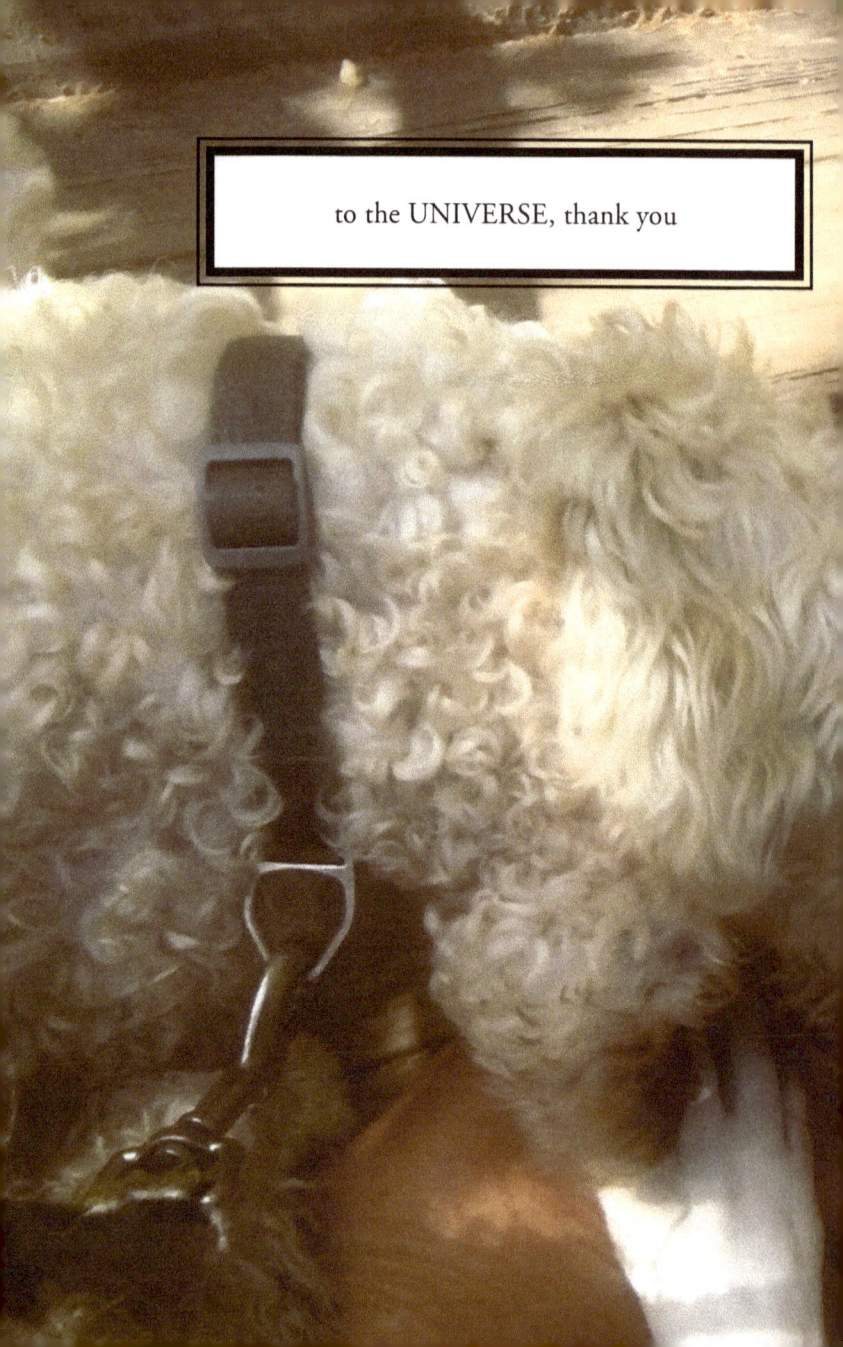
to the UNIVERSE, thank you

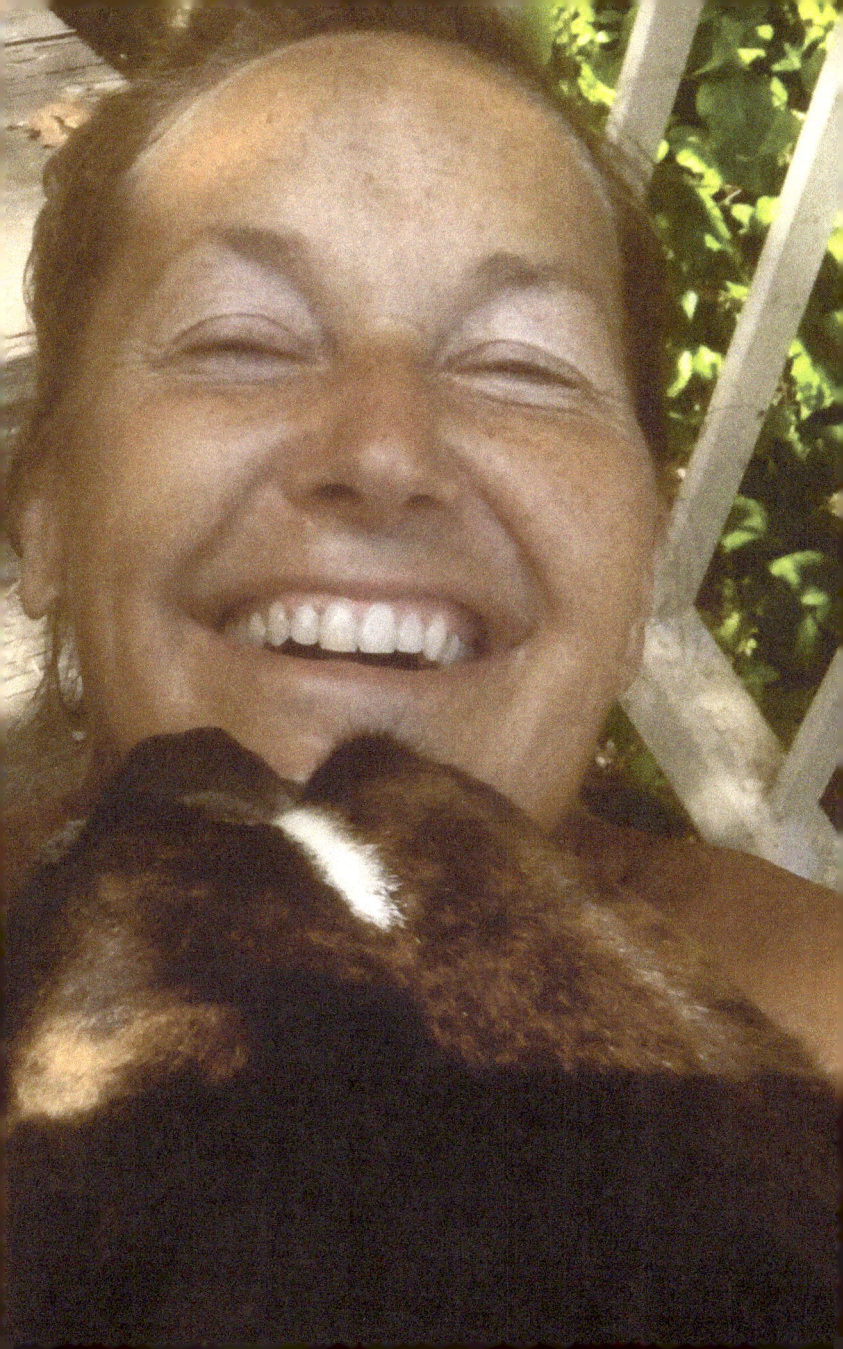

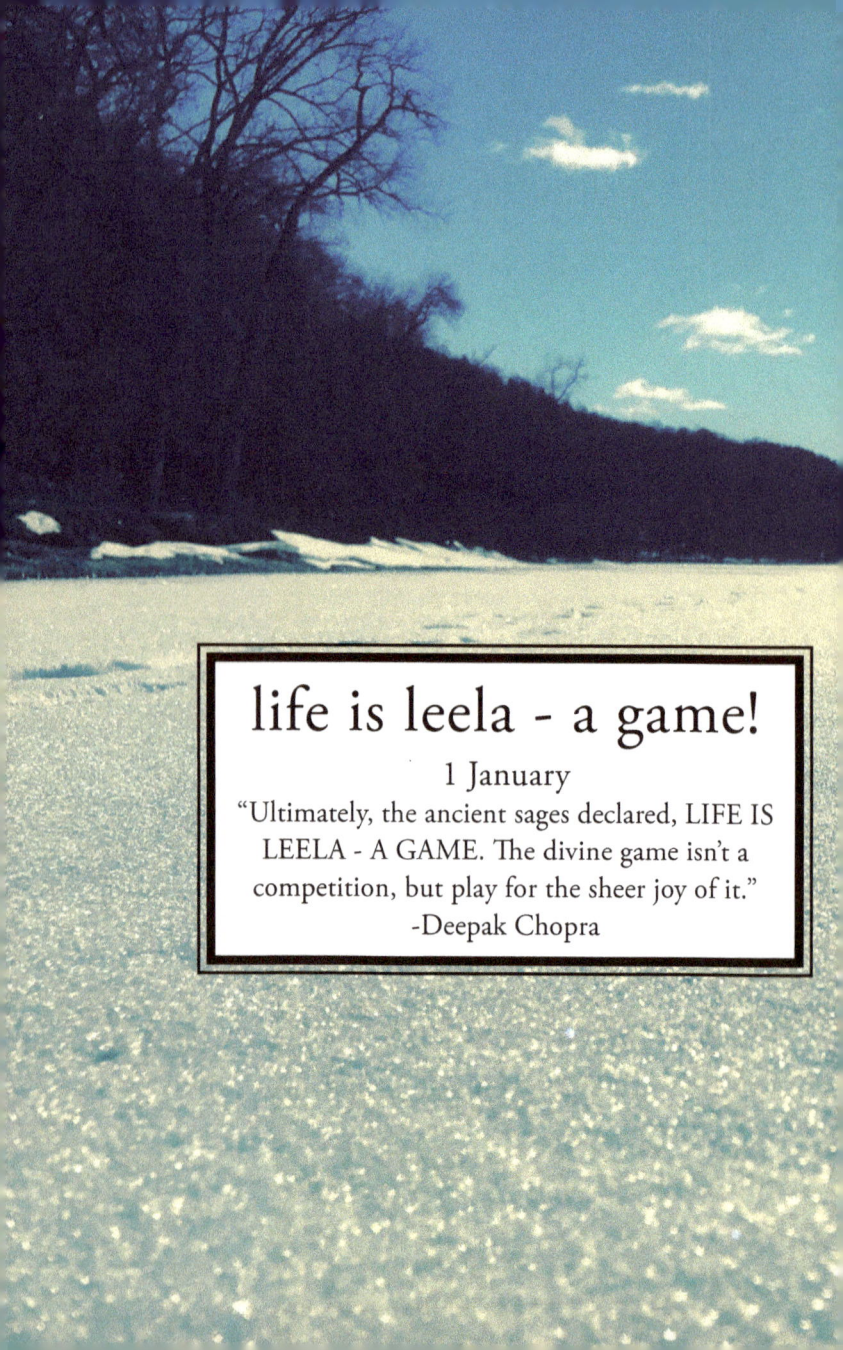

life is leela - a game!

1 January

"Ultimately, the ancient sages declared, LIFE IS LEELA - A GAME. The divine game isn't a competition, but play for the sheer joy of it."
-Deepak Chopra

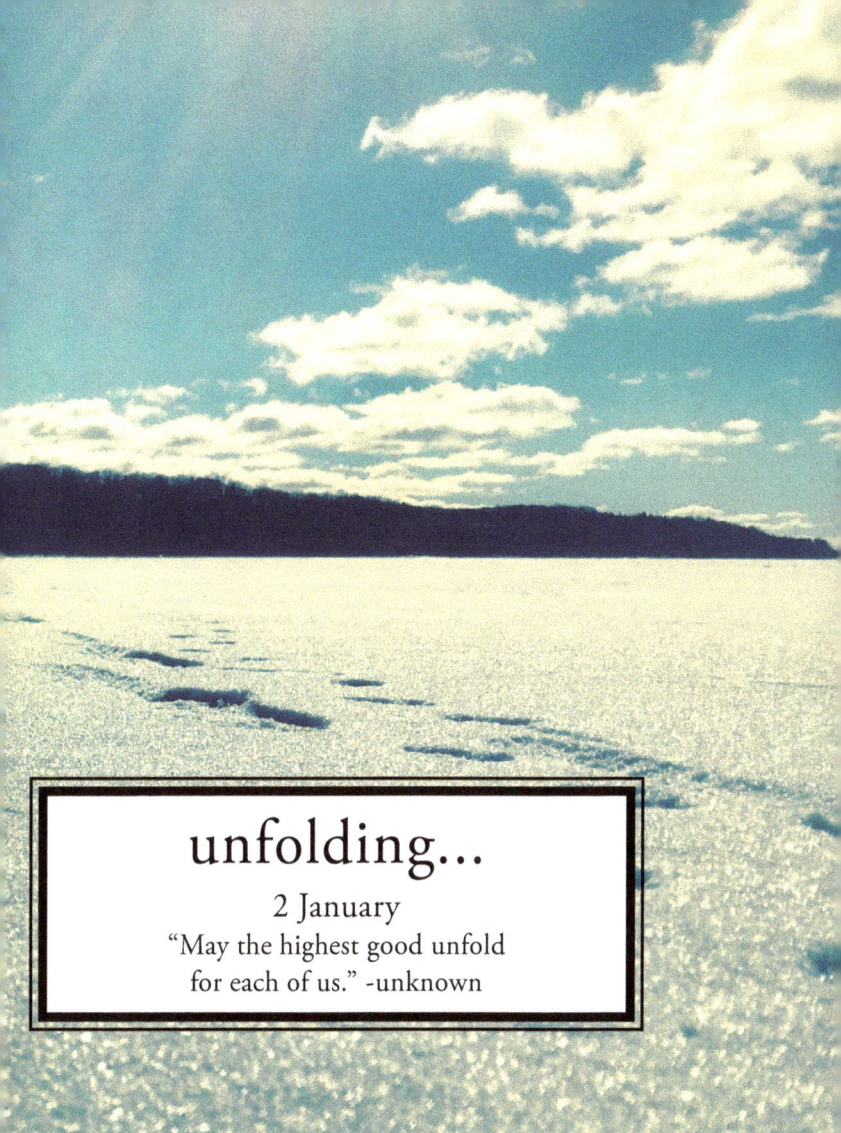

unfolding...

2 January
"May the highest good unfold for each of us." -unknown

happiness

3 January

"Just to breathe is always enough to be happy."
-Don Miguel Ruiz

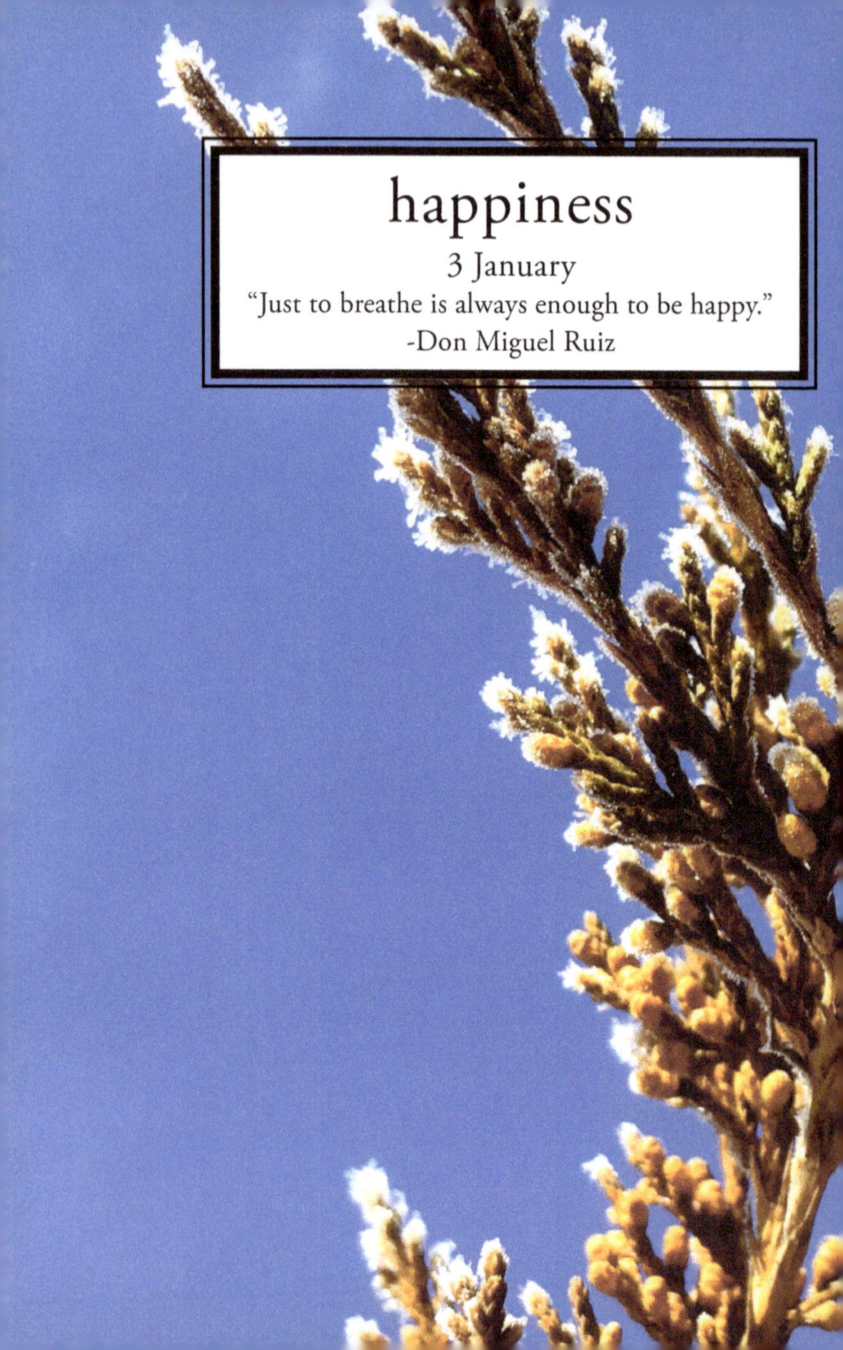

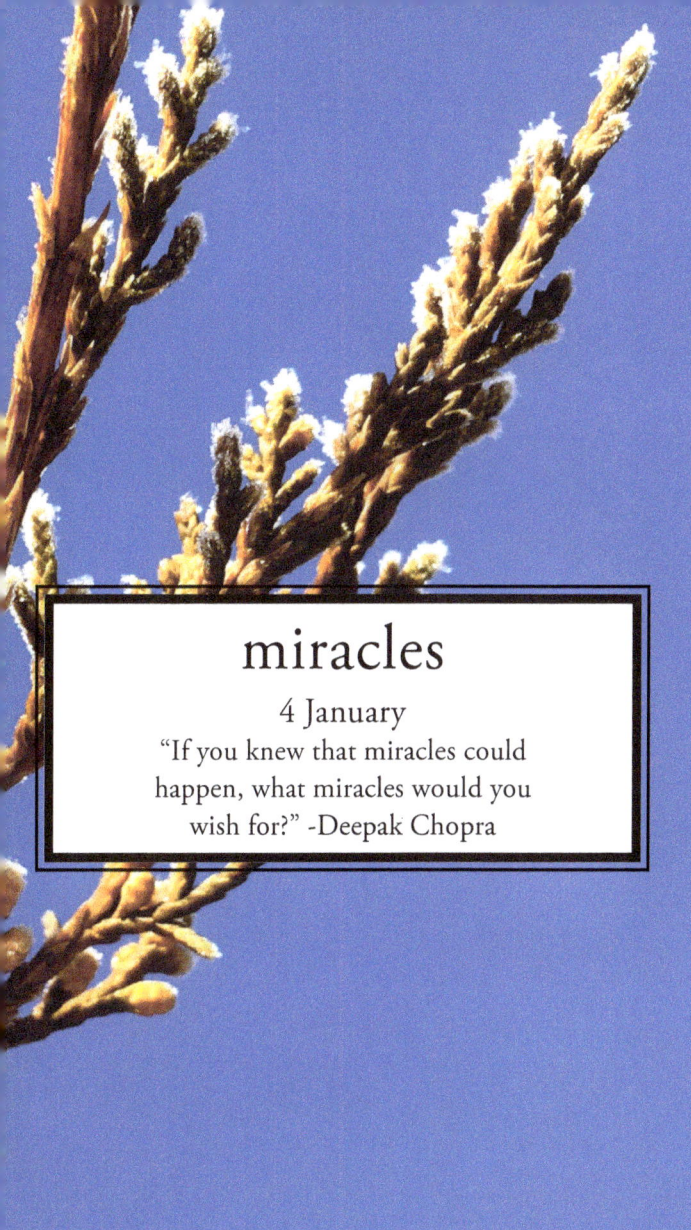

miracles

4 January
"If you knew that miracles could happen, what miracles would you wish for?" -Deepak Chopra

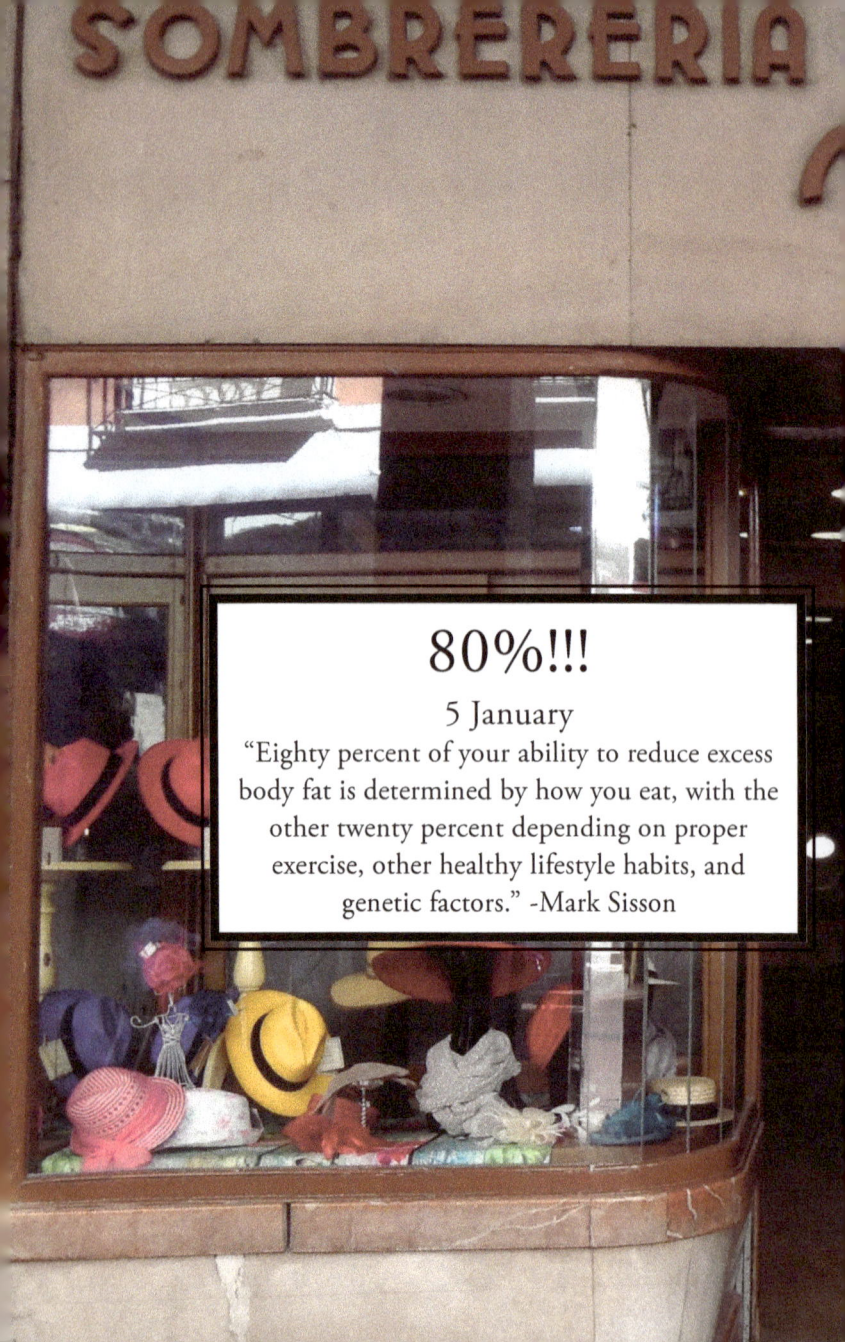

80%!!!

5 January

"Eighty percent of your ability to reduce excess body fat is determined by how you eat, with the other twenty percent depending on proper exercise, other healthy lifestyle habits, and genetic factors." -Mark Sisson

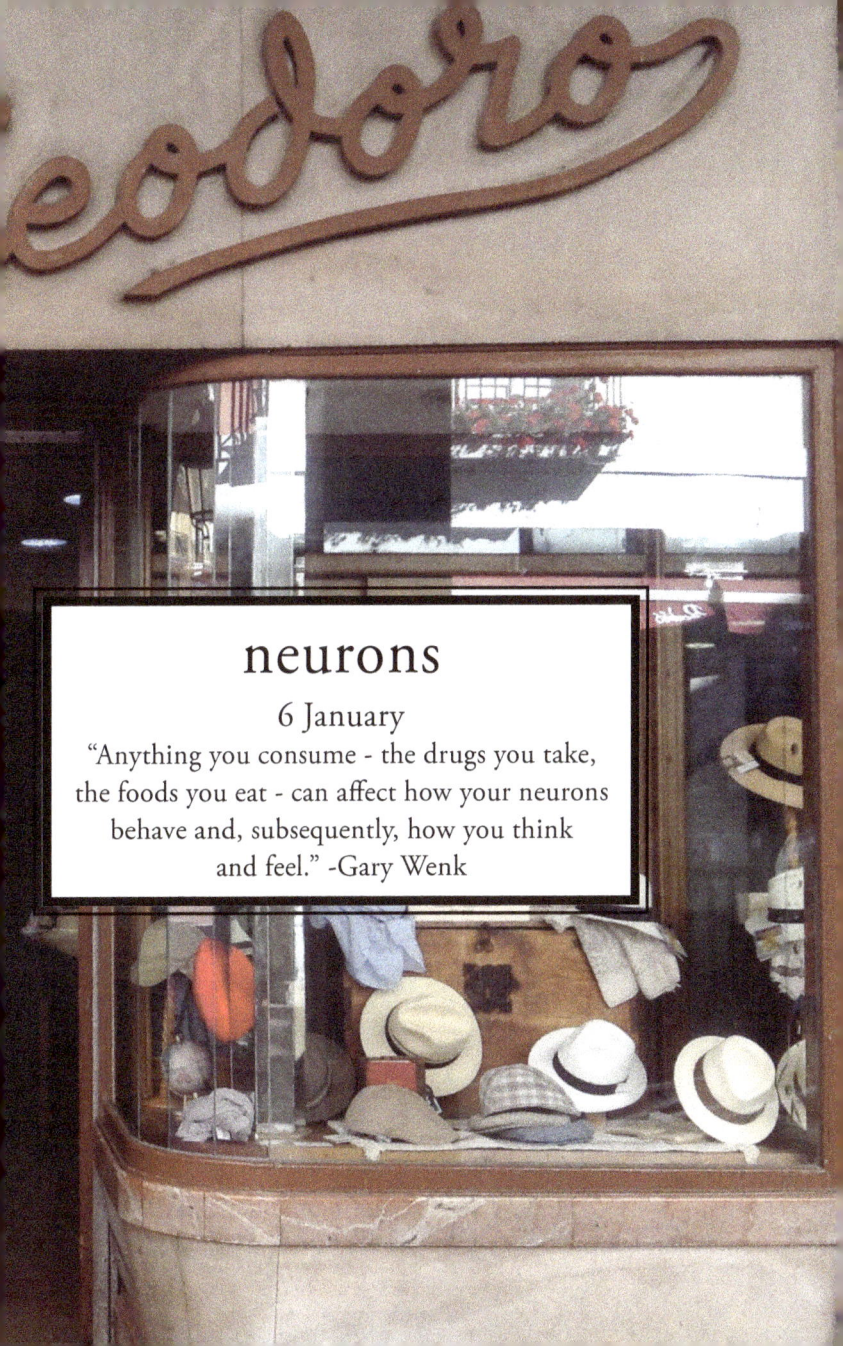

neurons

6 January
"Anything you consume - the drugs you take, the foods you eat - can affect how your neurons behave and, subsequently, how you think and feel." -Gary Wenk

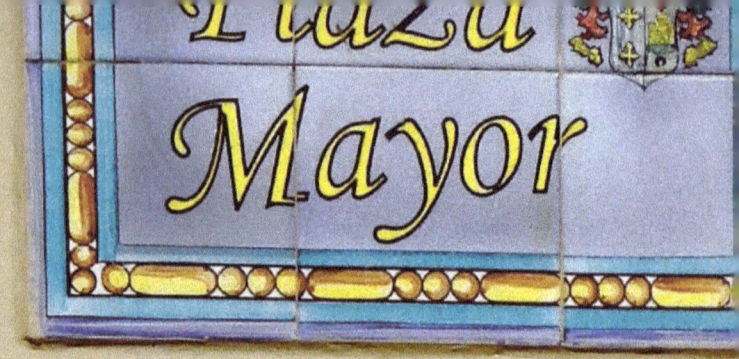

the WAY

7 January
How will I know where I am going
if I don't know my WAY?

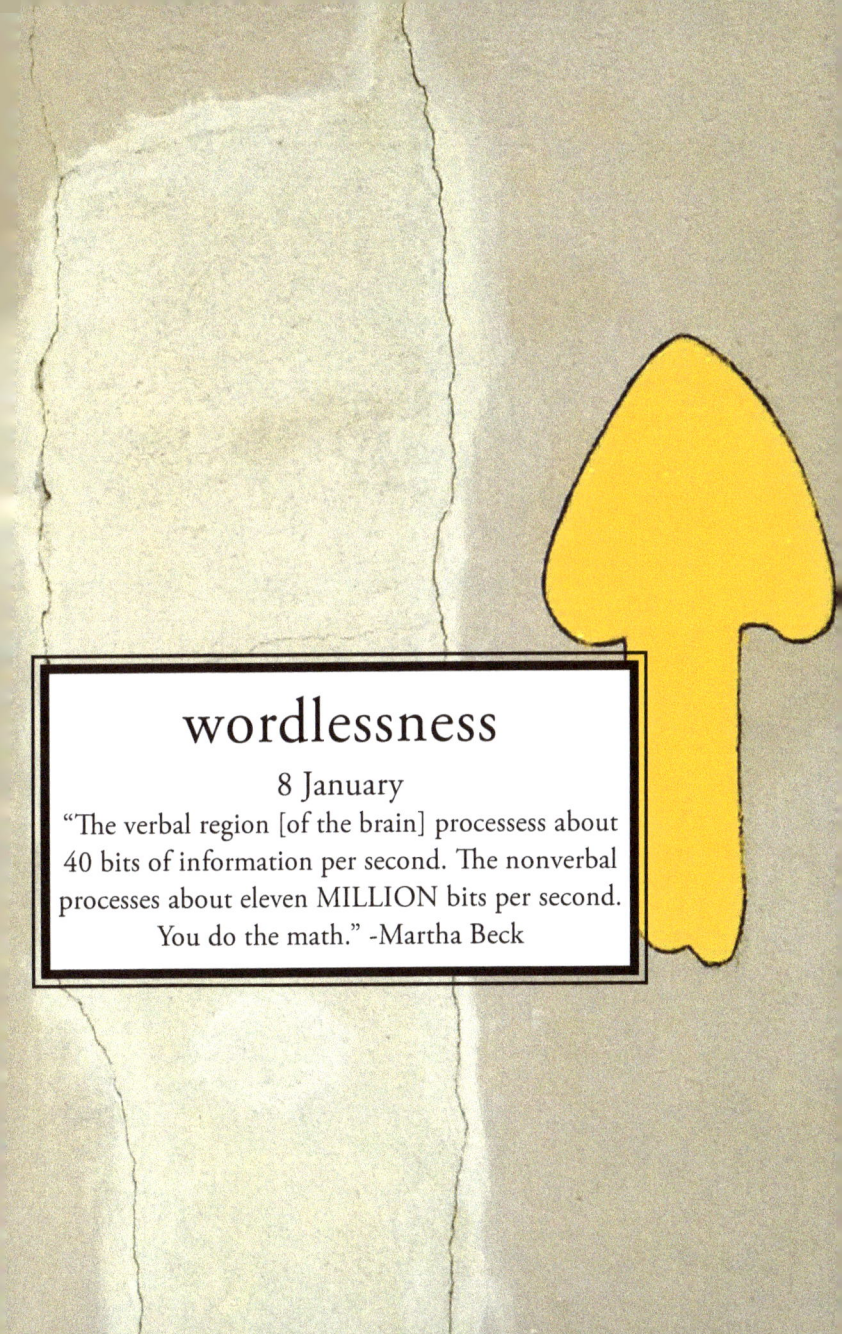

wordlessness

8 January

"The verbal region [of the brain] processess about 40 bits of information per second. The nonverbal processes about eleven MILLION bits per second. You do the math." -Martha Beck

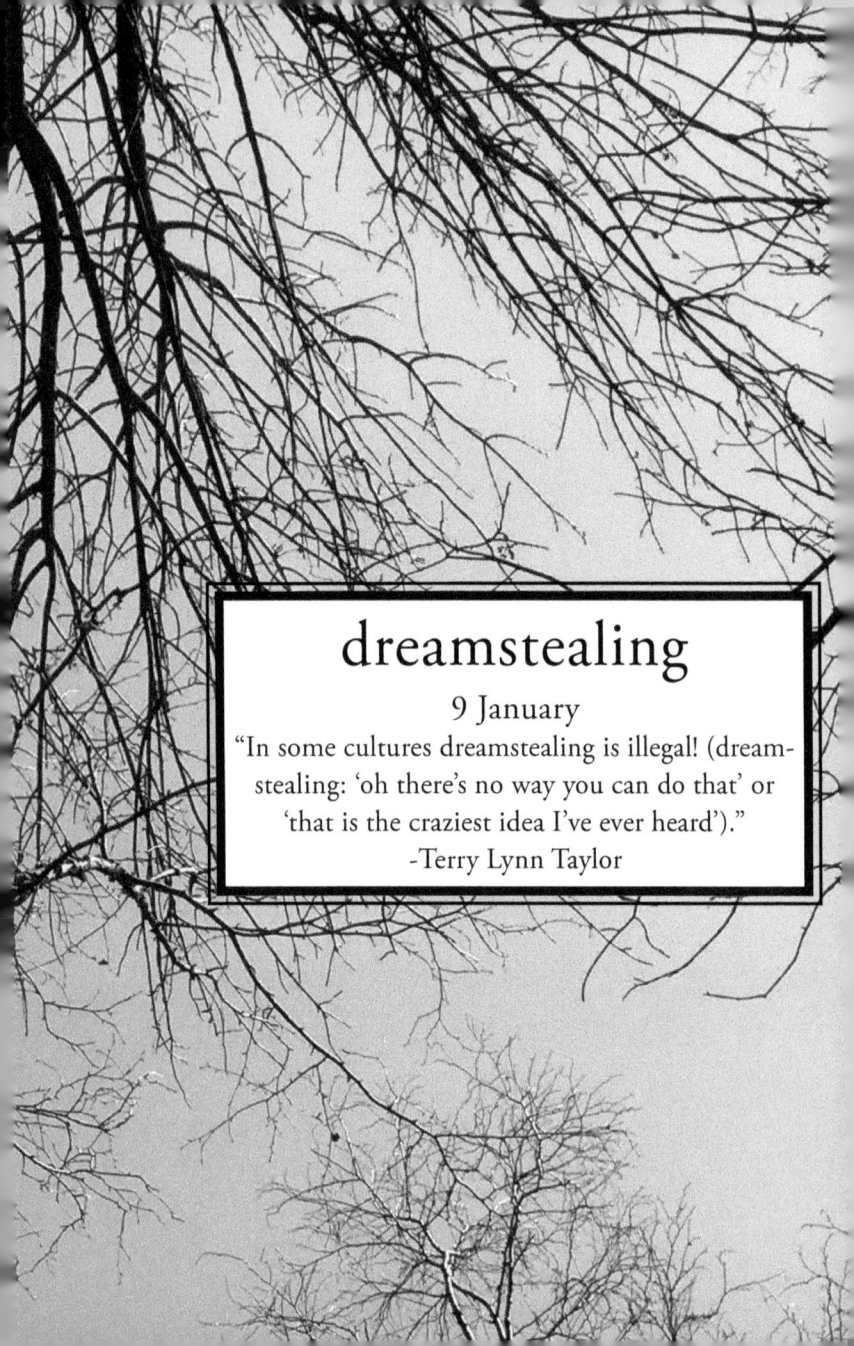

dreamstealing

9 January

"In some cultures dreamstealing is illegal! (dream-stealing: 'oh there's no way you can do that' or 'that is the craziest idea I've ever heard')."
-Terry Lynn Taylor

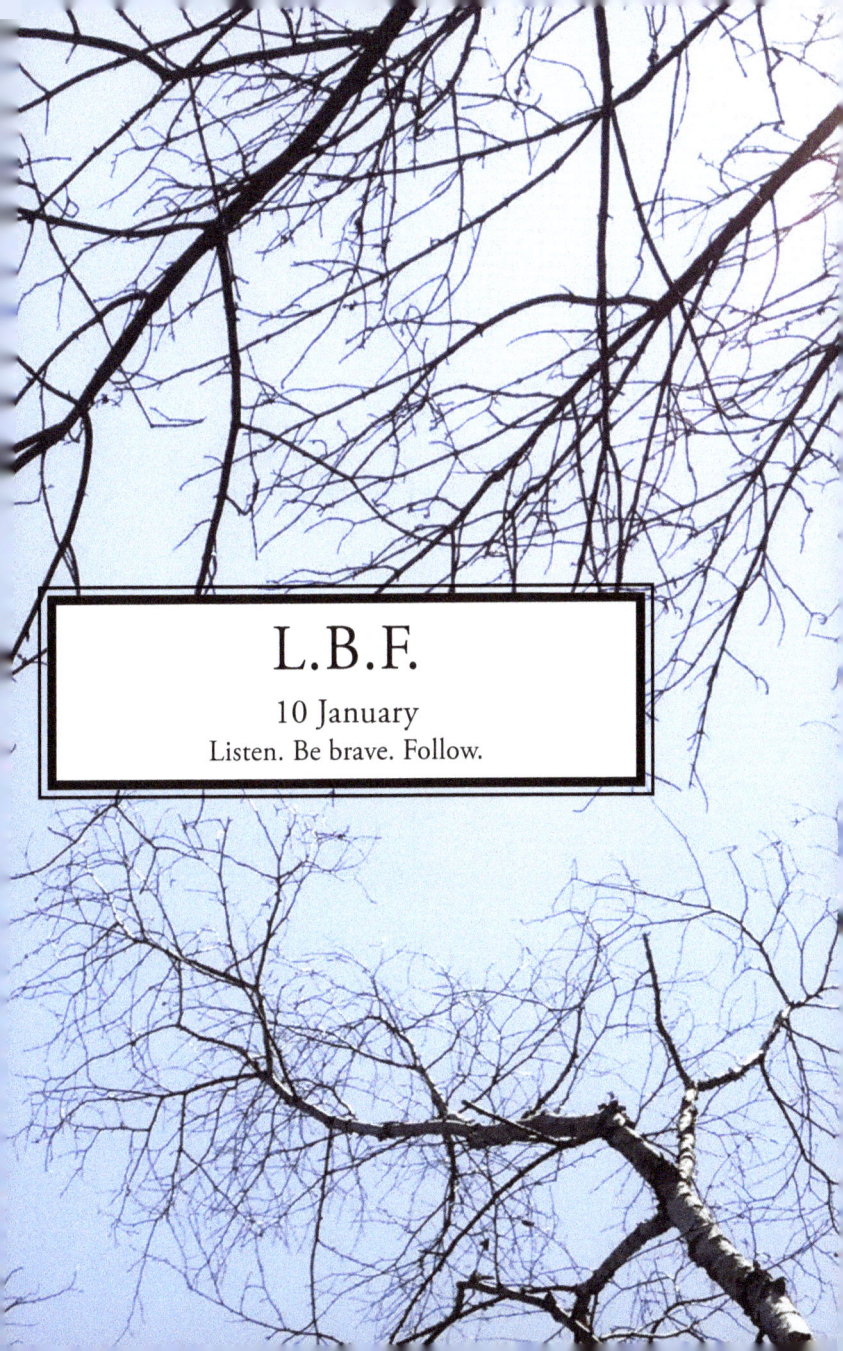

L.B.F.

10 January
Listen. Be brave. Follow.

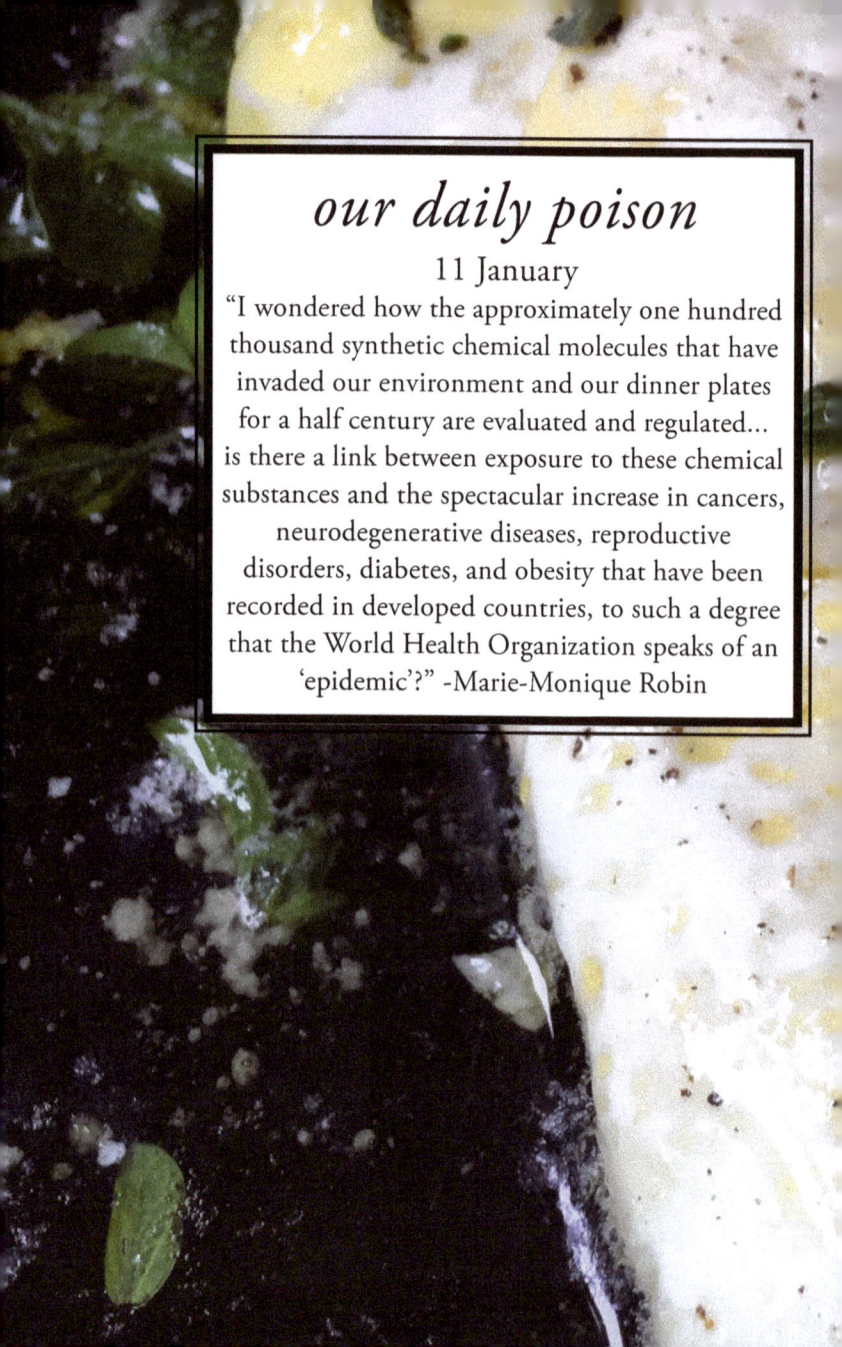

our daily poison
11 January

"I wondered how the approximately one hundred thousand synthetic chemical molecules that have invaded our environment and our dinner plates for a half century are evaluated and regulated... is there a link between exposure to these chemical substances and the spectacular increase in cancers, neurodegenerative diseases, reproductive disorders, diabetes, and obesity that have been recorded in developed countries, to such a degree that the World Health Organization speaks of an 'epidemic'?" -Marie-Monique Robin

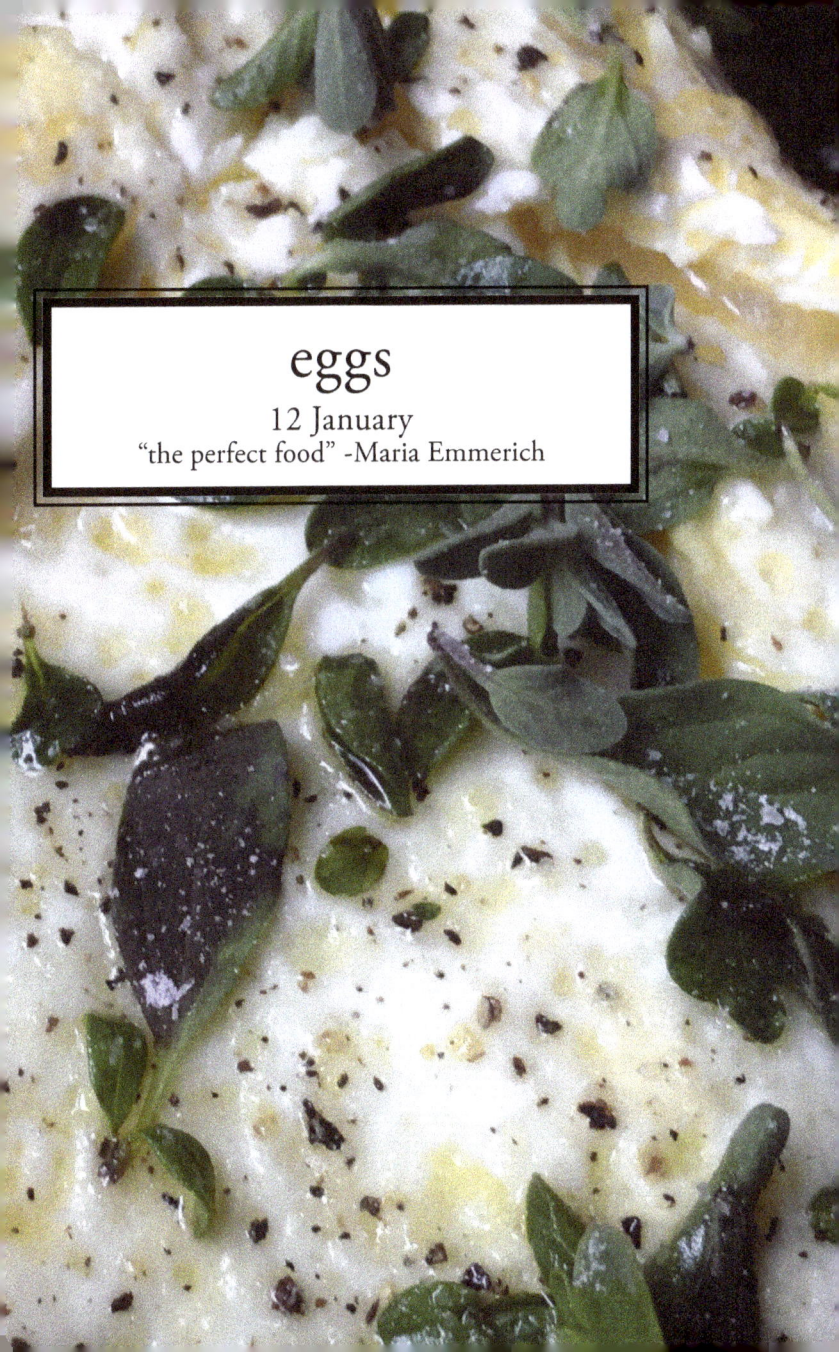

eggs
12 January
"the perfect food" -Maria Emmerich

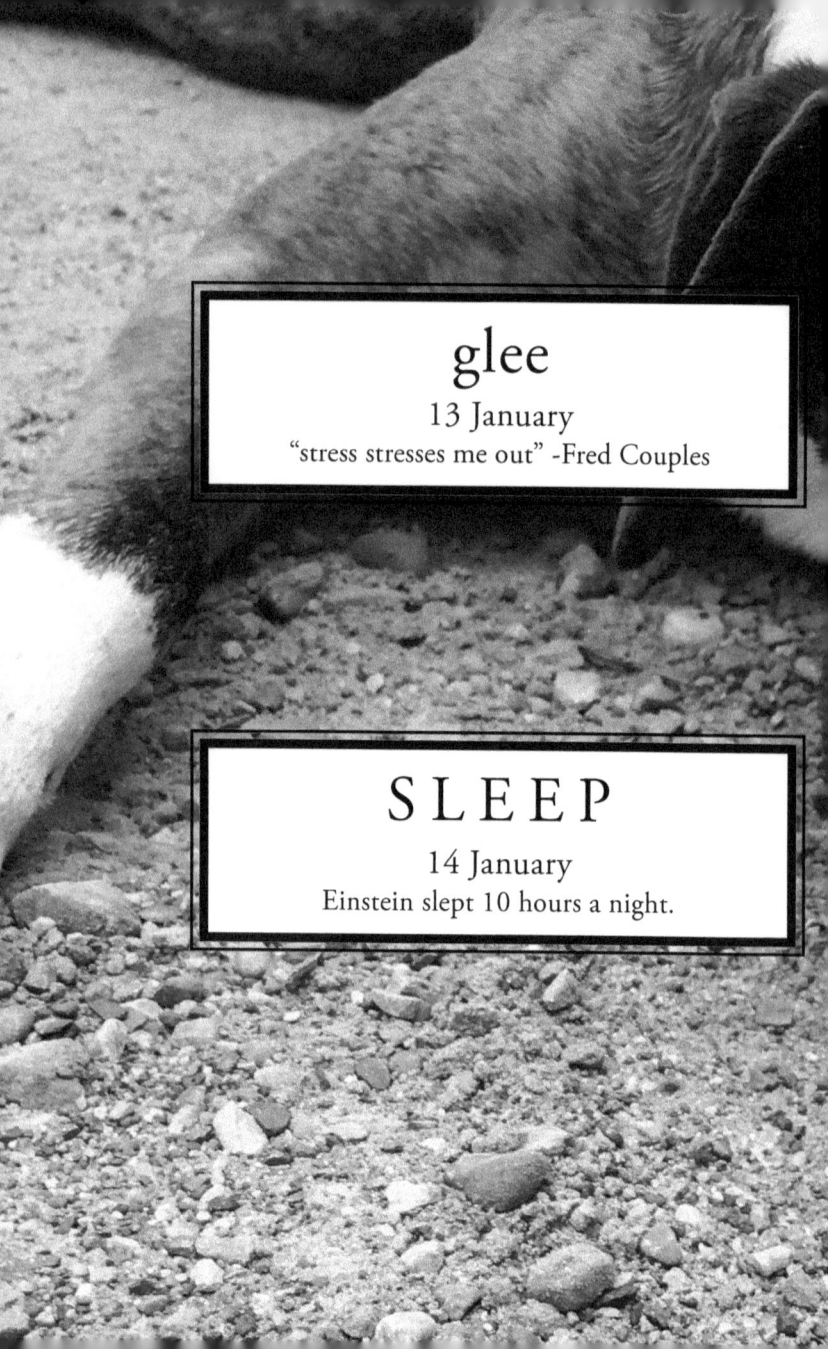

glee
13 January
"stress stresses me out" -Fred Couples

SLEEP
14 January
Einstein slept 10 hours a night.

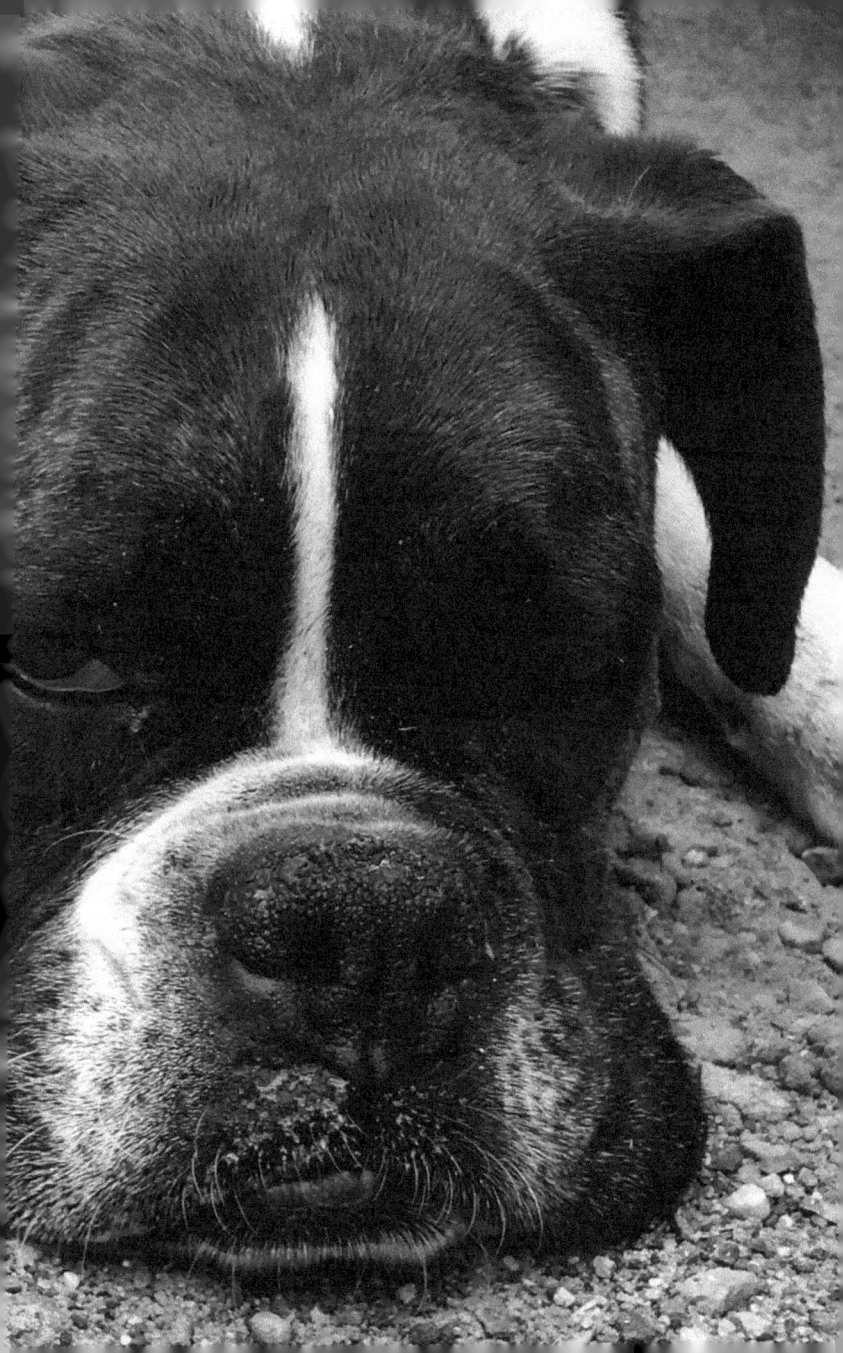

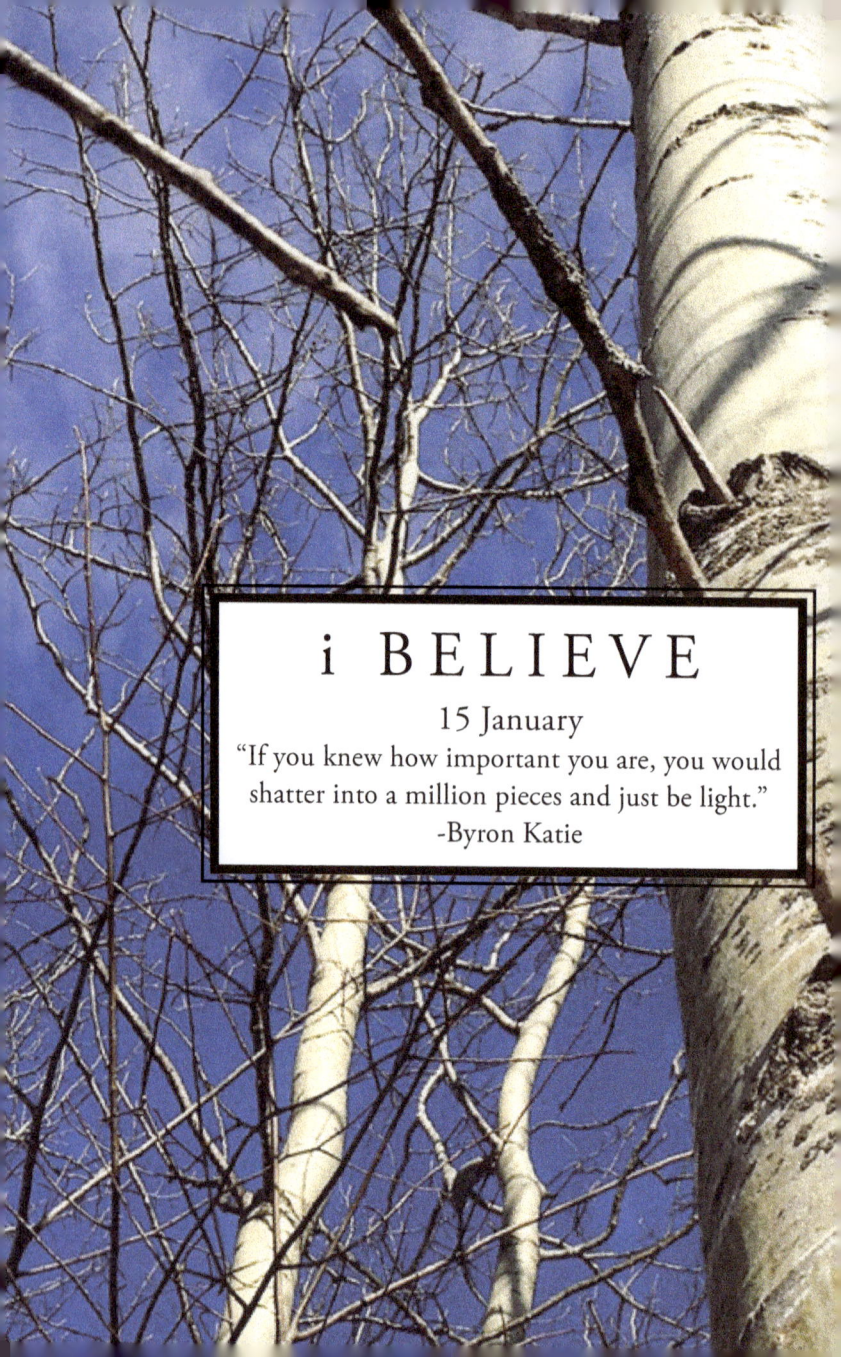

i BELIEVE

15 January
"If you knew how important you are, you would shatter into a million pieces and just be light."
-Byron Katie

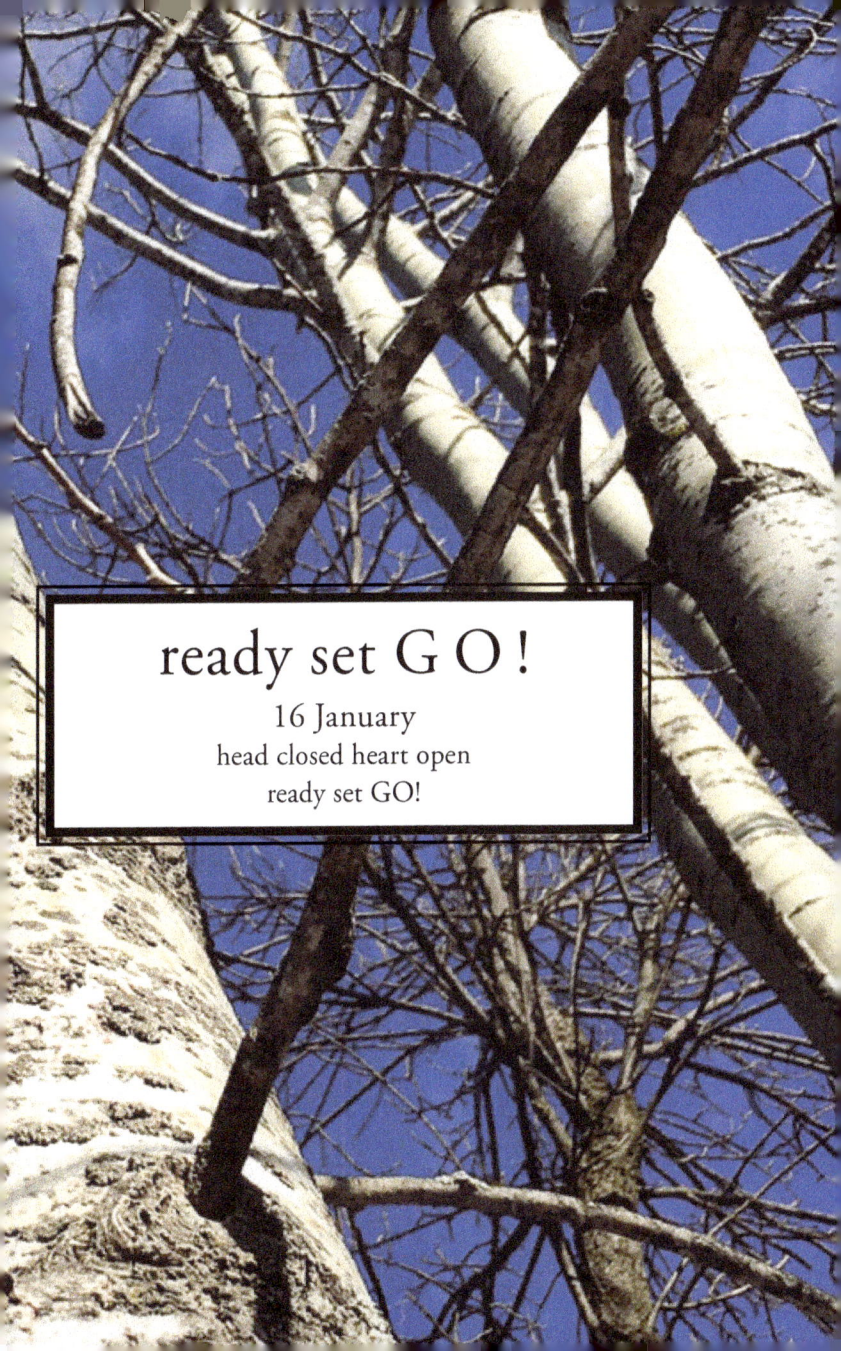

ready set G O !

16 January
head closed heart open
ready set GO!

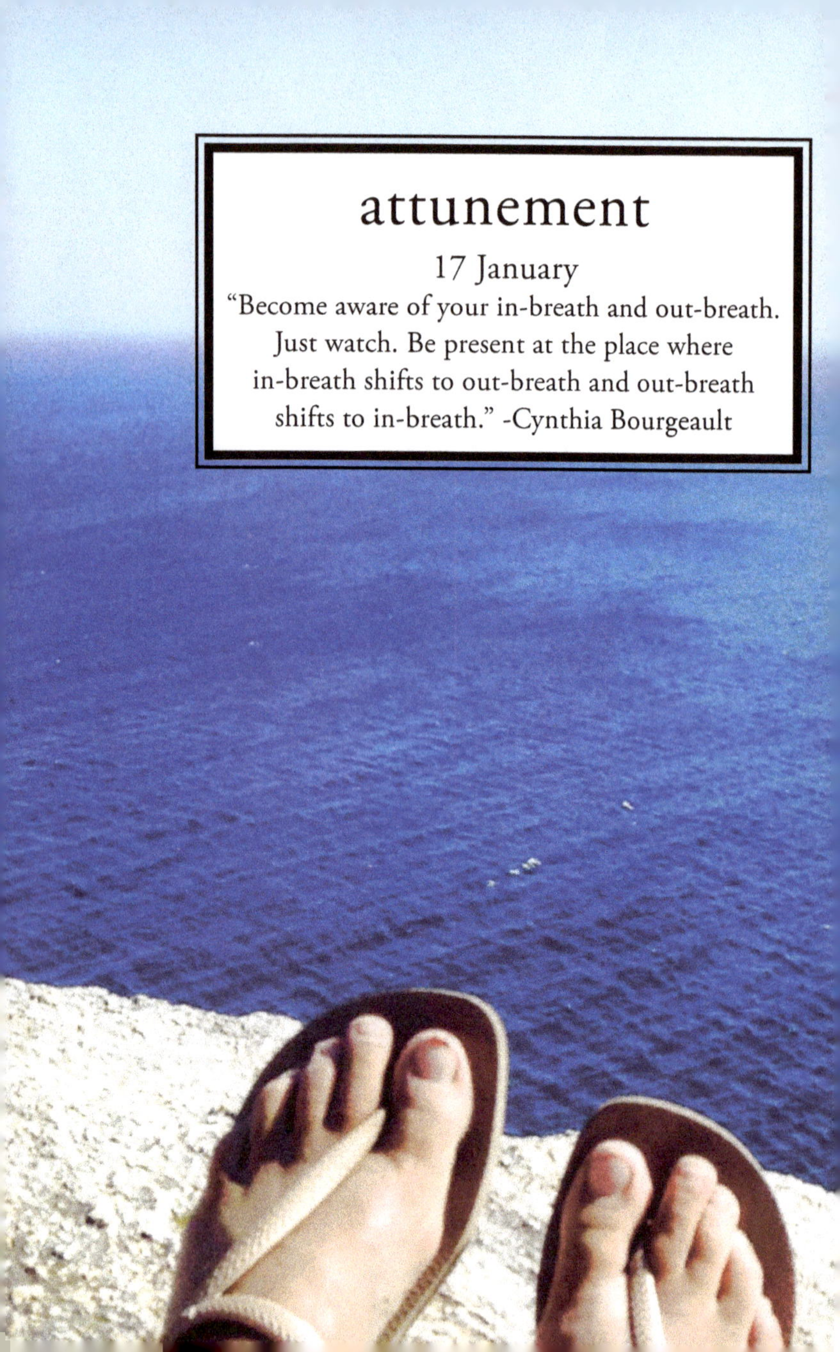

attunement

17 January

"Become aware of your in-breath and out-breath. Just watch. Be present at the place where in-breath shifts to out-breath and out-breath shifts to in-breath." -Cynthia Bourgeault

secret

18 January
"I discovered the secret of the sea in meditation
upon a dewdrop."
-Kahlil Gibran

optimistic

19 January

"If you keep resting your mind on good events and conditions, pleasant feelings, the things you do get done, physical pleasures, and your good intentions and qualities, then over time your brain will take a different shape, one with strength and resilience hardwired into it, as well as a realistically optimistic outlook, a positive mood, and a sense of worth." -Rick Hanson PhD

infinite bliss!

20 January

dear thoughts,
please quiet down.
thank you

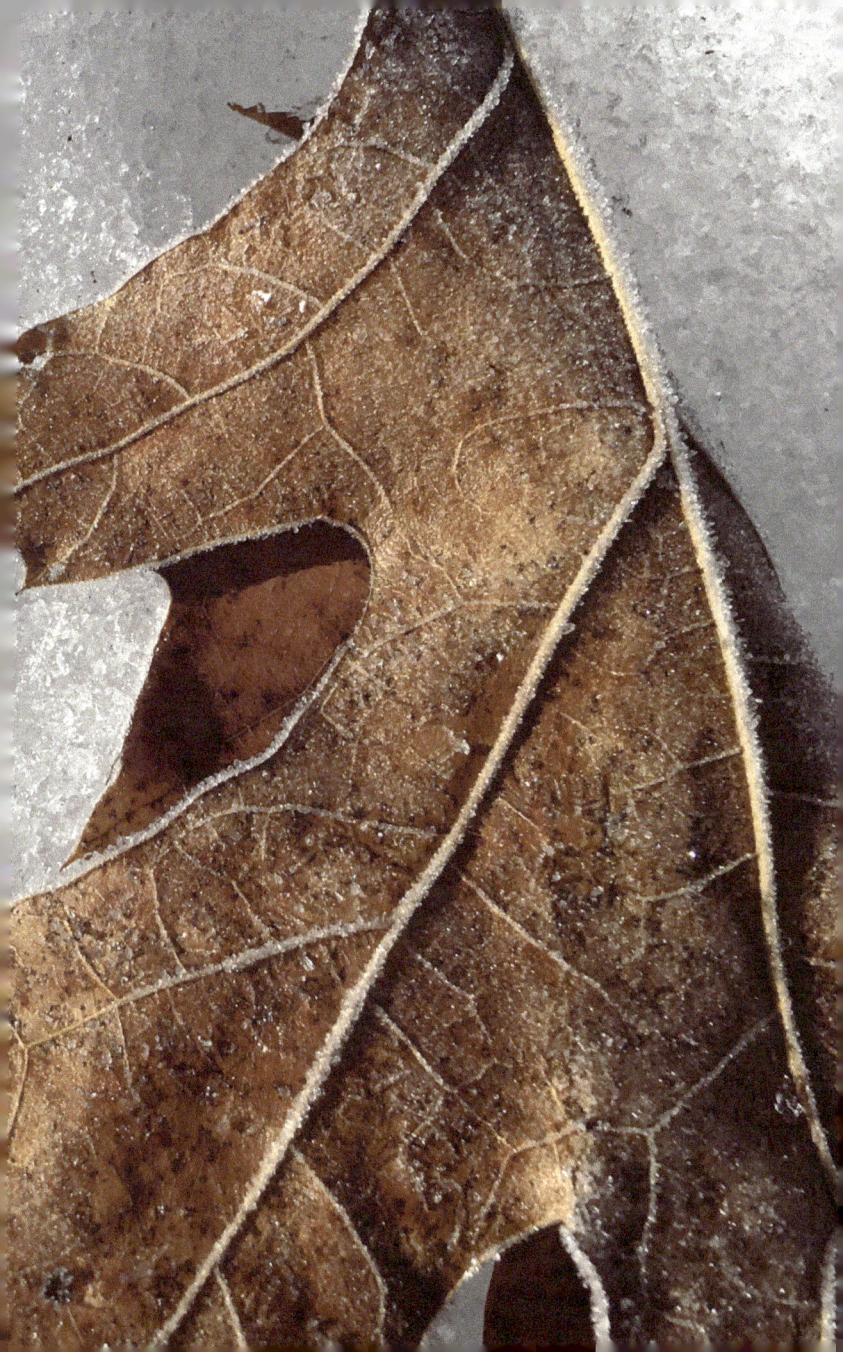

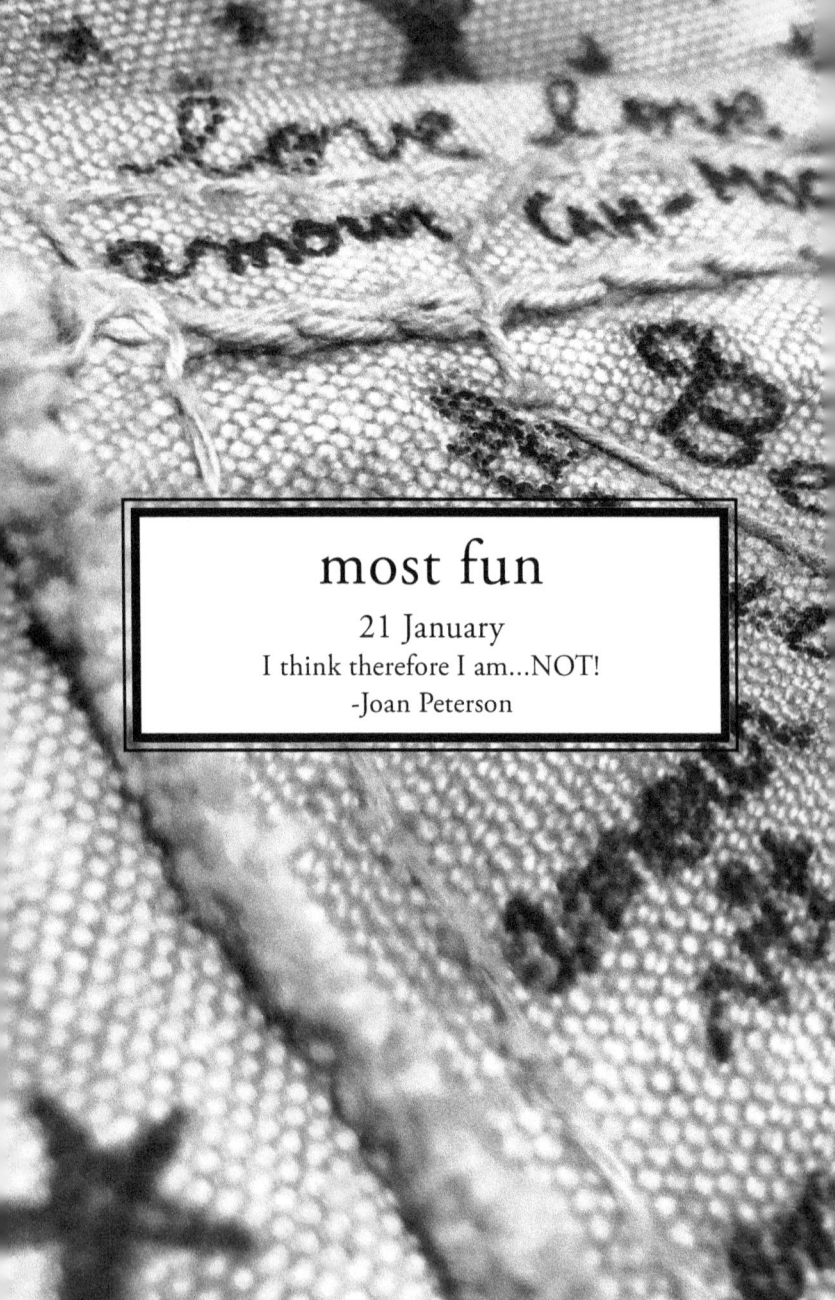

most fun

21 January
I think therefore I am...NOT!
-Joan Peterson

dreamgenie

22 January

dream: a strongly desired goal or purpose; something that fully satisfies a wish

genie: a magic spirit believed to take human form and serve the person who calls it

eat meat & herbs

23 January
"eat meat and herbs" -Maria Emmerich

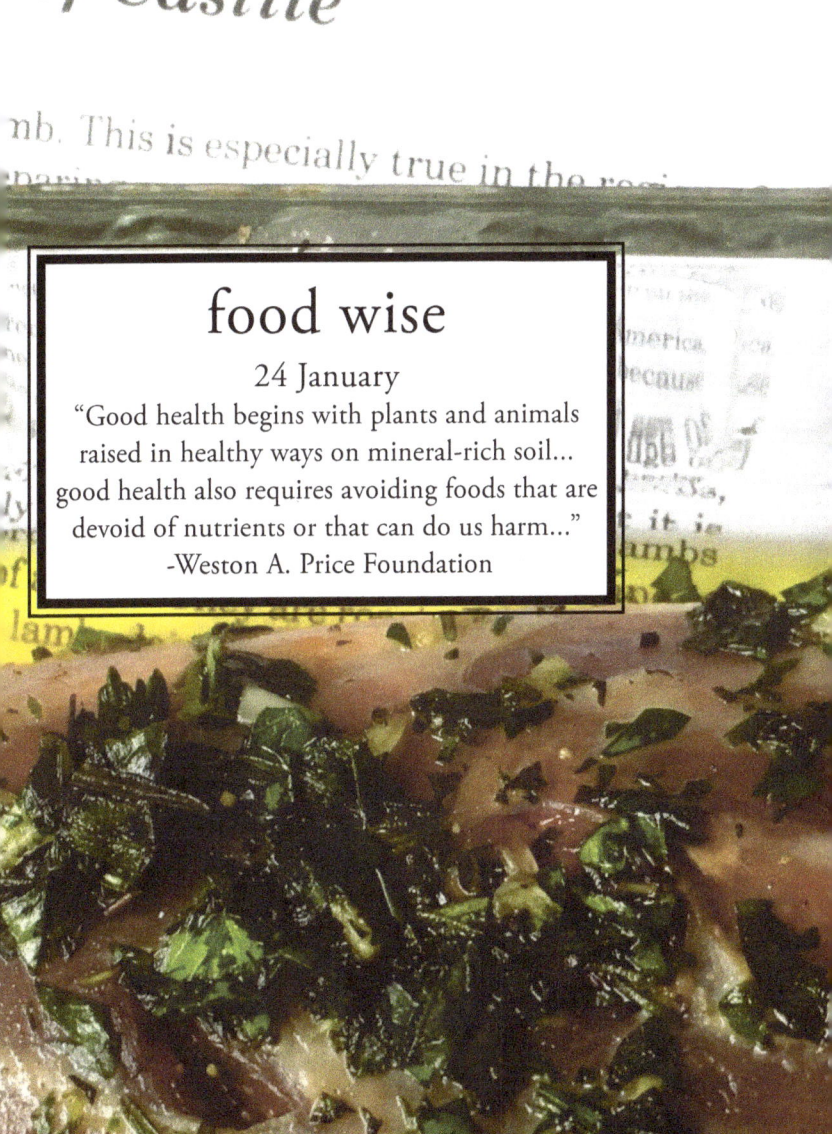

mb with Herbs of Castile

food wise

24 January

"Good health begins with plants and animals raised in healthy ways on mineral-rich soil... good health also requires avoiding foods that are devoid of nutrients or that can do us harm..."
-Weston A. Price Foundation

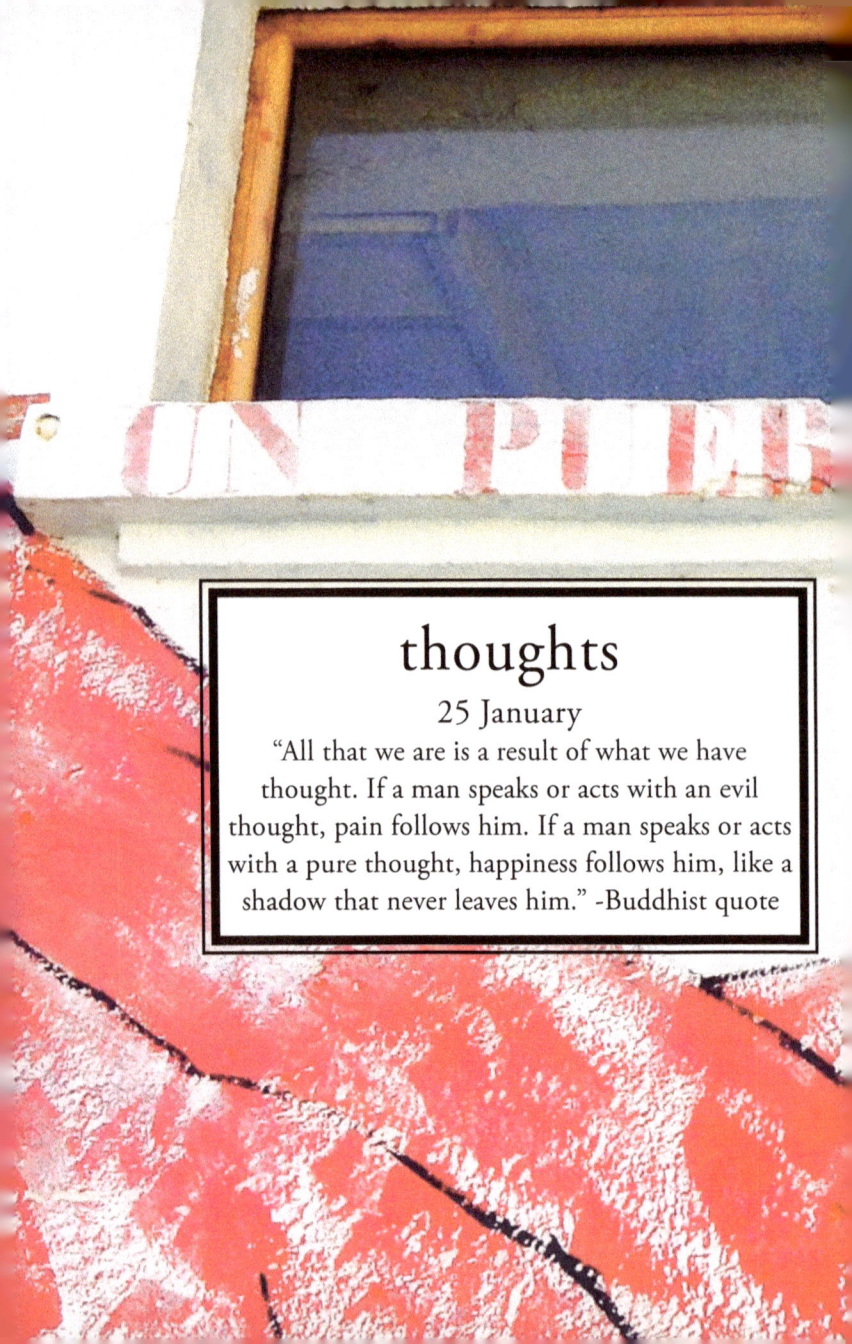

thoughts

25 January

"All that we are is a result of what we have thought. If a man speaks or acts with an evil thought, pain follows him. If a man speaks or acts with a pure thought, happiness follows him, like a shadow that never leaves him." -Buddhist quote

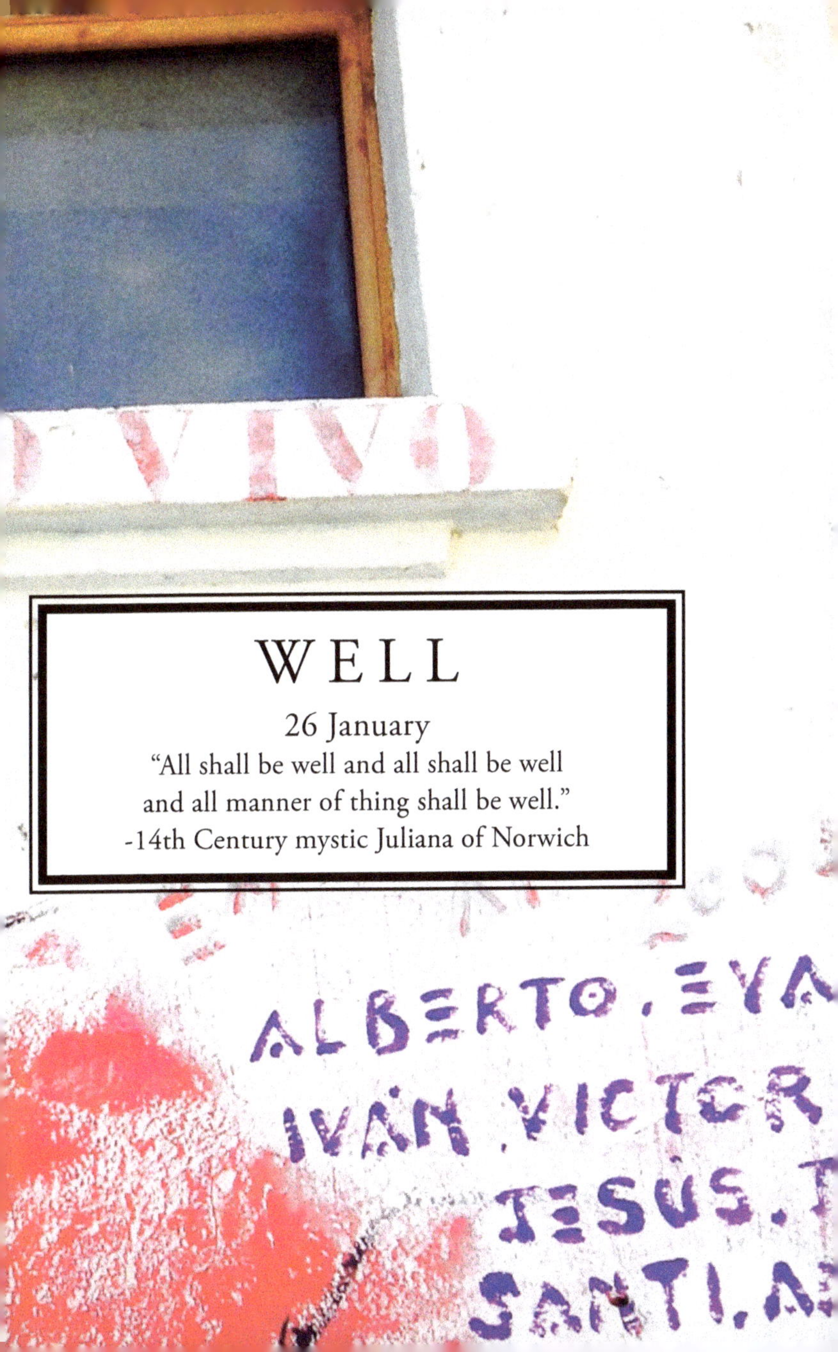

WELL

26 January
"All shall be well and all shall be well
and all manner of thing shall be well."
-14th Century mystic Juliana of Norwich

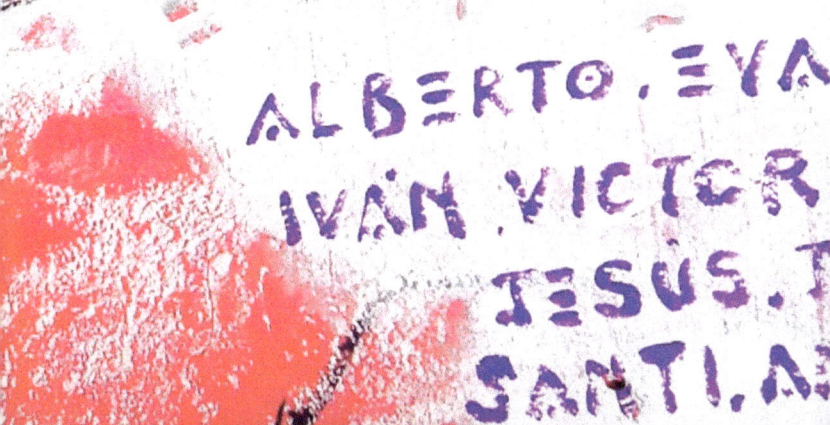

time time time time
time time time time
time time time time

27 January

"Live as though you have all the time in the world." -Deepak Chopra

feelings

28 January

"By taking just a few extra seconds to stay with a positive experience - even the comfort in a single breath - you'll help turn a passing mental state into a lasting neural structure."
-Rick Hanson PhD

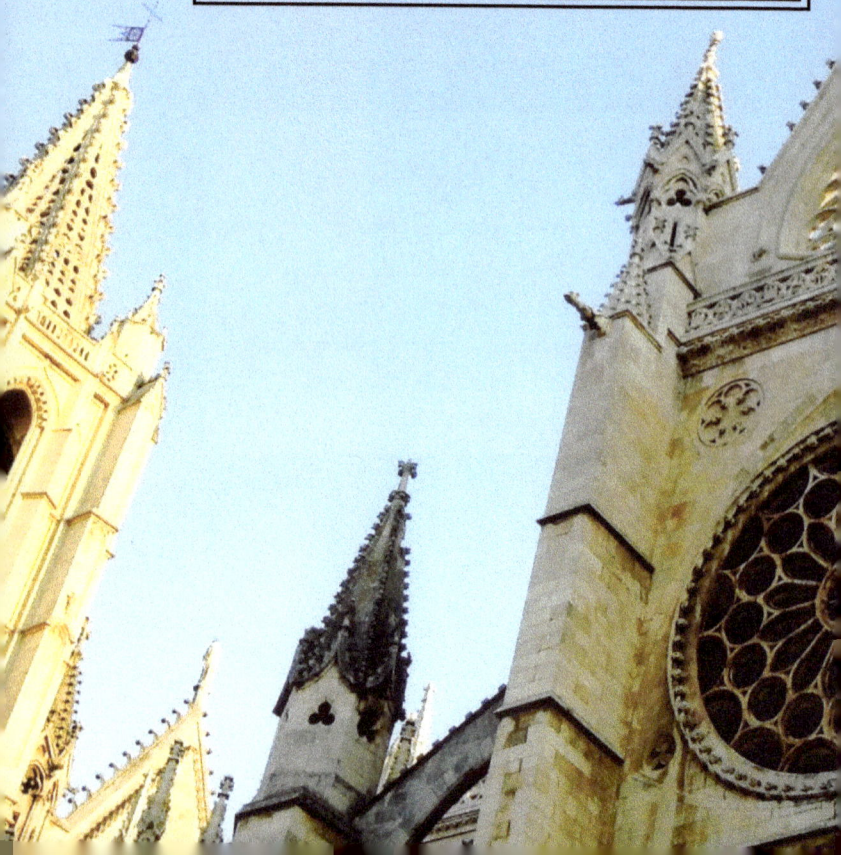

everything
29 January
"Everything which you can conceive and accept is yours! Entertain no doubt. Refuse to accept worry or hurry or fear. That which knows and does everything is inside you and harkens to the slightest whisper." -Wayne Dyer

FAITH

30 January
"Faith is what makes all things possible.
Faith is what sustains the human spirit.
Believe it and you will see it." -Jean Slatter

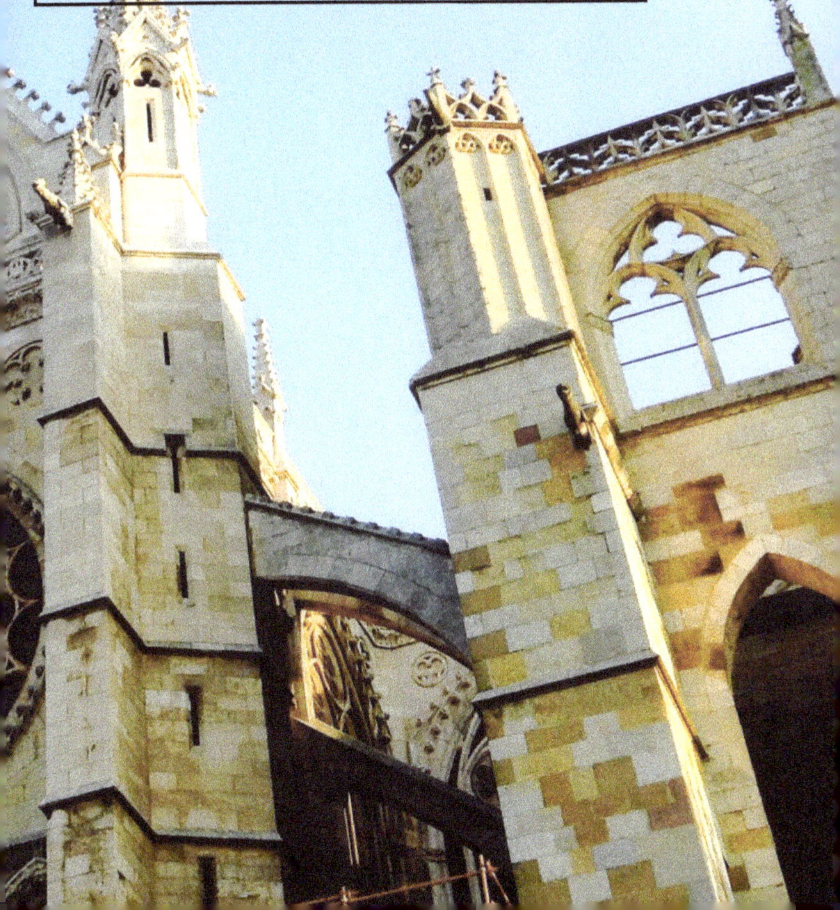

hallelujah

31 January
desire = destiny
-Martha Beck

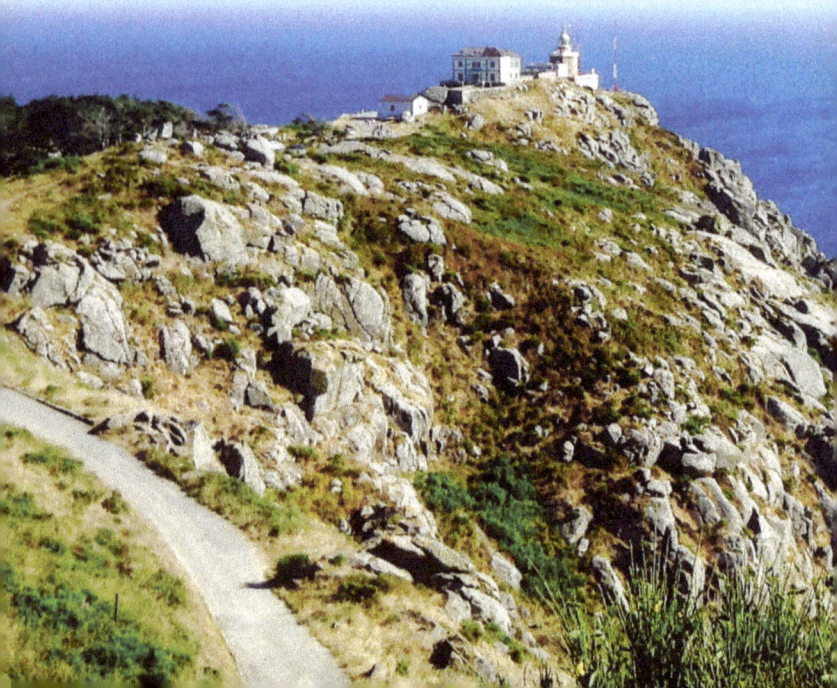

i choose

1 February
i choose MIRACLES

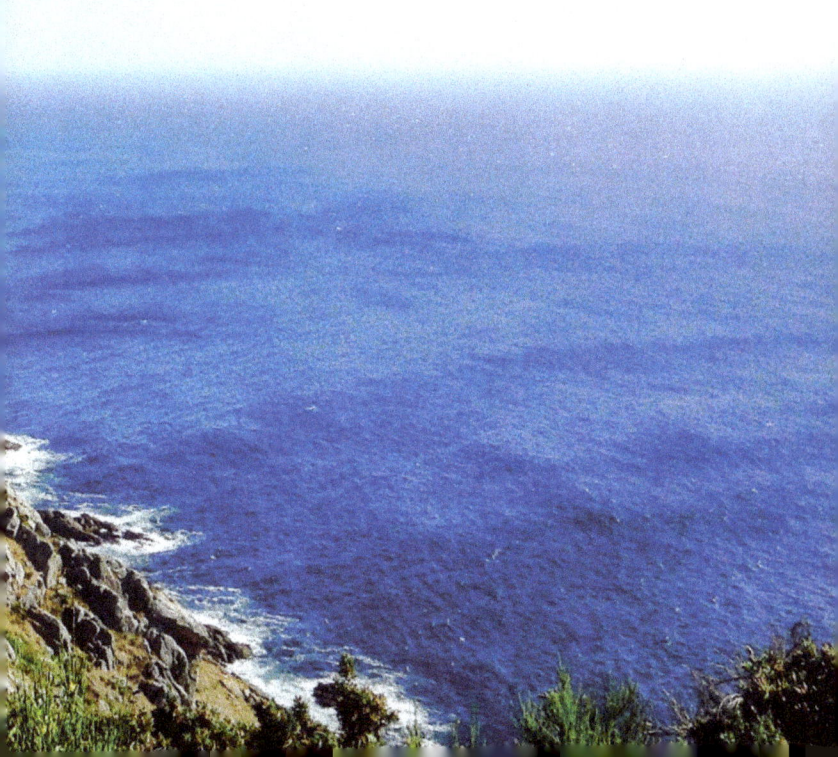

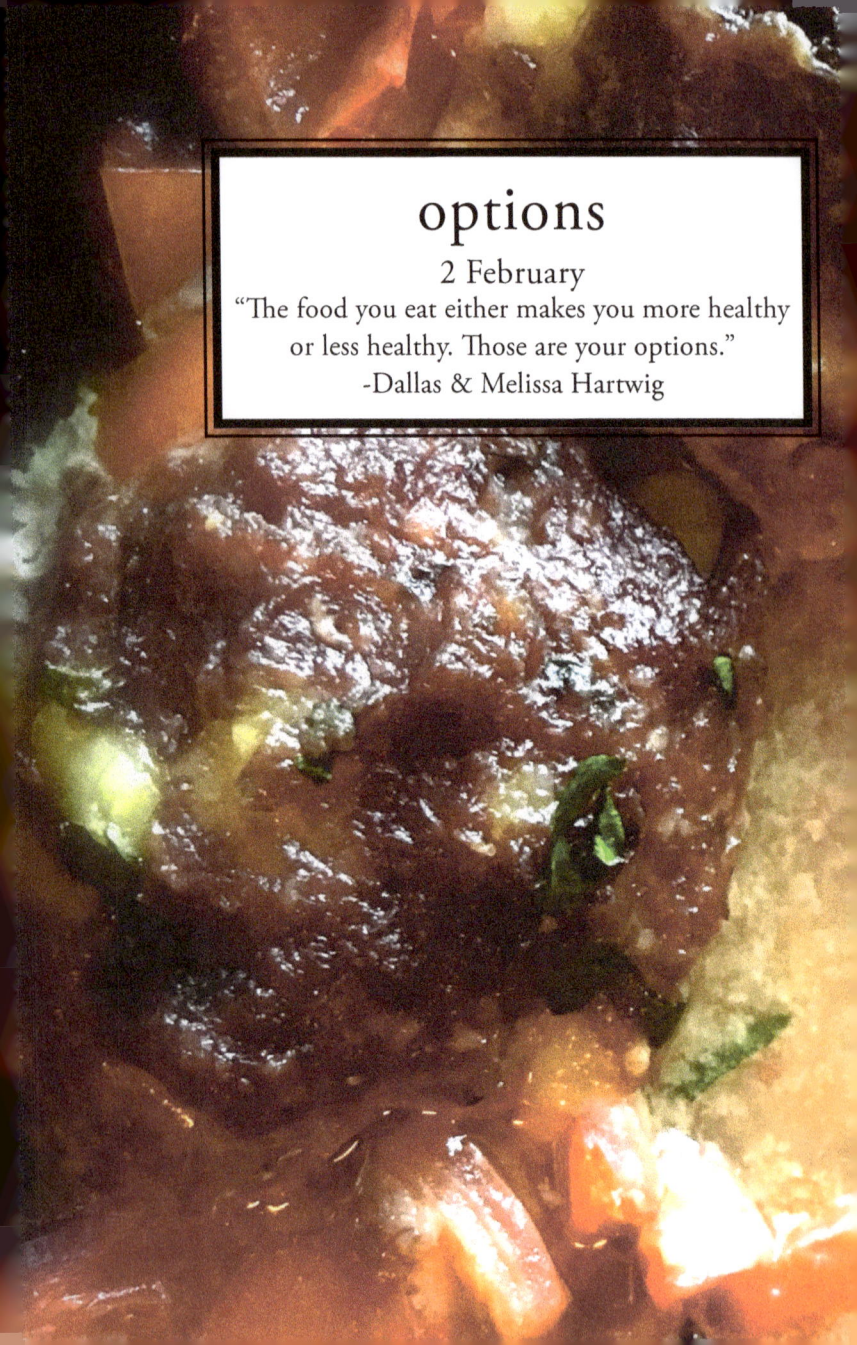

options

2 February
"The food you eat either makes you more healthy or less healthy. Those are your options."
-Dallas & Melissa Hartwig

i know it's TRUE

3 February

"Malnutrition could be one of the main reasons why many people are overweight...the body, in its deepest inner wisdom, may know that it is missing some essential nutrients. It sends messages to the appropriate parts of the brain, setting up hunger and craving, despite plenty of calories already eaten, in the hope of getting missing nutrients."

-Richard Shames, MD &
Karilee Halo Shames, RN, PhD

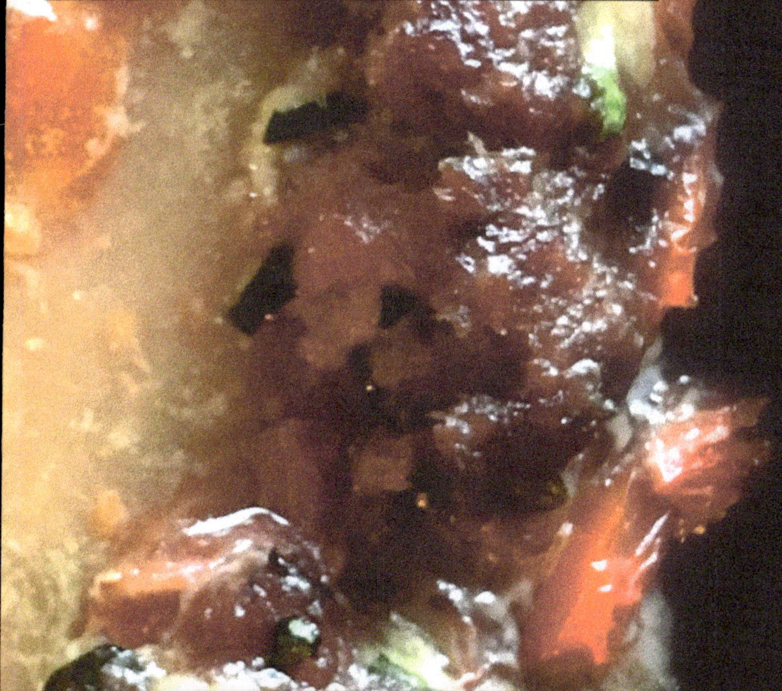

eudaimonia

4 February

eudaimonia: 'true' or 'real' happiness; the sort of happiness worth seeking or having; virtues guarantee a happy life...everything the soul endeavors or endures under the guidance of wisdom ends in happiness (Meno 88C)...health of a soul; when a soul has been properly cared for and perfected it possesses the virtues; life is not worth living if the soul is ruined by wrong doing; a person who is not virtuous cannot be happy and a person with virtue cannot fail to be happy... virtues such as self-control, courage, justice, piety, wisdom and related qualities of mind and soul are absolutely crucial if a person is to lead a good and happy life (Socrates).

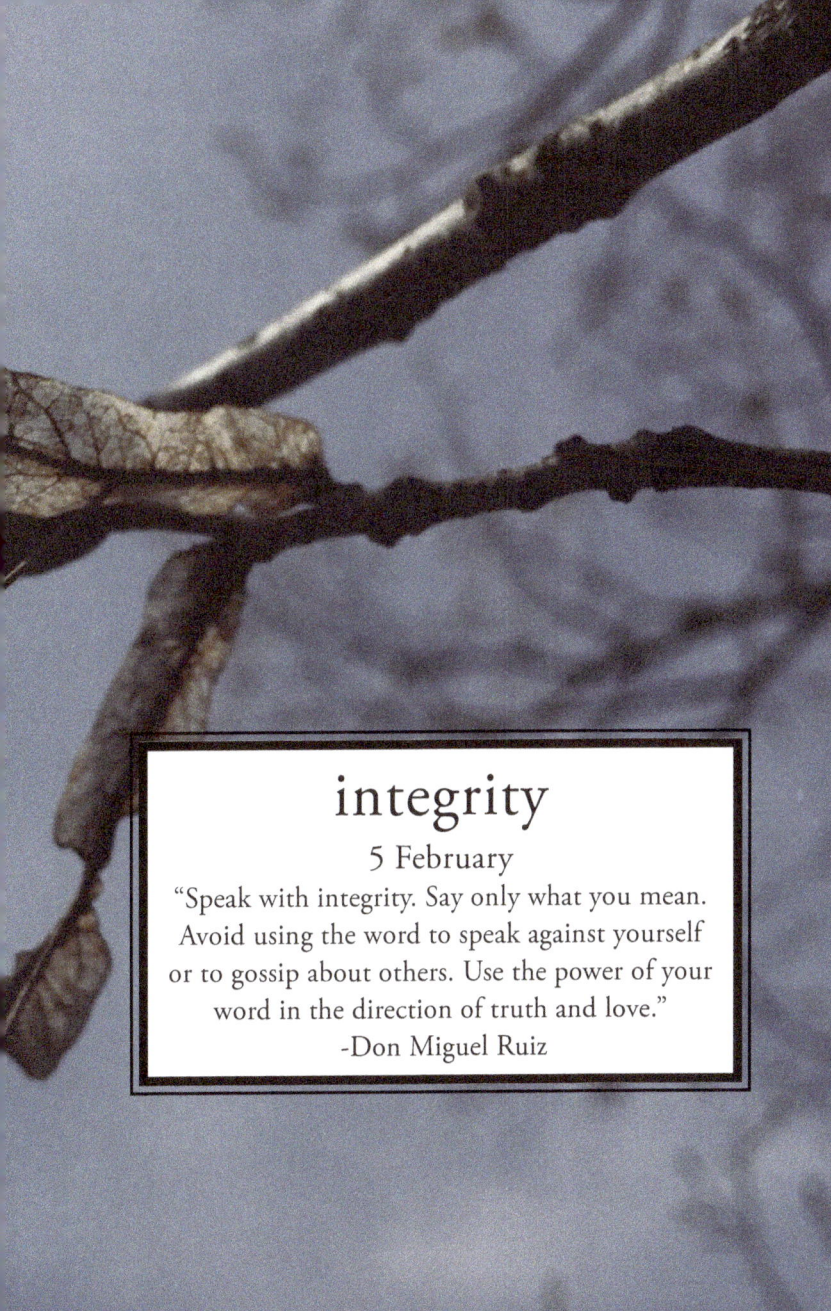

integrity
5 February
"Speak with integrity. Say only what you mean. Avoid using the word to speak against yourself or to gossip about others. Use the power of your word in the direction of truth and love."
-Don Miguel Ruiz

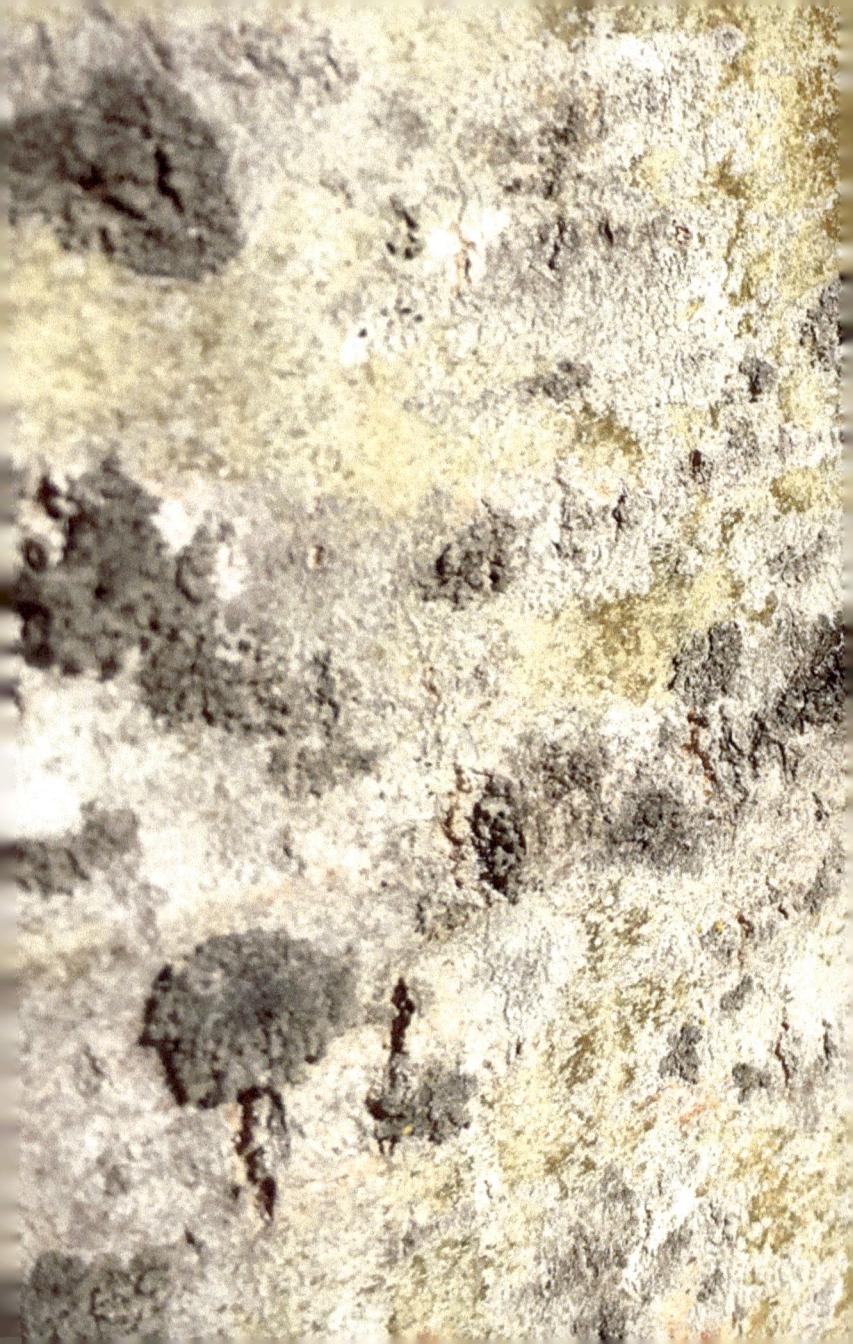

knock knock

6 February
"Go to your bosom knock there and
ask your heart what it doth know."
-William Shakespeare

feeling free

7 February
"Picture a place where there is nothing to fear
and all your dreams have come true...
If you do nothing more than to choose whatever
feels most freeing moment by moment you will
fulfill your best destiny." -Martha Beck

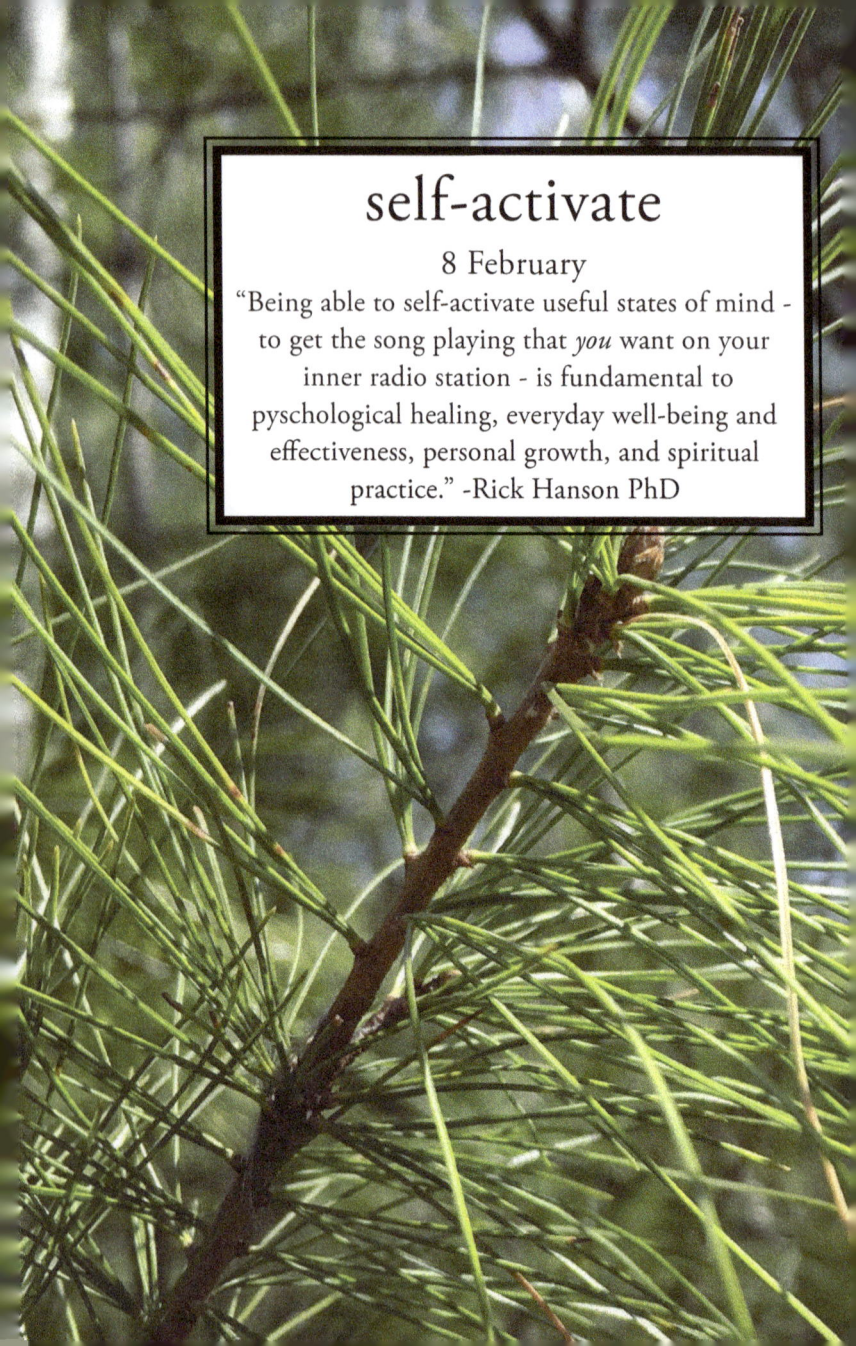

self-activate

8 February

"Being able to self-activate useful states of mind - to get the song playing that *you* want on your inner radio station - is fundamental to pyschological healing, everyday well-being and effectiveness, personal growth, and spiritual practice." -Rick Hanson PhD

higher

9 February

"The higher your aims and vaster your desires, the more energy you will have for their fulfillment. Desire the good of all and the universe will work with you." -Sri Nisargadatta Maharaj

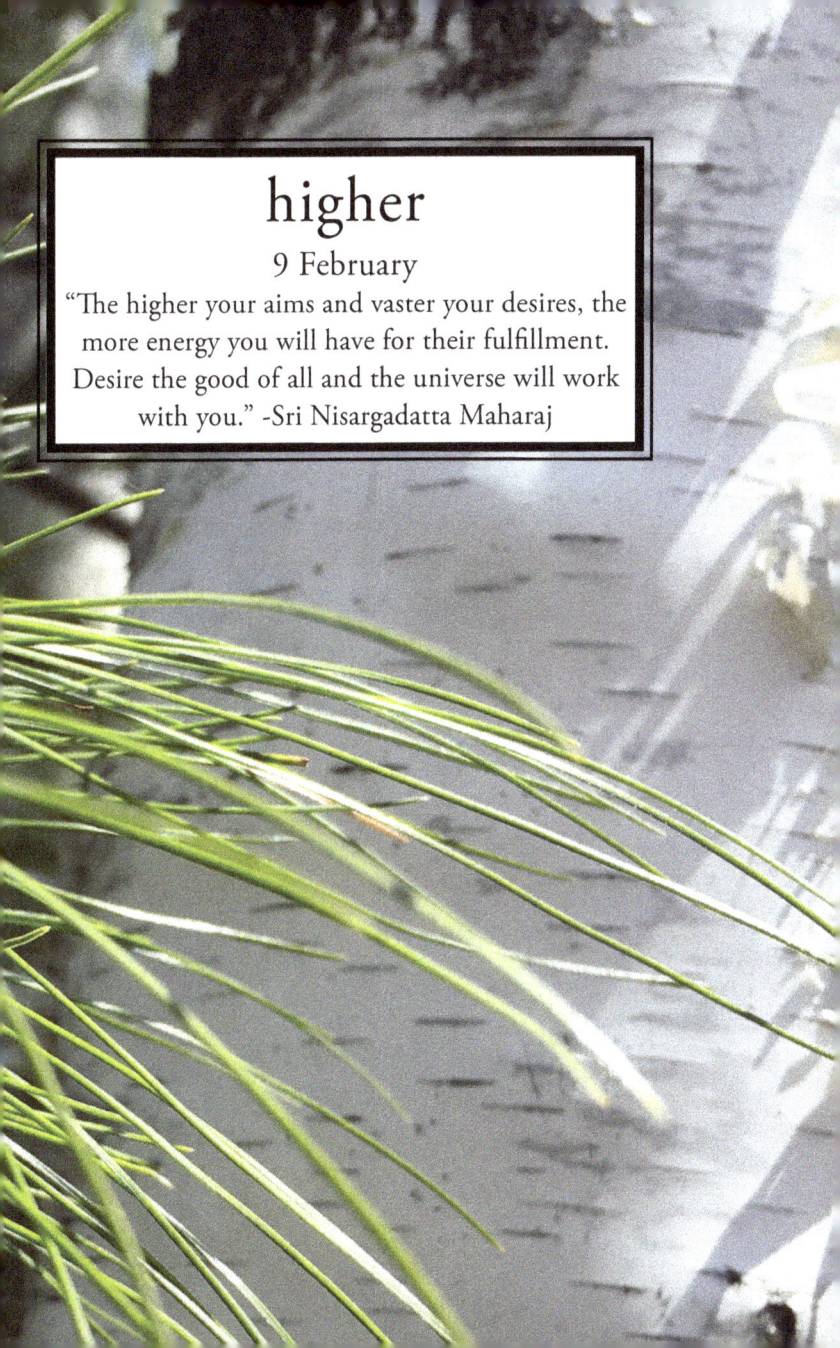

joy & freshness!

10 February

"If you take good care of yourself you help everyone, you stop being a source of suffering to the world, and you become a reservoir of joy and freshness. Here and there are people who know how to take good care of themselves who live joyfully and happily. They are our strongest support. Everything they do, they do for everyone." -Thich Nhat Hanh

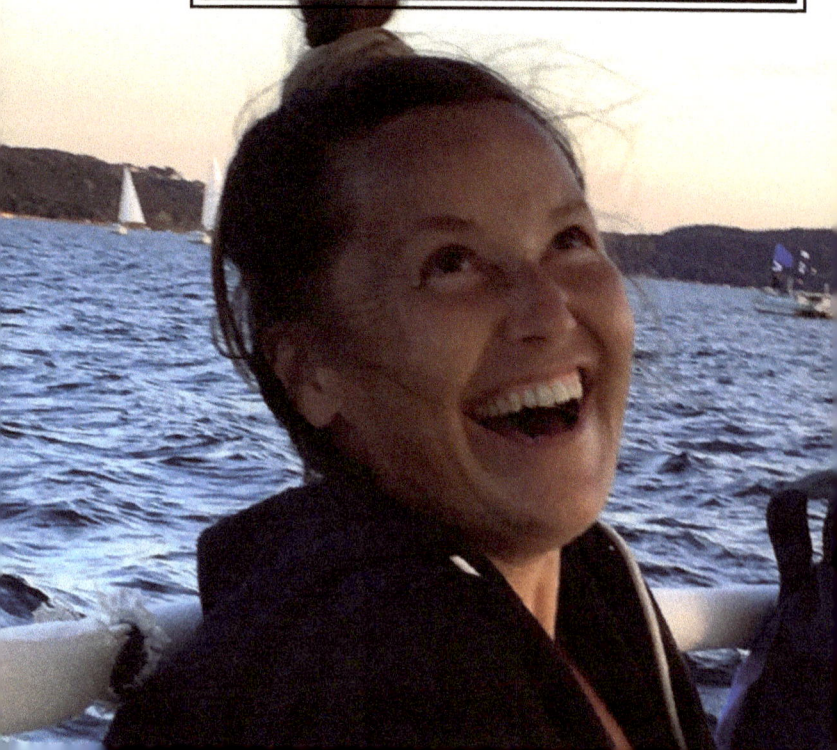

epigenetic

11 February

"Epigenetic translates to upon the gene. Epigenetic researchers study how our genes react to our behavior, and they've found that just about everything we eat, think, breathe, or can do, directly or indirectly, trickle down to affect its performance in some way. These effects are carried forward into the next gerneration where they can be magnified." -Catherine Shanahan MD & Luke Shanahan

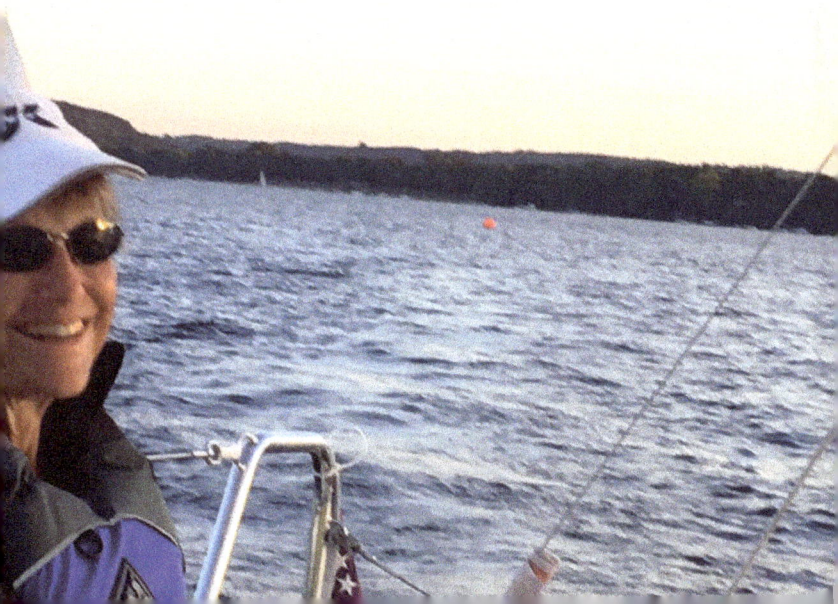

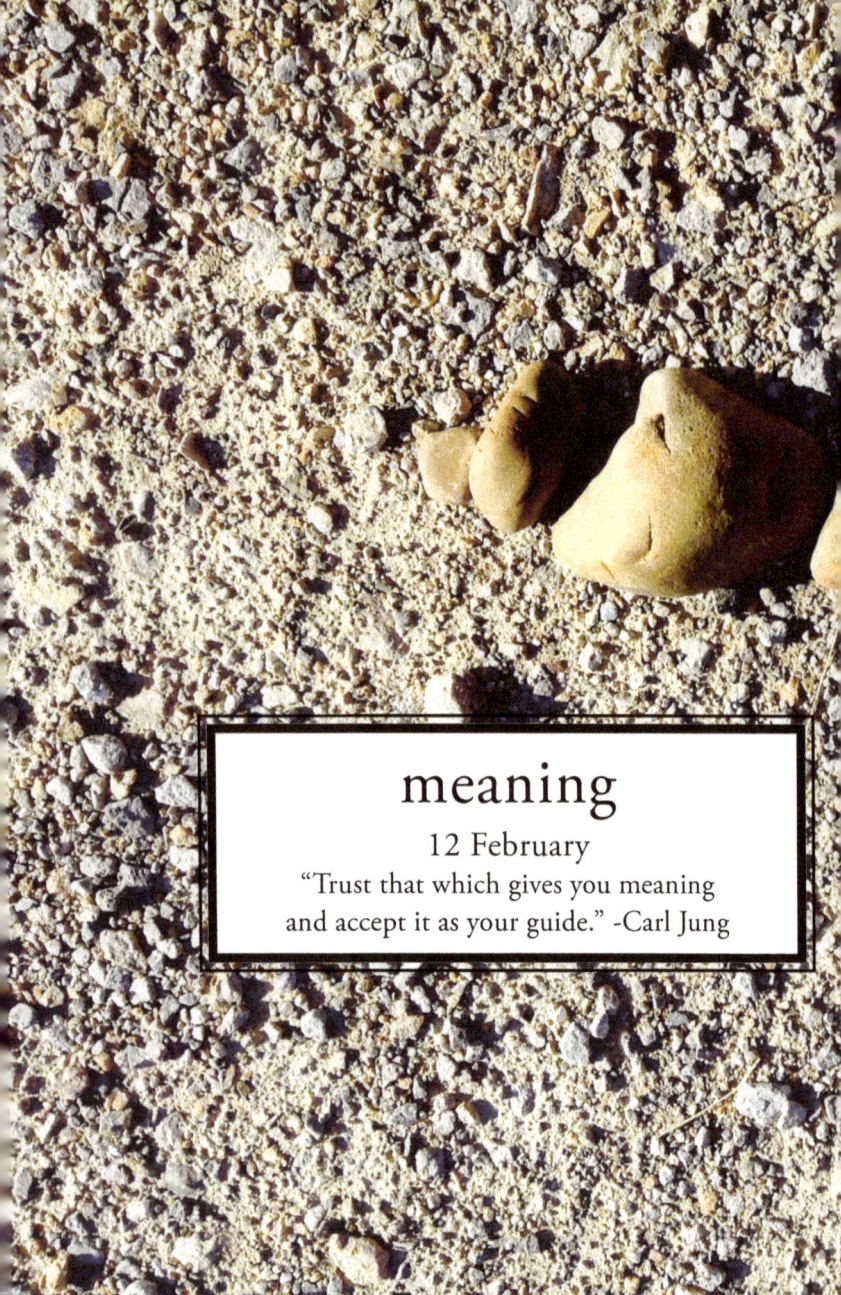

meaning

12 February
"Trust that which gives you meaning and accept it as your guide." -Carl Jung

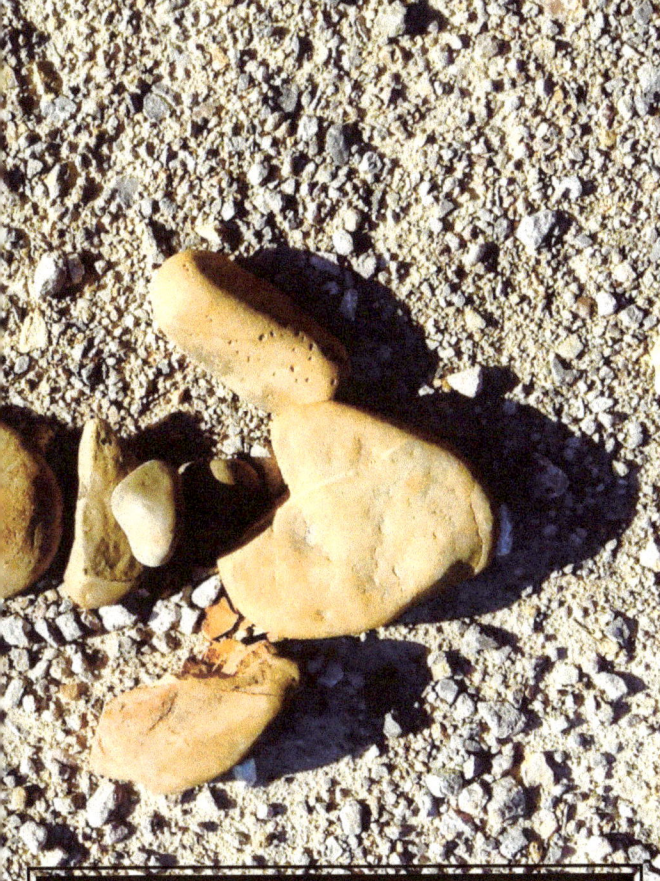

WOW!

13 February
"You have a unique gift to offer this world, and you are unique in the entire history of creation."
-Wayne Dyer

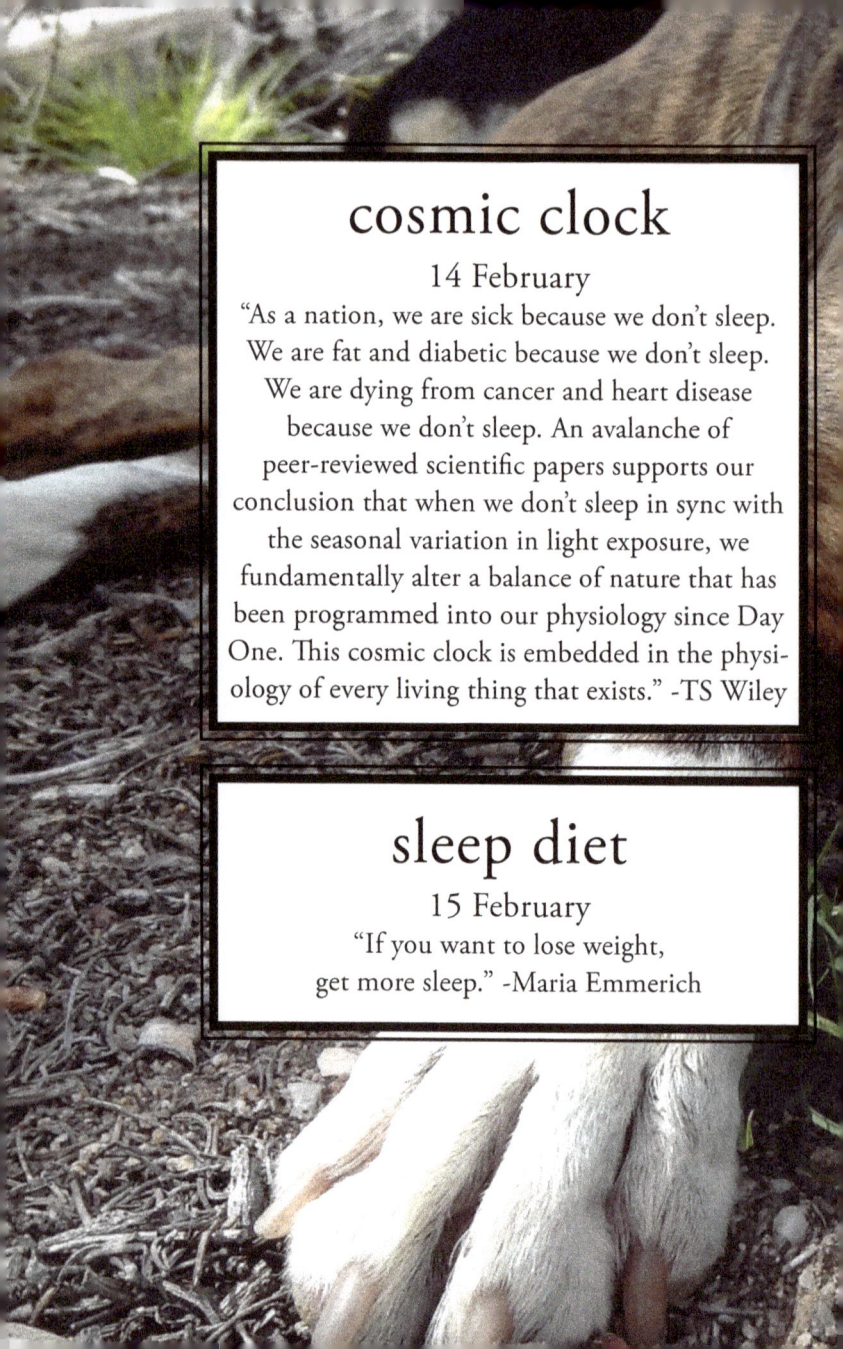

cosmic clock

14 February

"As a nation, we are sick because we don't sleep. We are fat and diabetic because we don't sleep. We are dying from cancer and heart disease because we don't sleep. An avalanche of peer-reviewed scientific papers supports our conclusion that when we don't sleep in sync with the seasonal variation in light exposure, we fundamentally alter a balance of nature that has been programmed into our physiology since Day One. This cosmic clock is embedded in the physiology of every living thing that exists." -TS Wiley

sleep diet

15 February

"If you want to lose weight, get more sleep." -Maria Emmerich

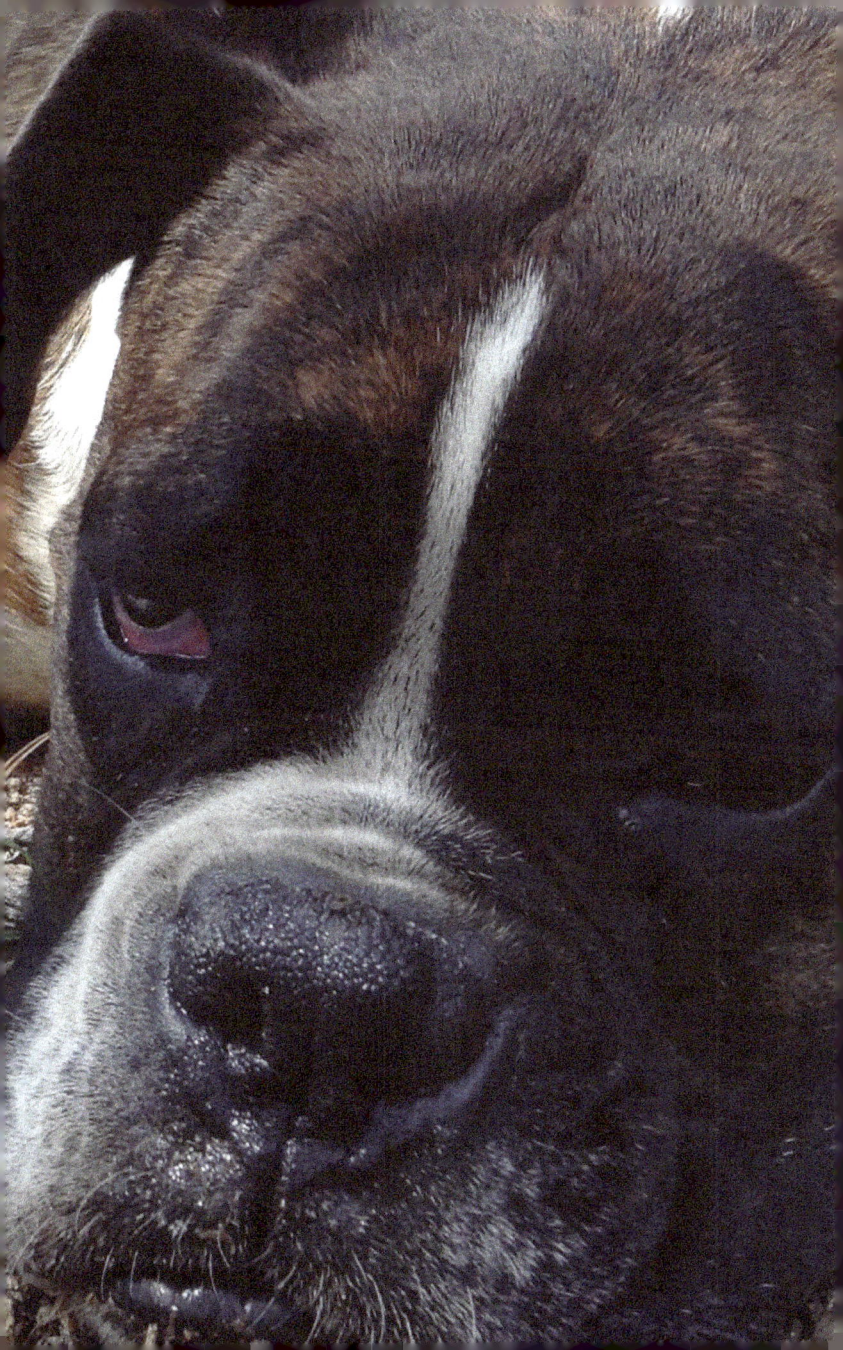

supermarket
16 February
"When you go into a supermarket in the United States, there is hardly any food!...There was not a lot, in most American supermarkets, that most French people would consider (traditionally at least) an *aliment* ('a nourishment')...the processed and prepared foods that filled up the aisles in a North American grocery store weren't real food, because, although they were edible, they weren't nourishing." -Karen Lebillon

protection
17 February
"It is whole food that heals, real food that protects, and traditional food that nourishes." -Katherine Erlich MD & Kelly Genzlinger CNC, CMTA

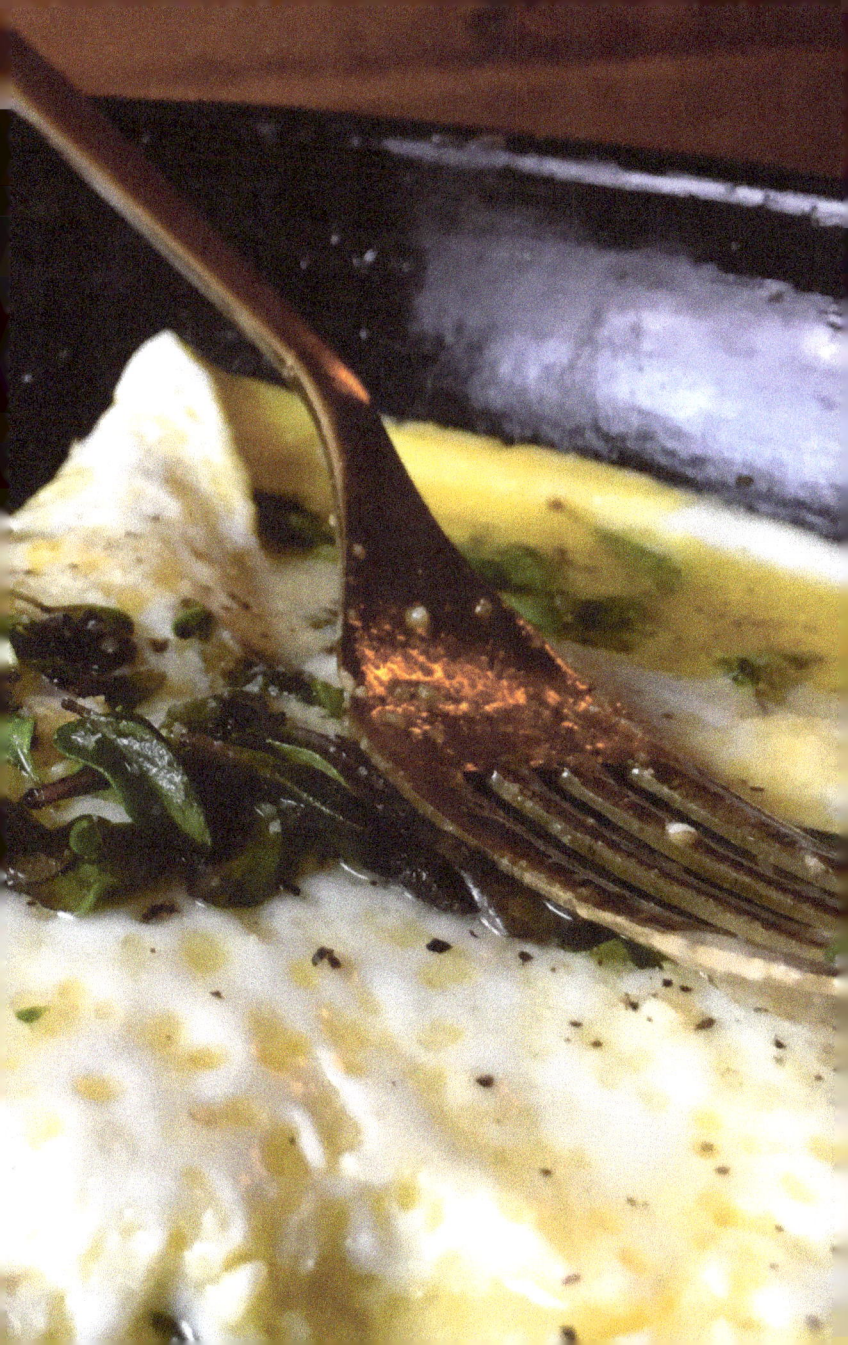

daring!

18 February
"If it's worth doing, it's worth daring."
-Martha Beck

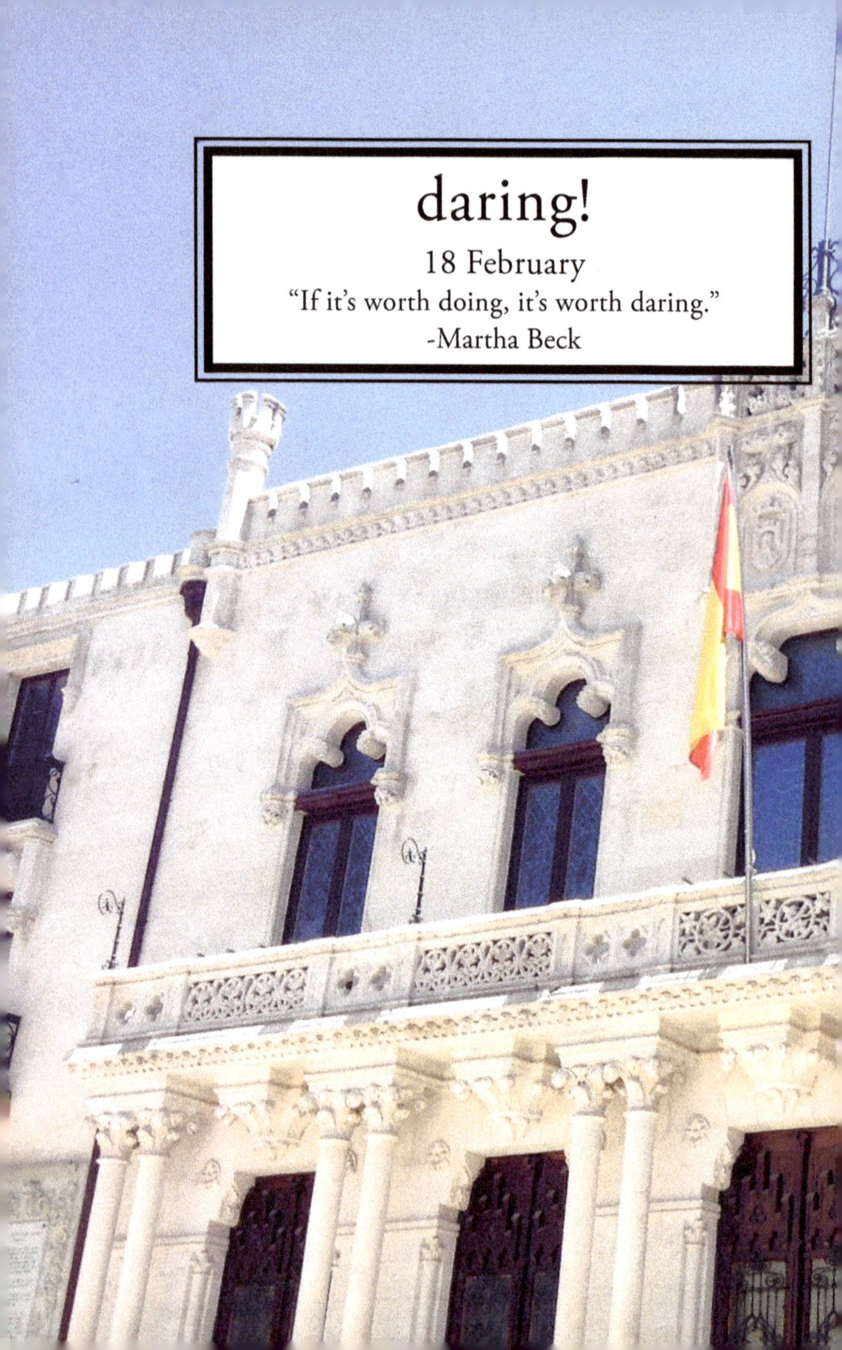

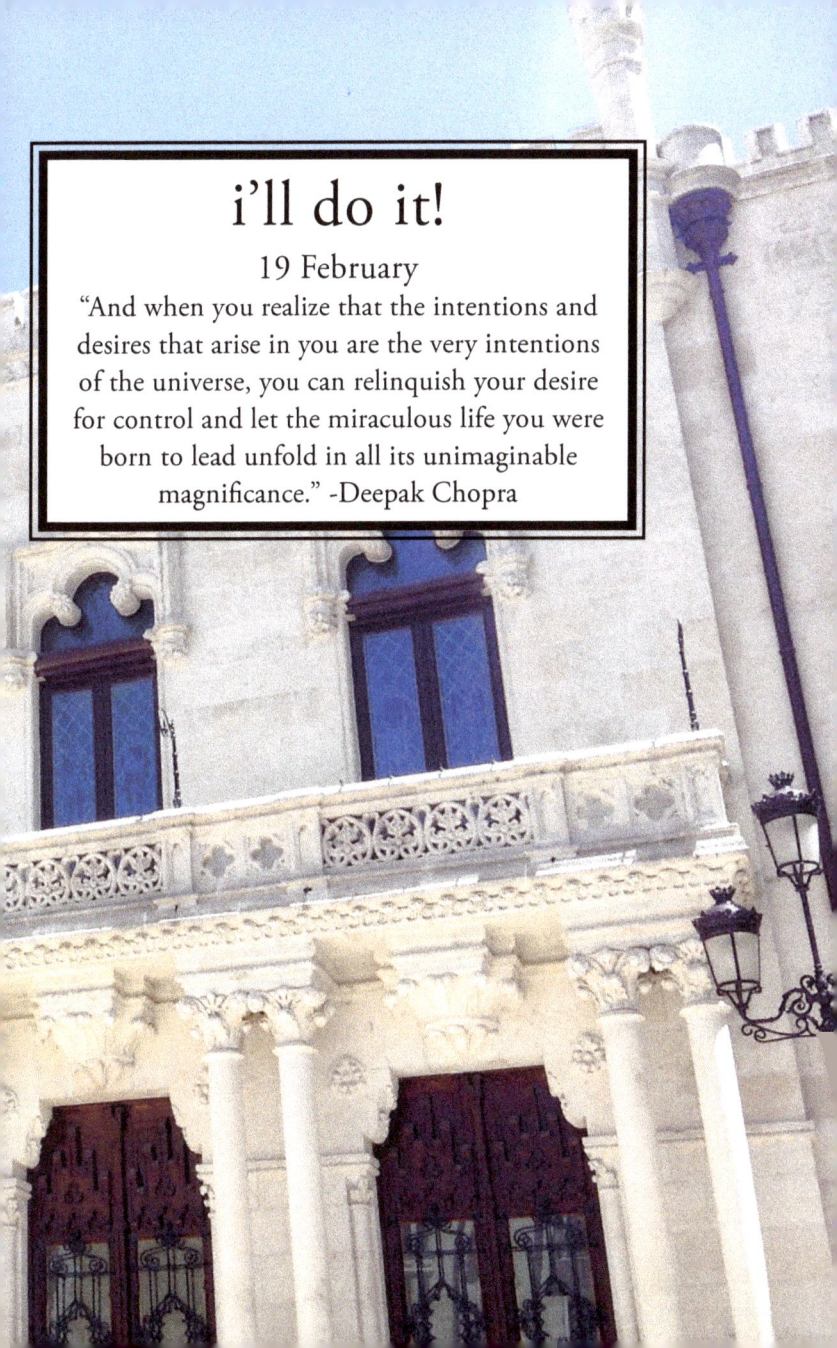

i'll do it!

19 February

"And when you realize that the intentions and desires that arise in you are the very intentions of the universe, you can relinquish your desire for control and let the miraculous life you were born to lead unfold in all its unimaginable magnificance." -Deepak Chopra

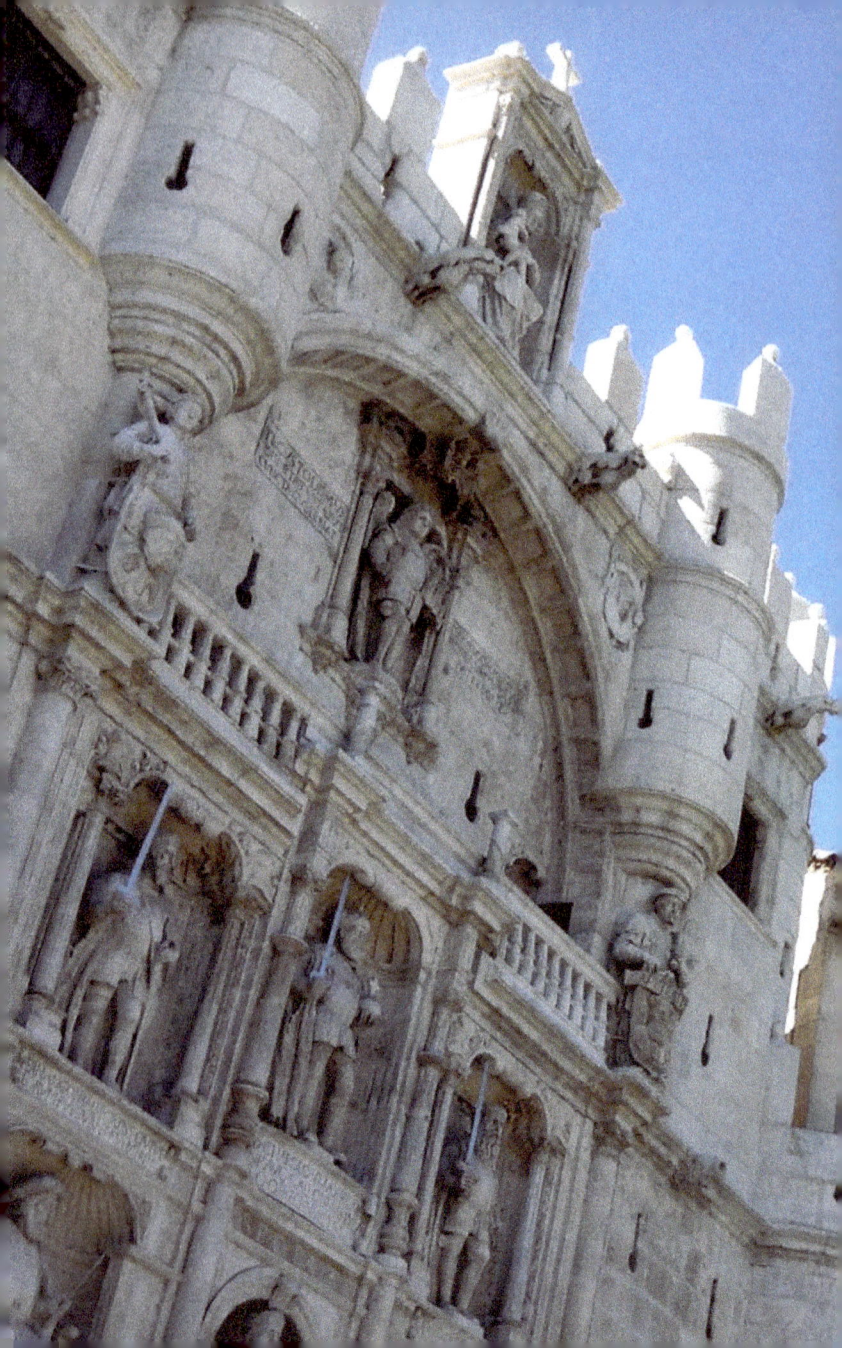

i choose joy

20 February
"Imagine that you can choose any emotional feeling you want to experience." -Deepak Chopra

heart

21 February
"With compassion in our heart: every thought every word every deed can bring about a miracle."
-Thich Nhat Hanh

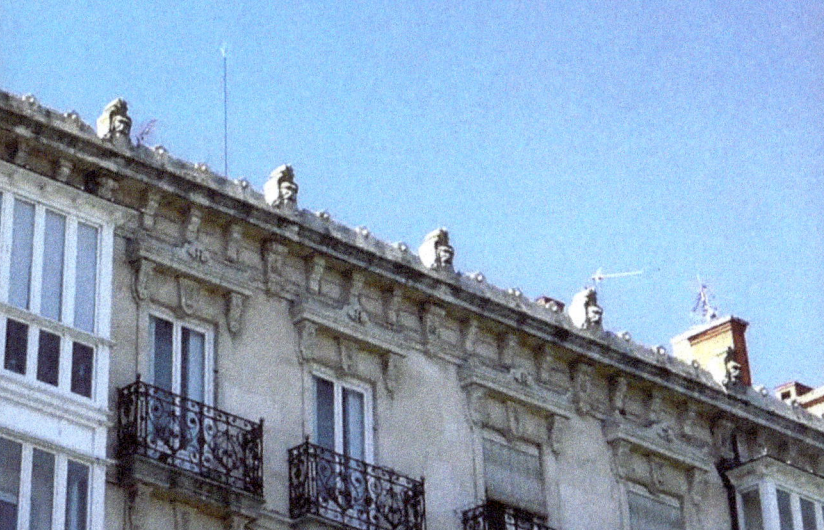

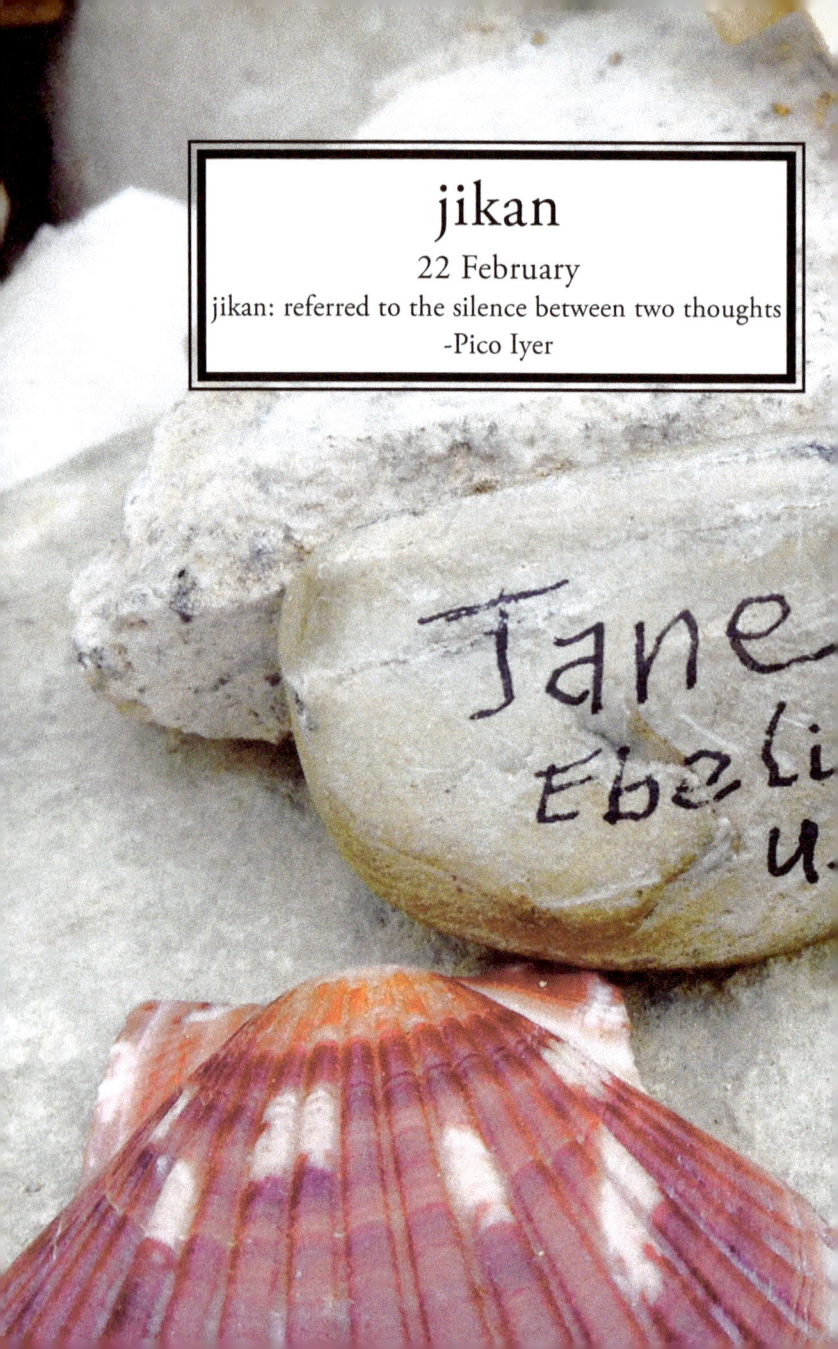

jikan
22 February
jikan: referred to the silence between two thoughts
-Pico Iyer

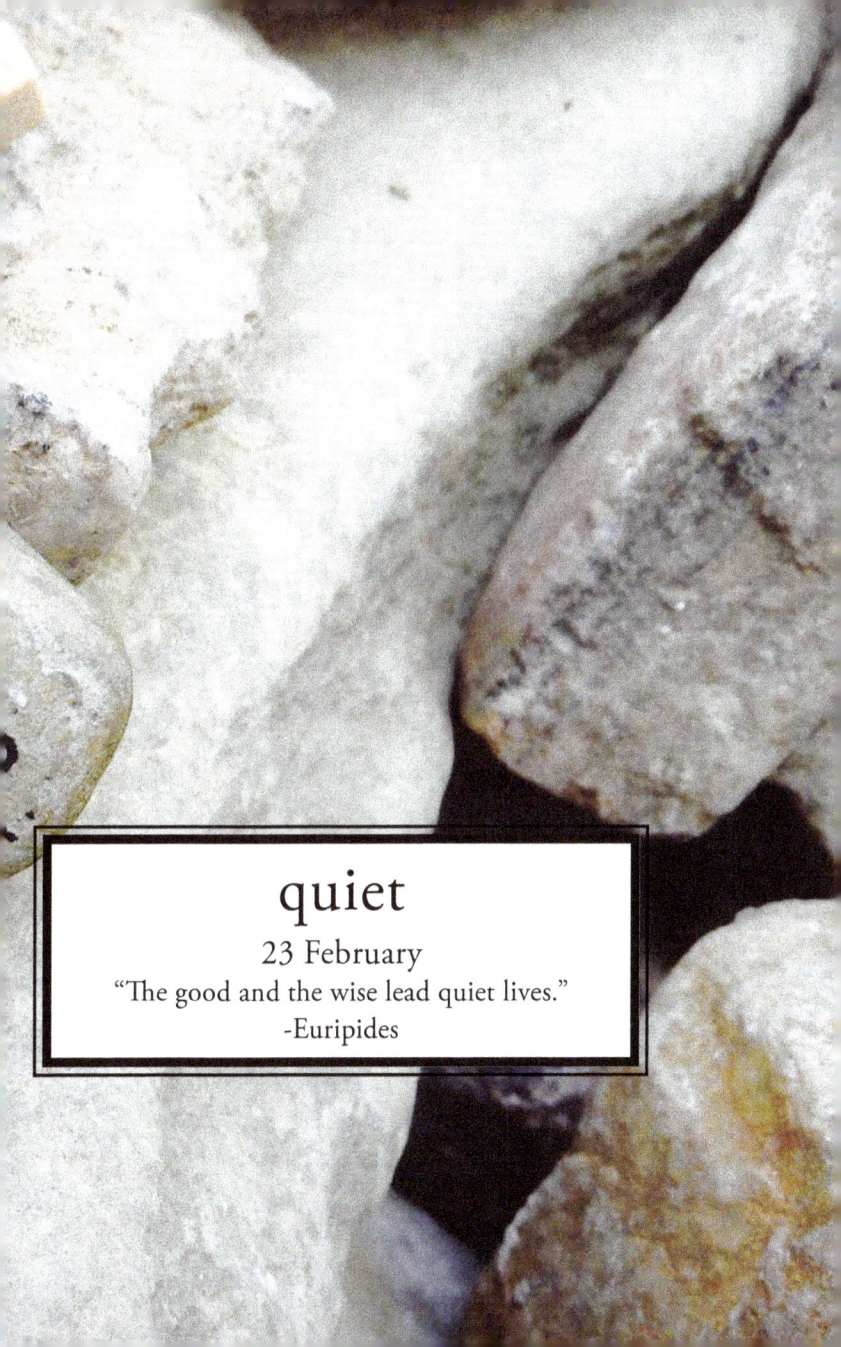

quiet

23 February
"The good and the wise lead quiet lives."
-Euripides

homeostasis
24 February

"Eating real food is the most painless way to keep blood sugar stable and avoid the cravings that come with overly processed factory foods... homeostasis - the system that regulates our weight (our appetites' on-off switch)."

-Christine Avanti

cholesterol
25 February

"Hopefully…[readers] don't bother about their cholesterol any longer…hopefully, everyone understands that eggs, cream, butter and fatty meat are healthy foods that they should prefer for industrially processed food with their dozens of added chemicals, the effects about which we know very little." -Uffe Ravnskov, MD, PhD

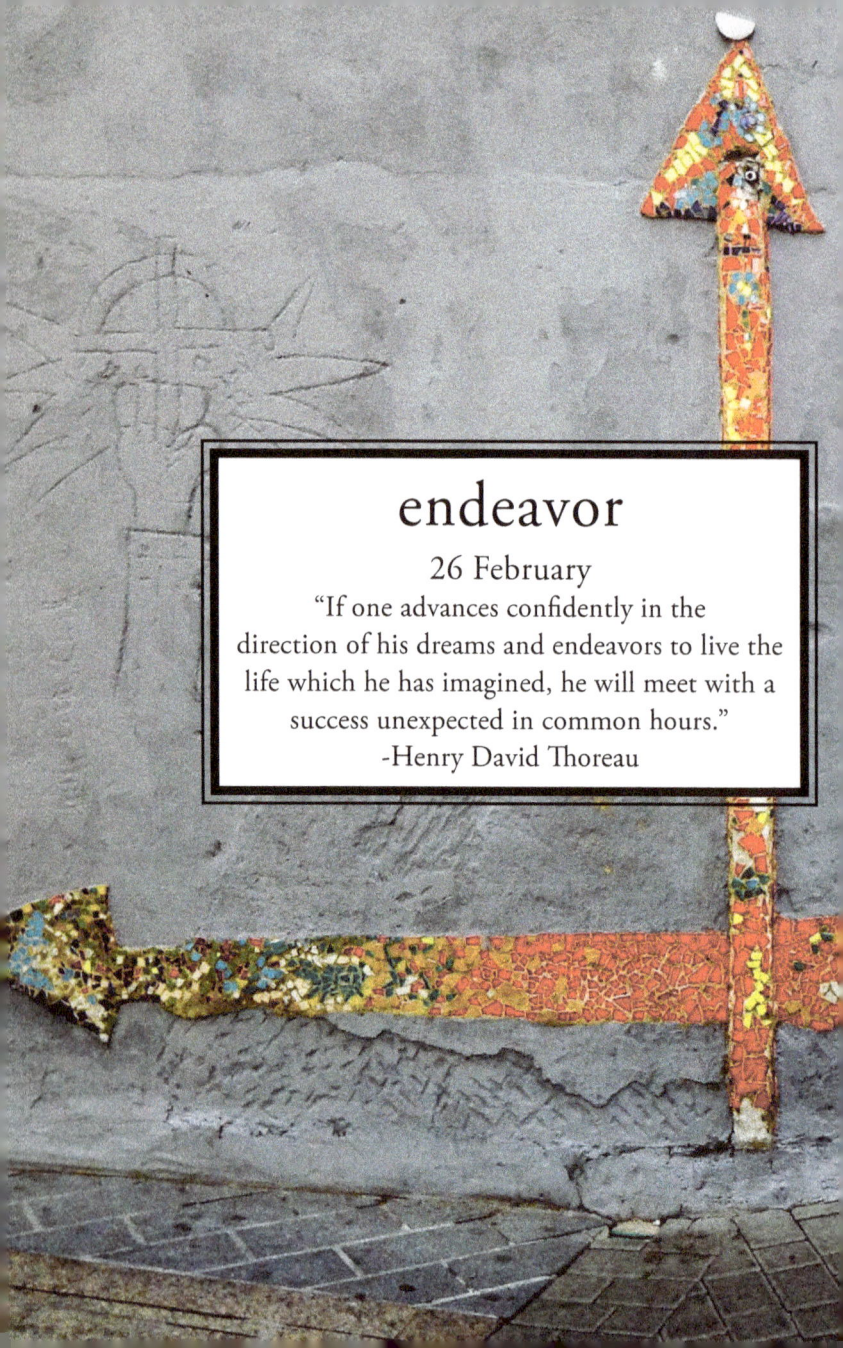

endeavor

26 February

"If one advances confidently in the direction of his dreams and endeavors to live the life which he has imagined, he will meet with a success unexpected in common hours."
-Henry David Thoreau

choices

27 February

"When you make choices from freedom, the result is more freedom. Once you accept that, you can receive everything you desire by simply recognizing that you already have everything you want." -James Twyman

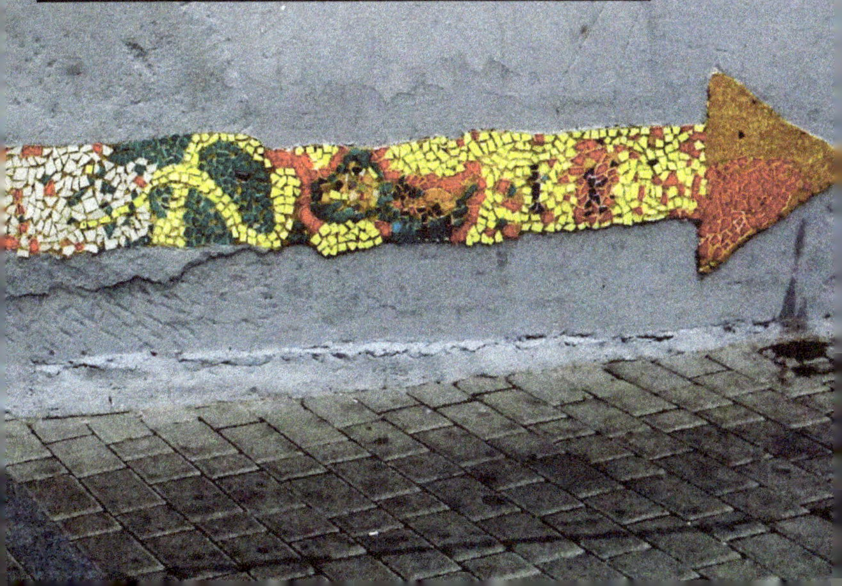

riches!
28 February
"Dismiss whatever insults your own soul and your very flesh shall be a great poem and have the richest fluency not only in its words but in the silent lines of its lips and face and between the lashes of your eyes and in every motion and joint of your body." -Walt Whitman

30 to 50 years!
1 March
"The way you think, the way you behave, the way you eat, can influence your life by 30 to 50 years."
-Deepak Chopra

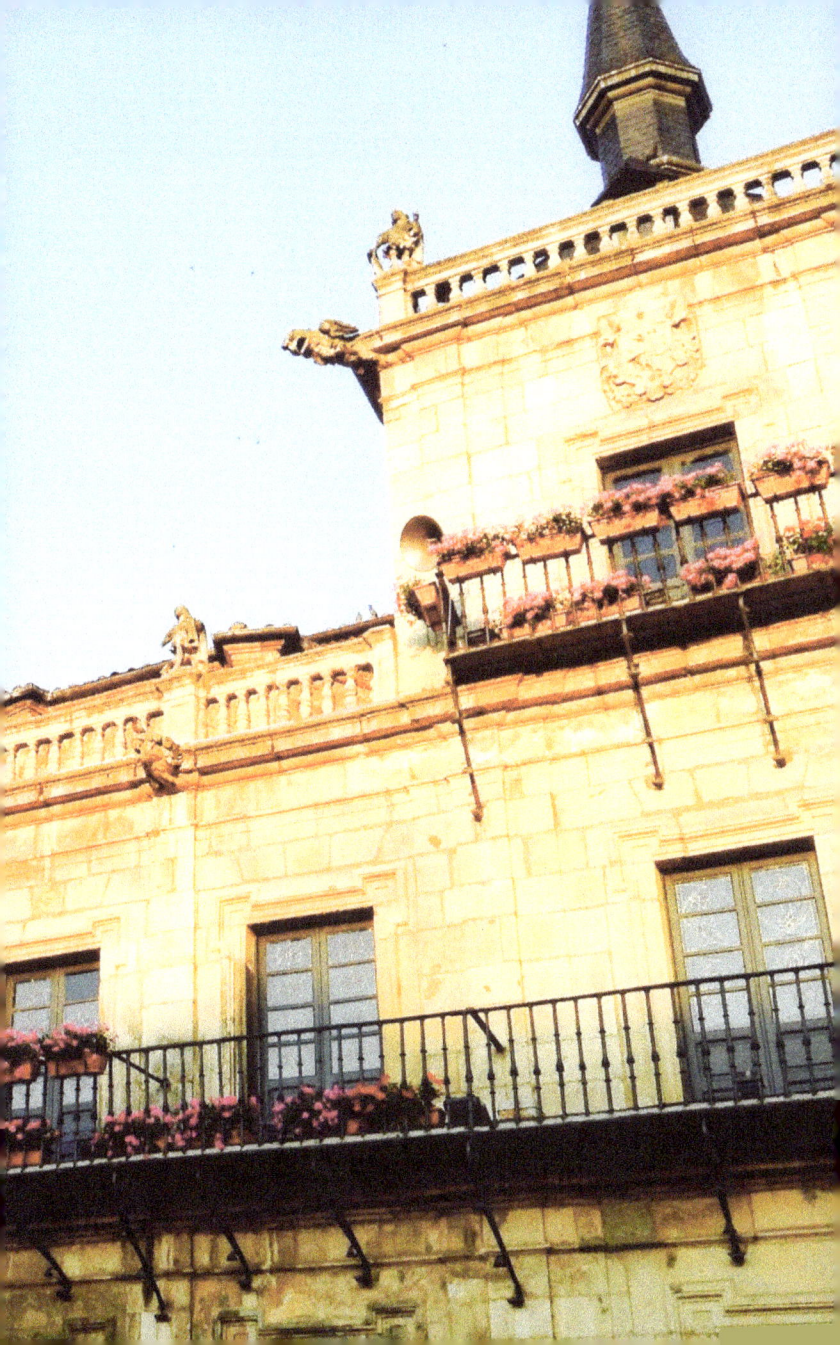

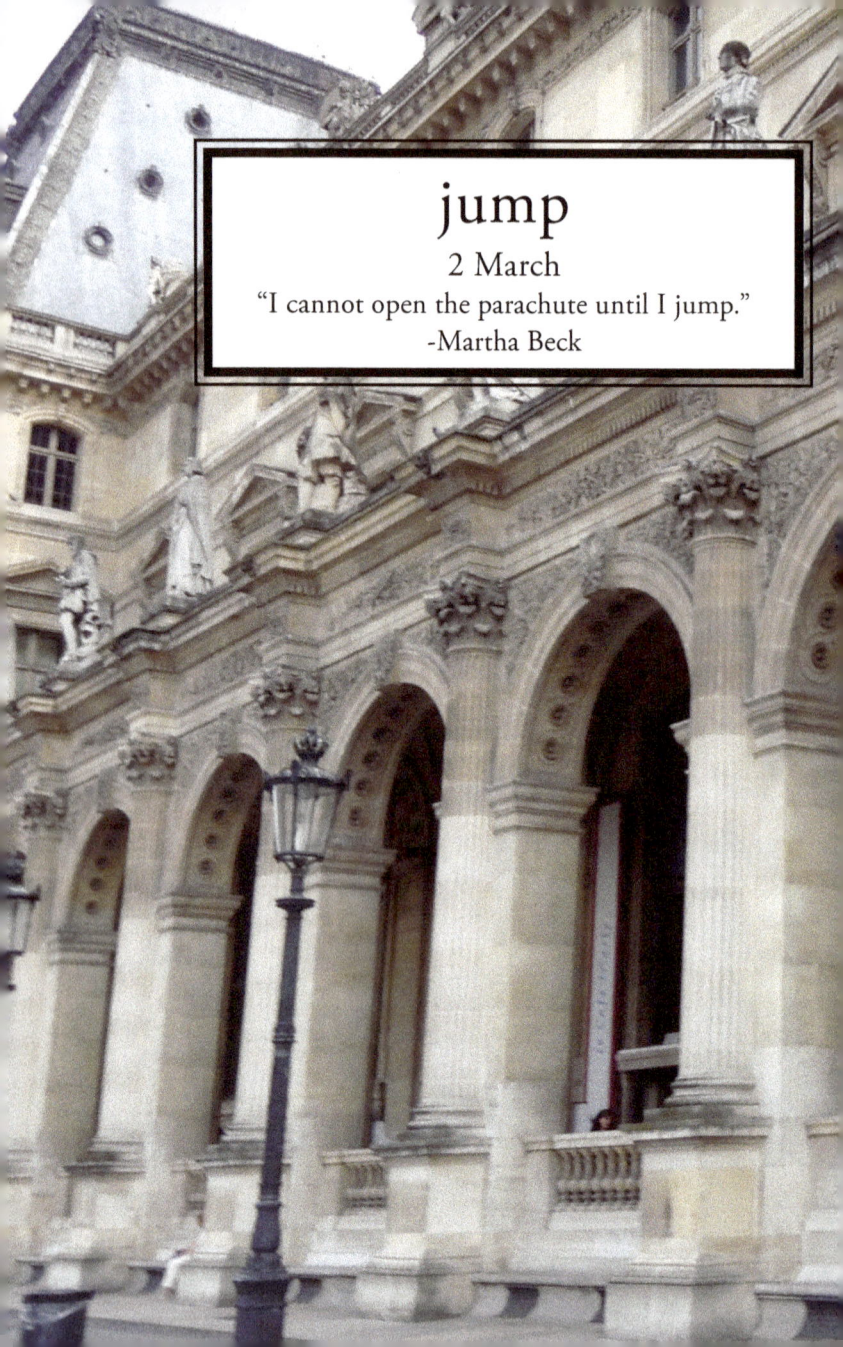

jump
2 March
"I cannot open the parachute until I jump."
-Martha Beck

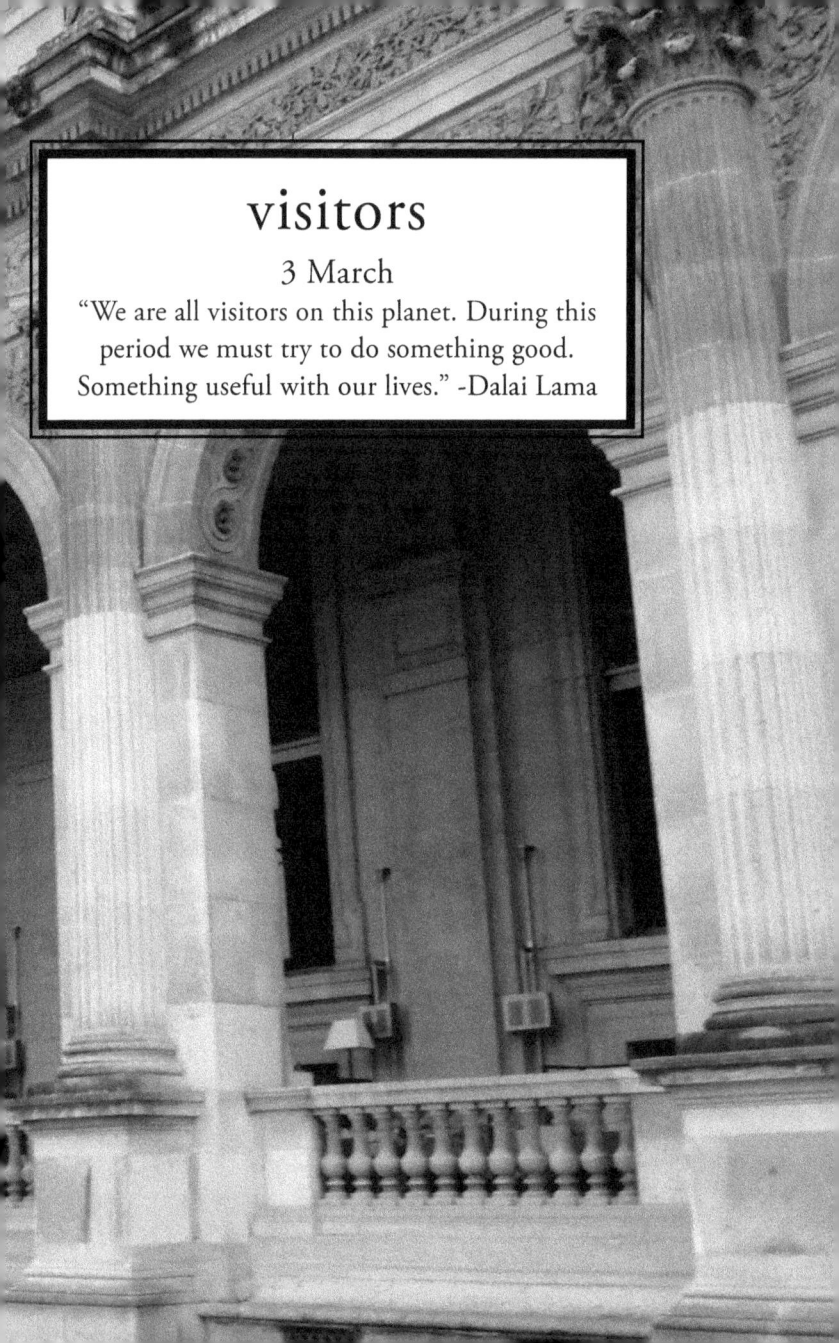

visitors

3 March

"We are all visitors on this planet. During this period we must try to do something good. Something useful with our lives." -Dalai Lama

happiness of life

4 March

"The happiness of your life depends on the quality of your thoughts." -Marcus Aurelius

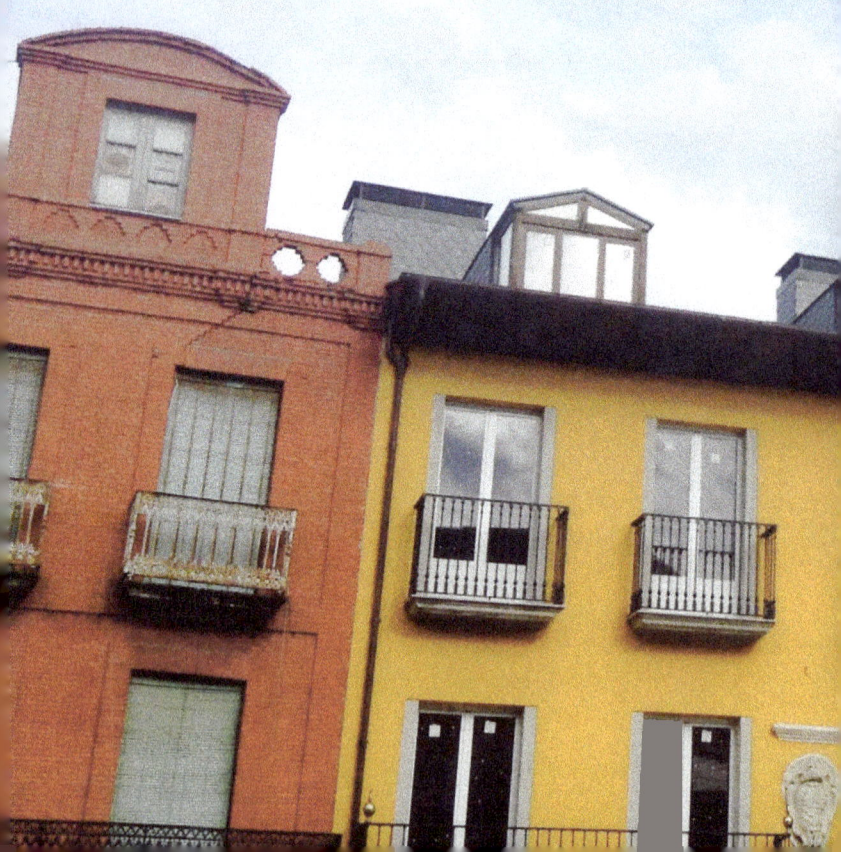

"taking in the good"

5 March

"The brain is a physical system that, like a muscle, gets stronger the more you exercise it. So make taking in the good a regular part of your life. This will be deliberate at first, but it will become increasingly automatic. Hardly thinking about it, you'll be weaving good experiences into your brain." -Rick Hanson PhD

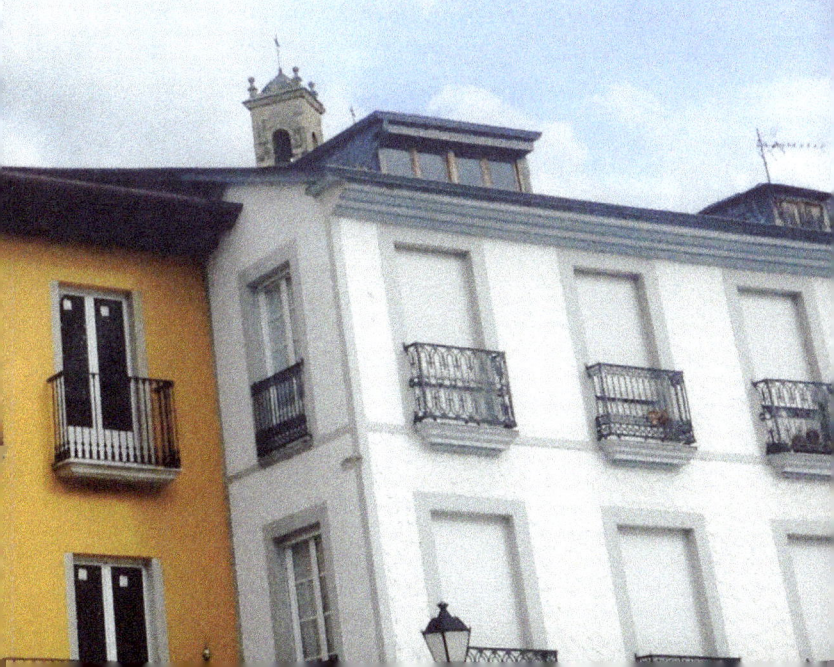

perfect balance
6 March
"You've created everything in your life, including what doesn't serve you well. Once you do accept it, though, you'll also be able to accept happiness, abundance, and perfect balance." -James Twyman

purpose
7 March
"What makes you feel happy capable on purpose?"
-Martha Beck

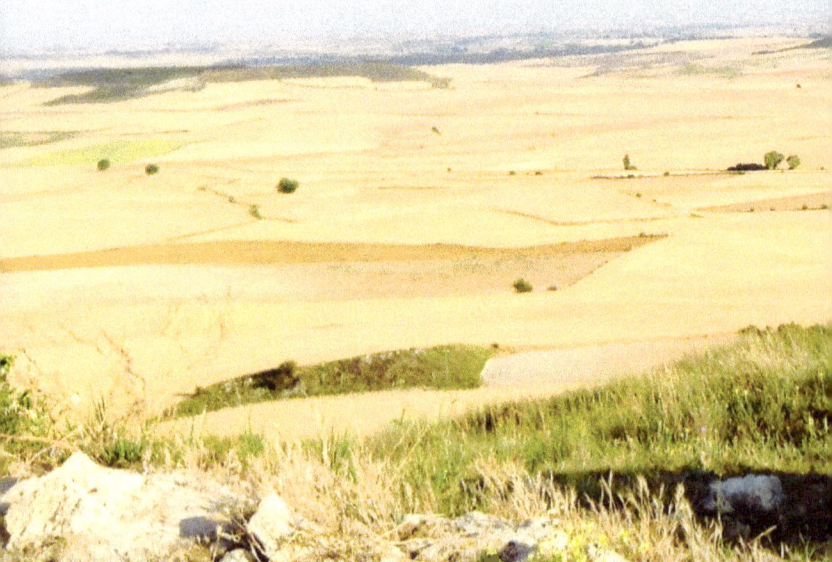

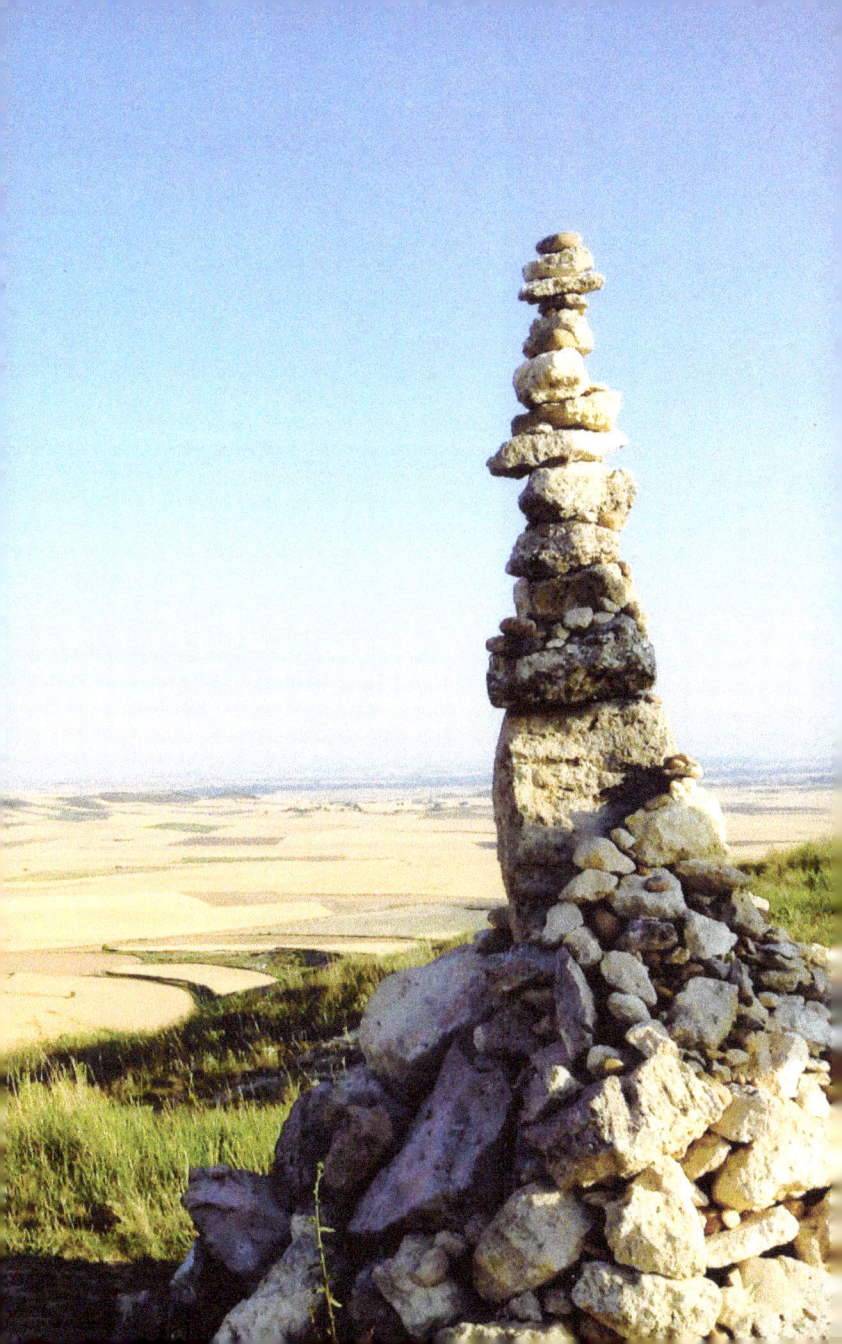

2,000,000 cells

8 March

"Your body manufactures 2,000,000 red blood cells every second; just look at what you ate and drank in the past 24 hours to see what your new red blood cells are made of!" -Paul Chek

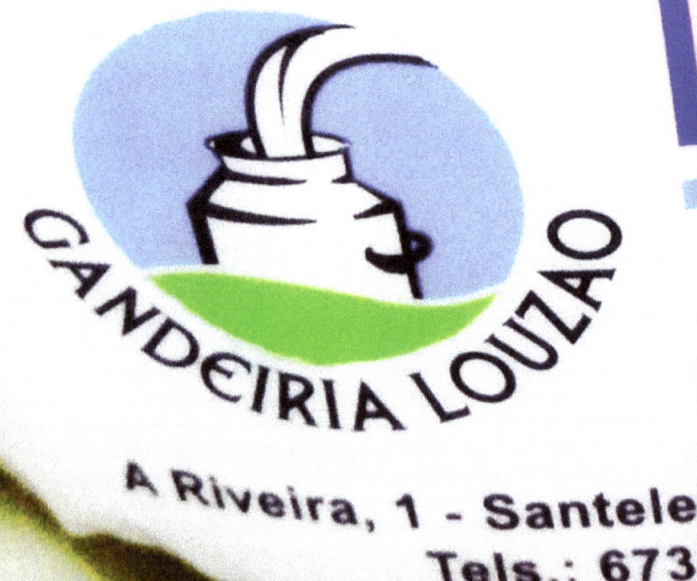

happy fat!
9 March
"The saturated fats you consume from grass-fed beef, poultry, pork, eggs, fish and seafood will not promote heart disease, cancer, or any chronic health problem. In fact, these foods can ensure your birthright - a long, healthy, and happy life."
-Loren Cordain

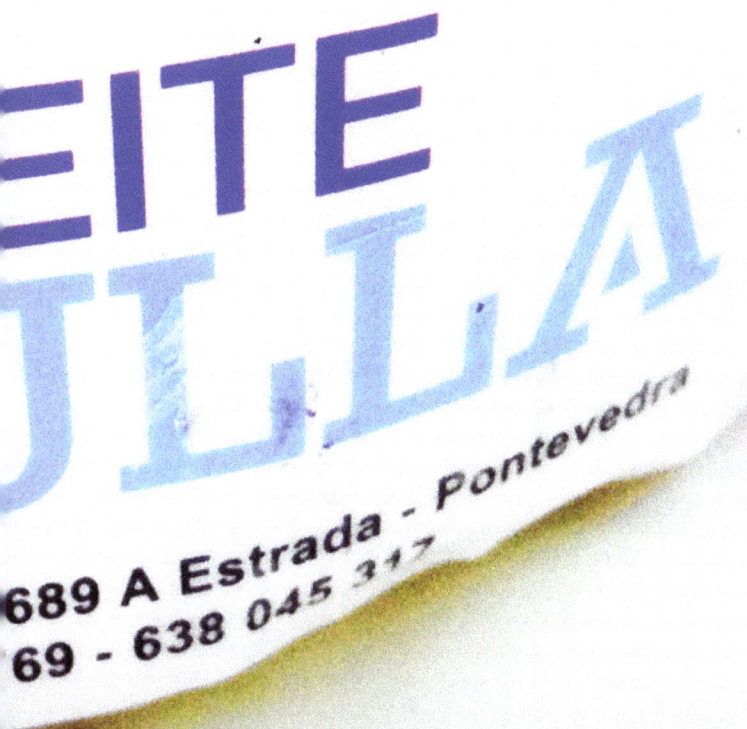

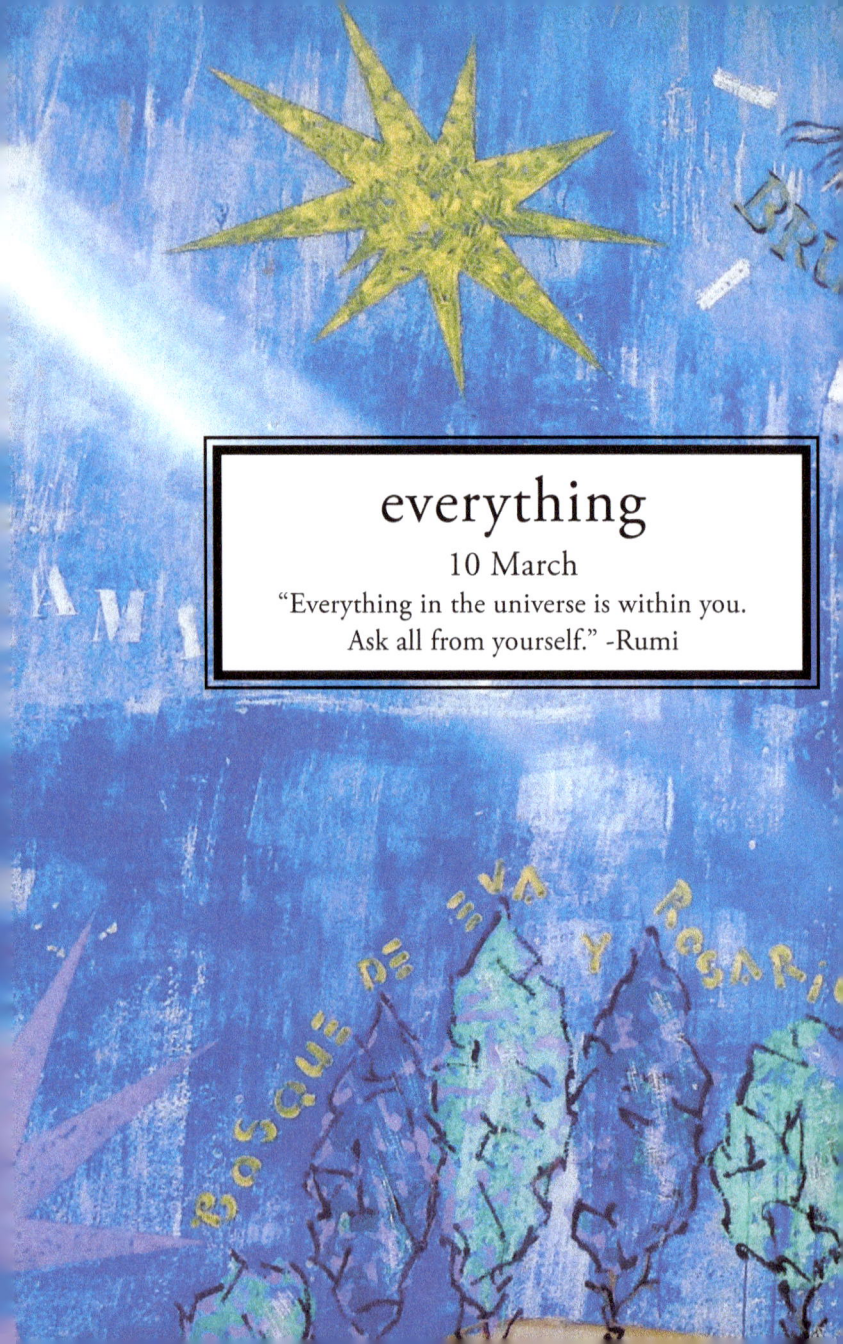

everything

10 March

"Everything in the universe is within you.
Ask all from yourself." -Rumi

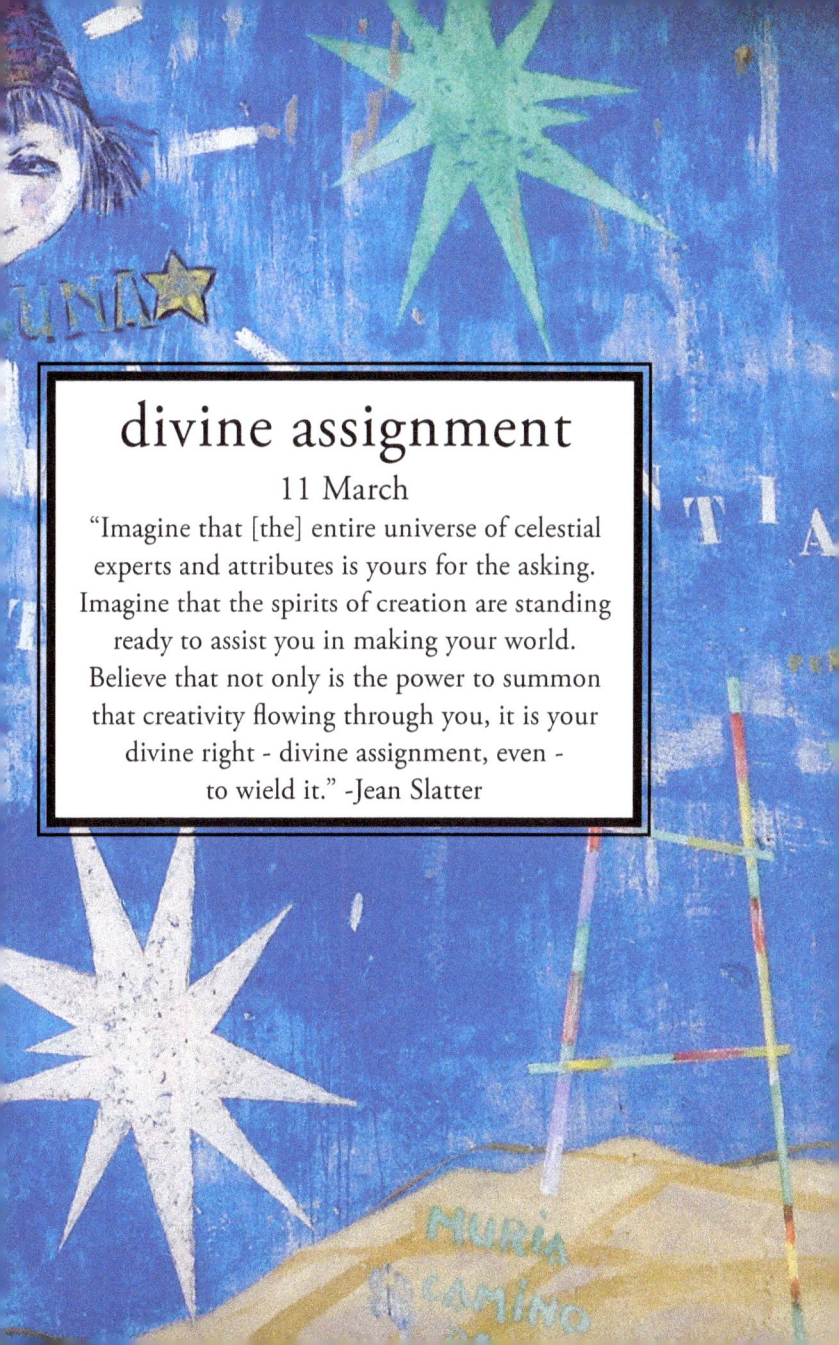

divine assignment
11 March

"Imagine that [the] entire universe of celestial experts and attributes is yours for the asking. Imagine that the spirits of creation are standing ready to assist you in making your world. Believe that not only is the power to summon that creativity flowing through you, it is your divine right - divine assignment, even - to wield it." -Jean Slatter

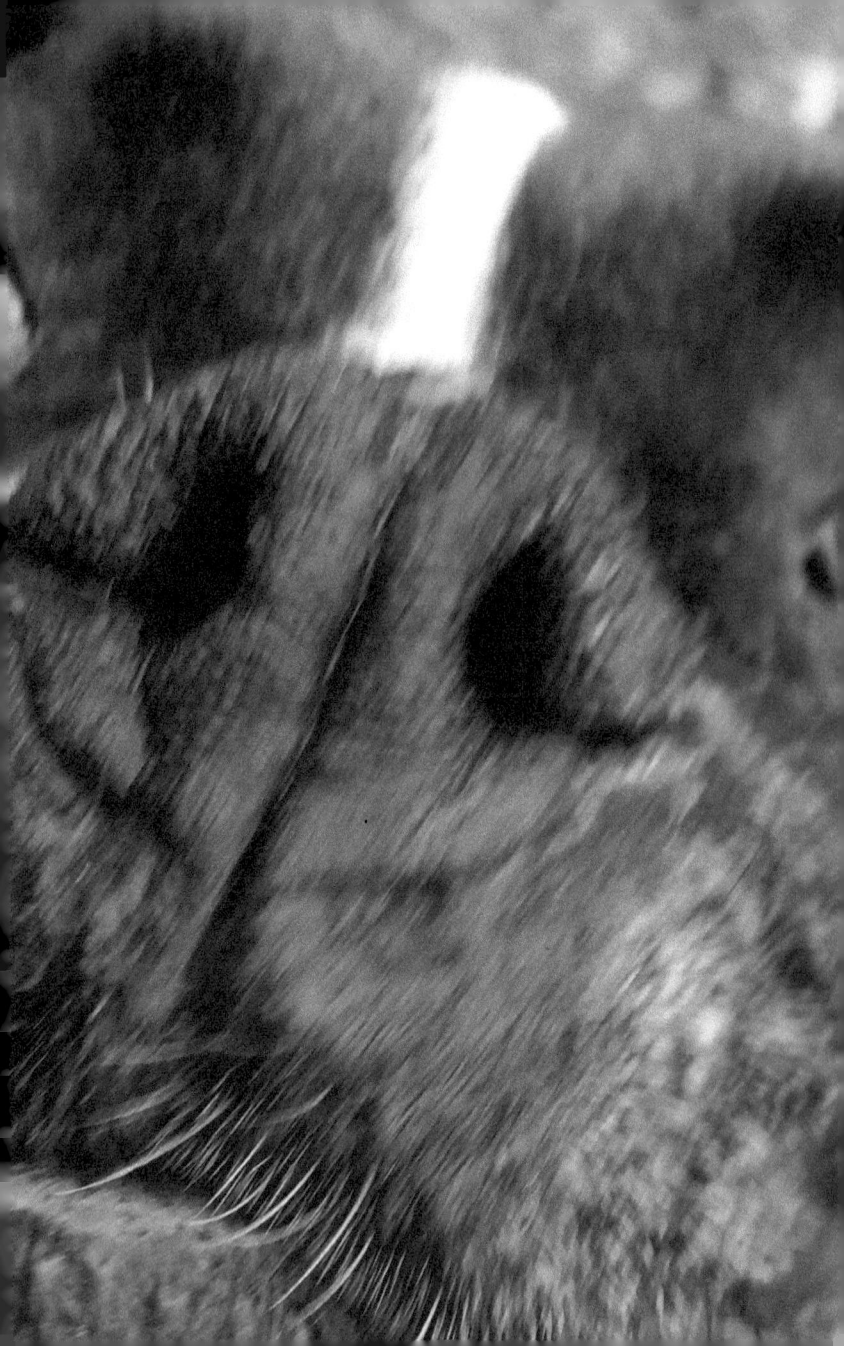

beam
12 March
"I will never force or strain. I will go where my joy leads me." -Deepak Chopra

happy molecules
13 March
"Happy thoughts create happy molecules. Your health is determined largely by the thoughts you have." -Wayne Dyer

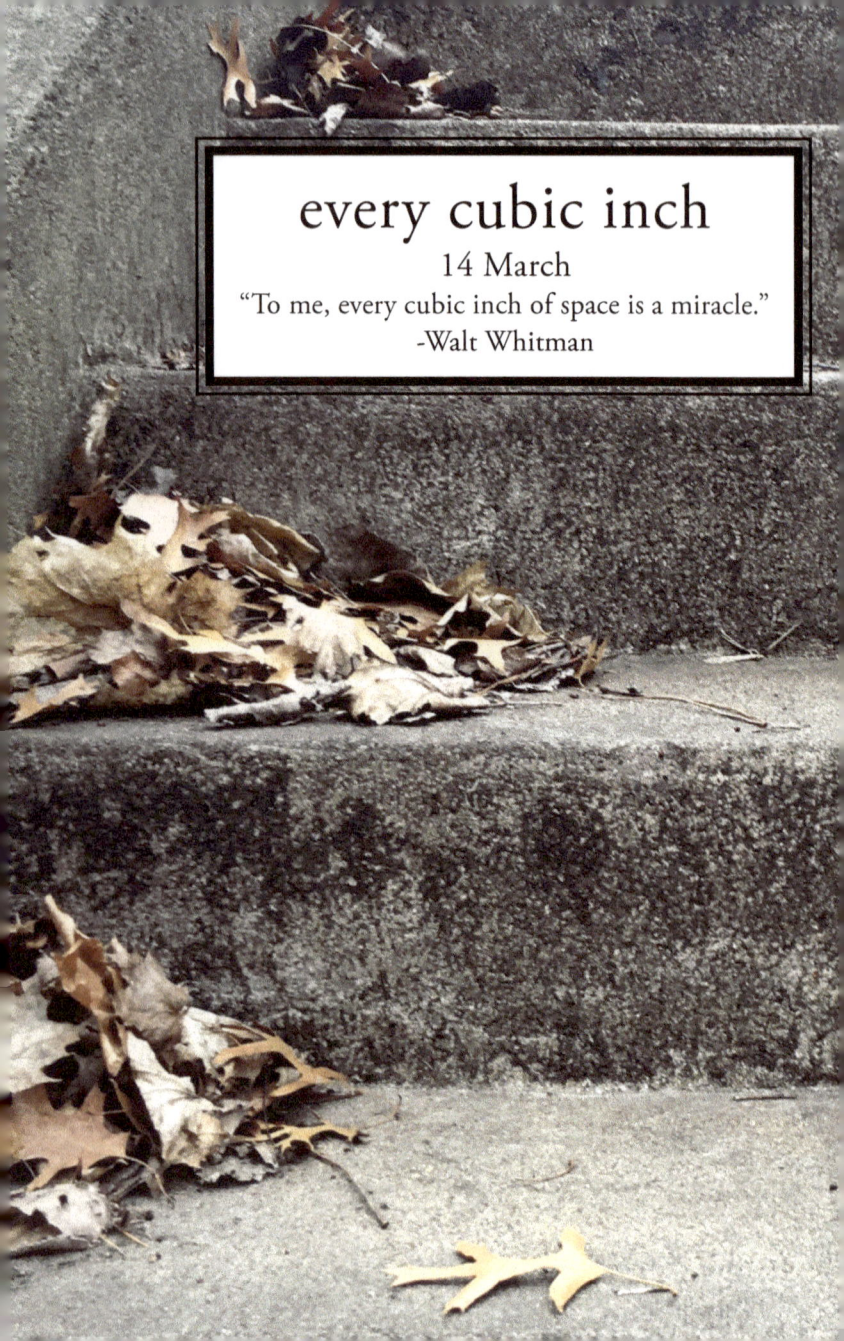

every cubic inch
14 March
"To me, every cubic inch of space is a miracle."
-Walt Whitman

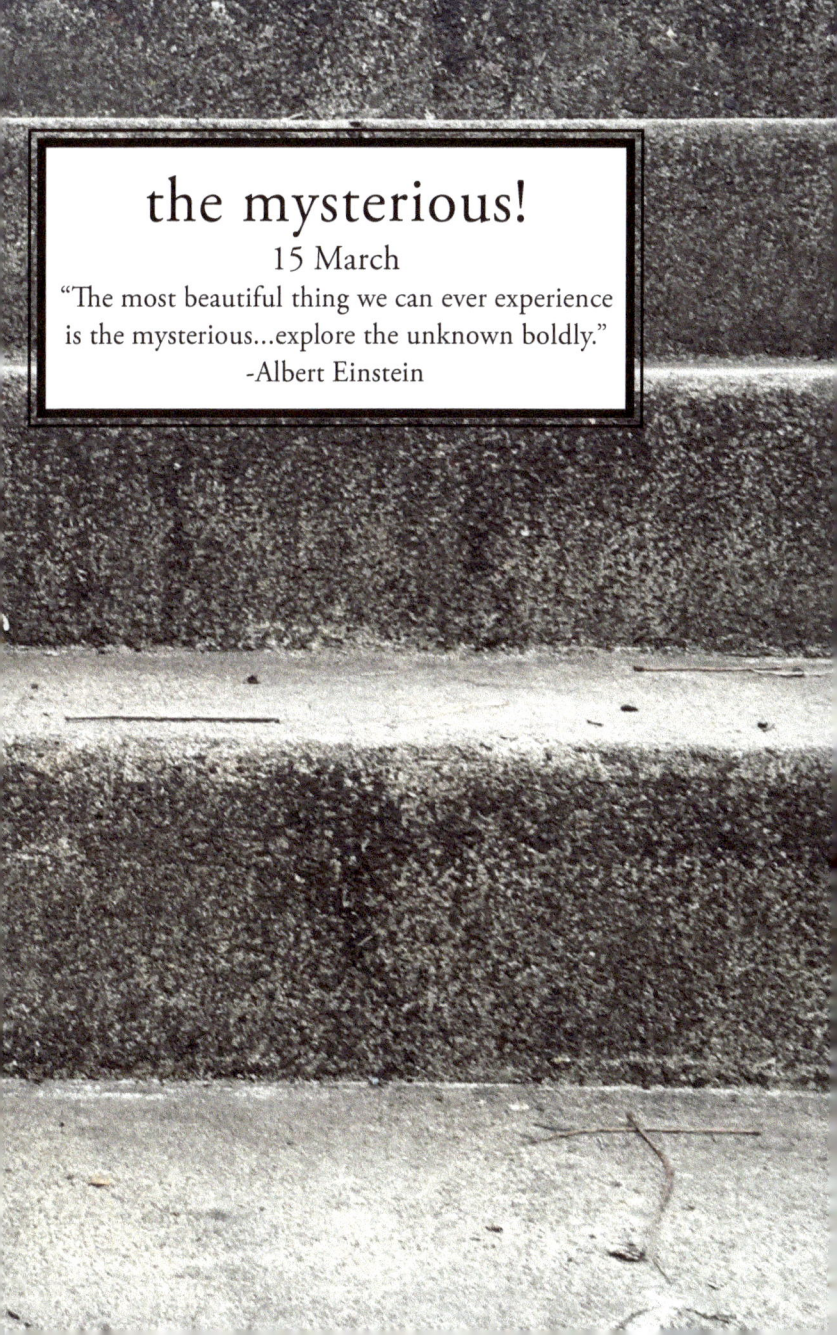

the mysterious!
15 March
"The most beautiful thing we can ever experience is the mysterious...explore the unknown boldly."
-Albert Einstein

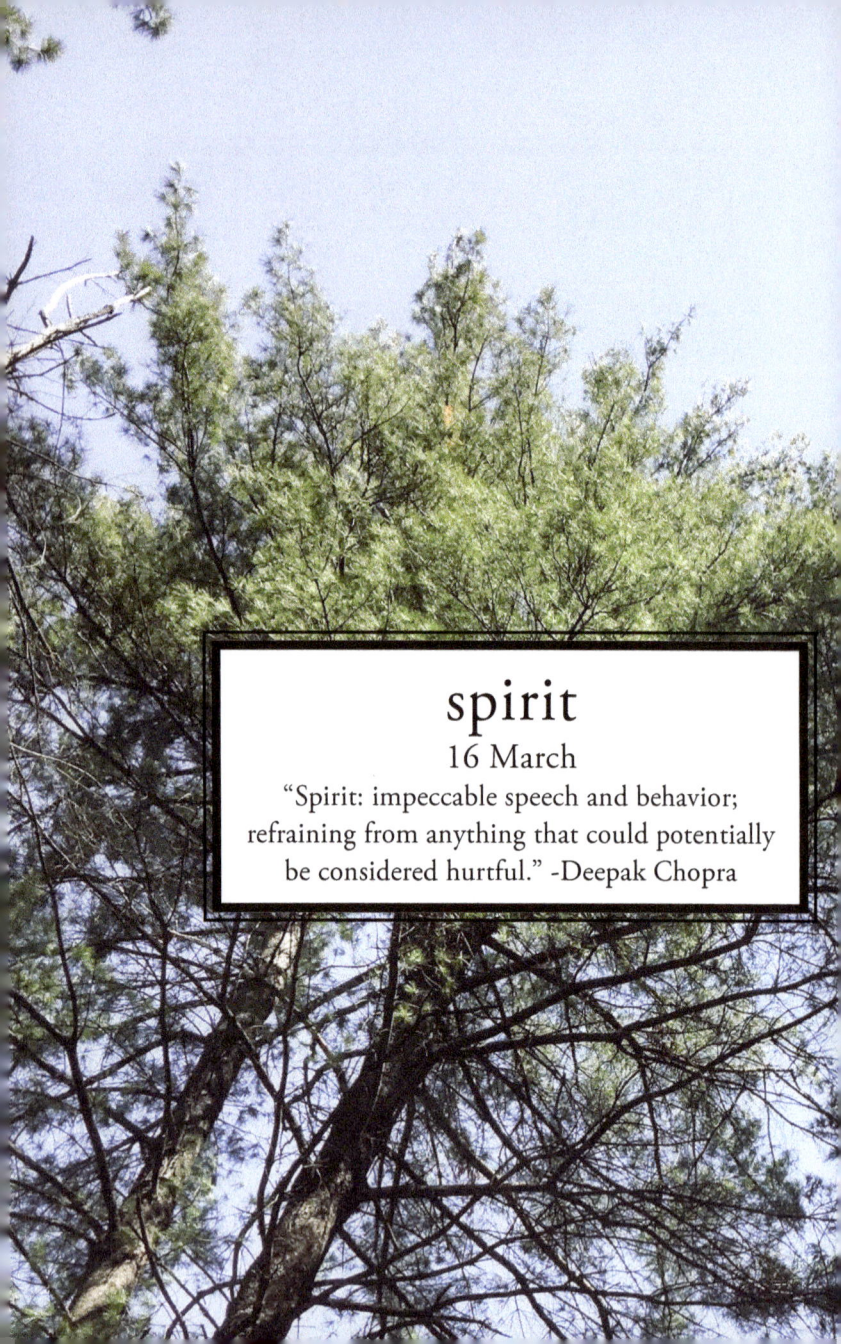

spirit
16 March
"Spirit: impeccable speech and behavior; refraining from anything that could potentially be considered hurtful." -Deepak Chopra

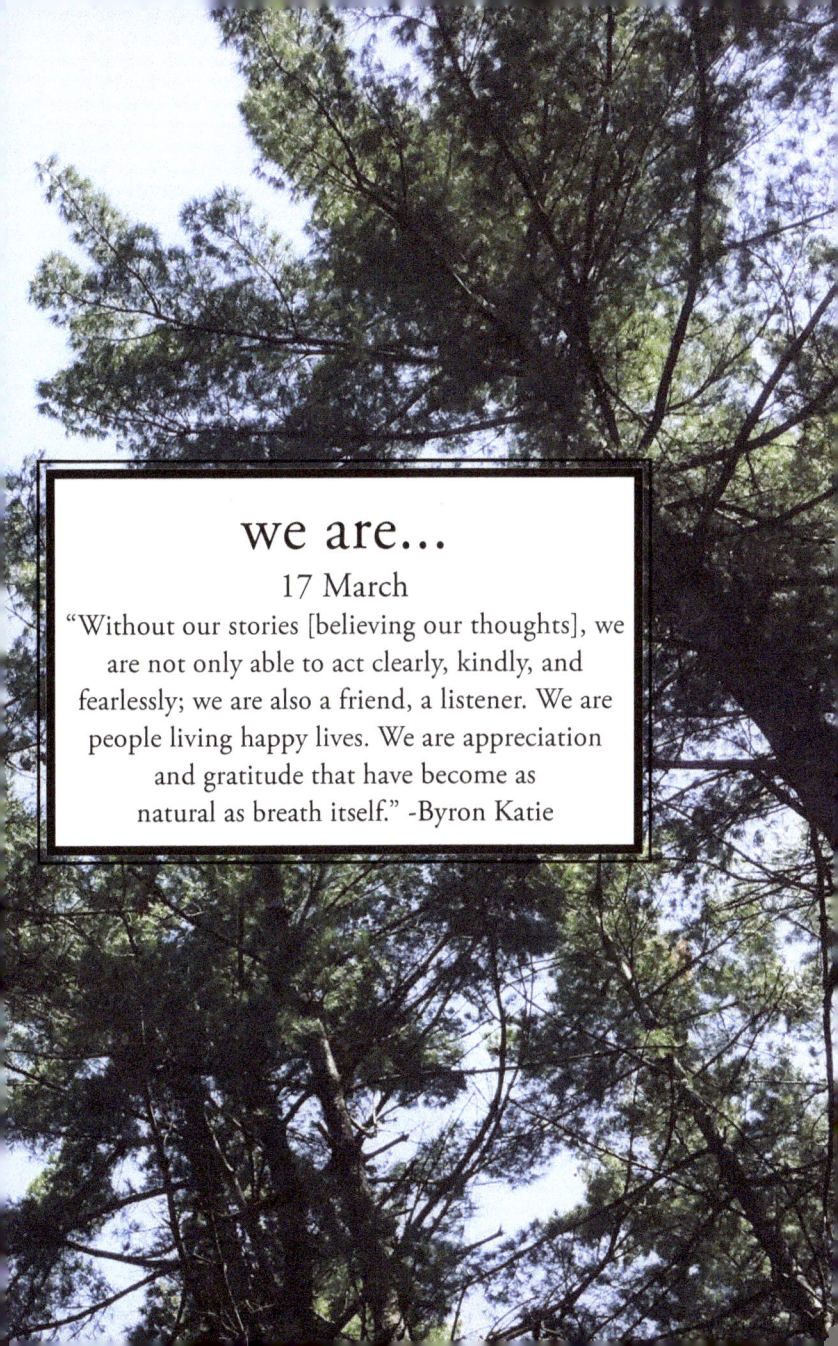

we are...
17 March
"Without our stories [believing our thoughts], we are not only able to act clearly, kindly, and fearlessly; we are also a friend, a listener. We are people living happy lives. We are appreciation and gratitude that have become as natural as breath itself." -Byron Katie

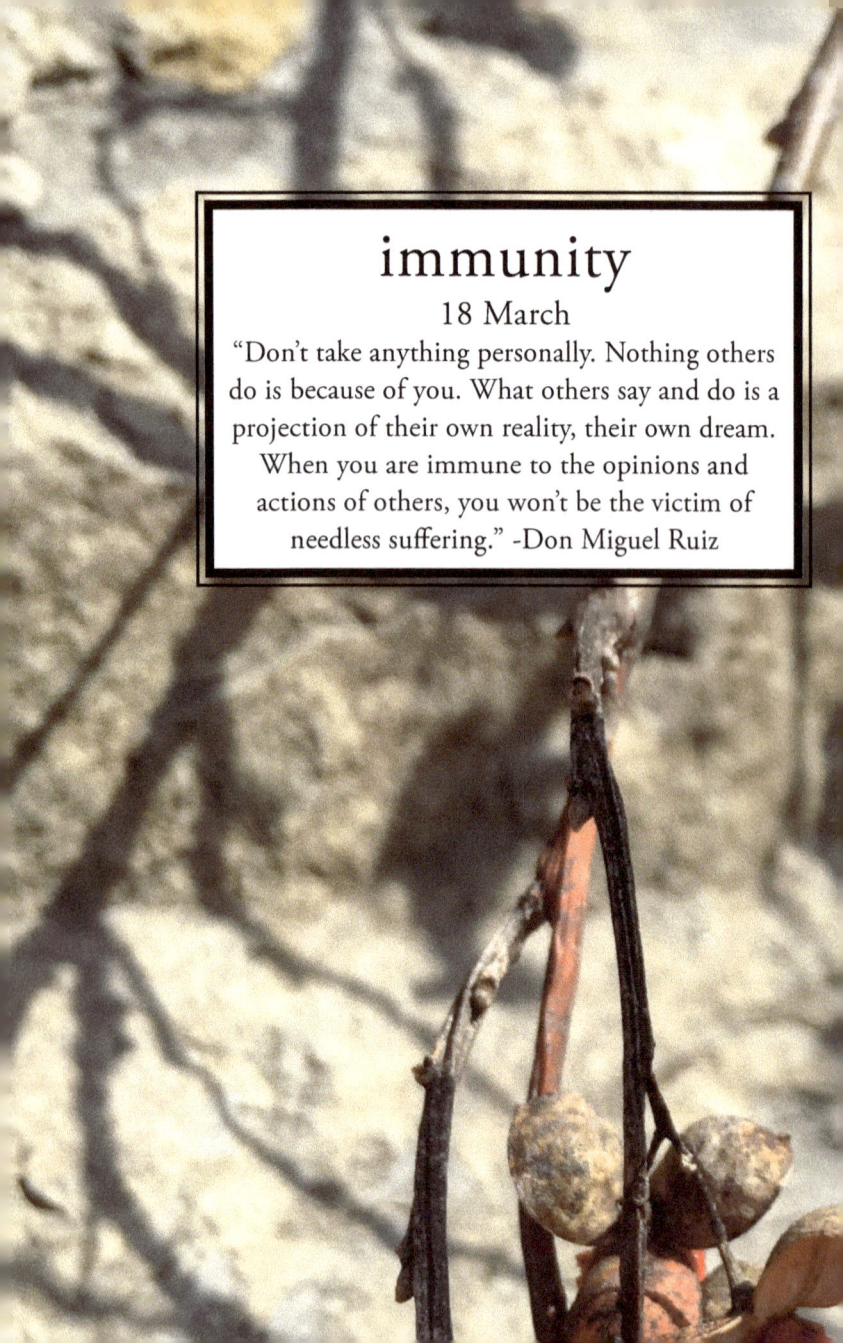

immunity
18 March

"Don't take anything personally. Nothing others do is because of you. What others say and do is a projection of their own reality, their own dream. When you are immune to the opinions and actions of others, you won't be the victim of needless suffering." -Don Miguel Ruiz

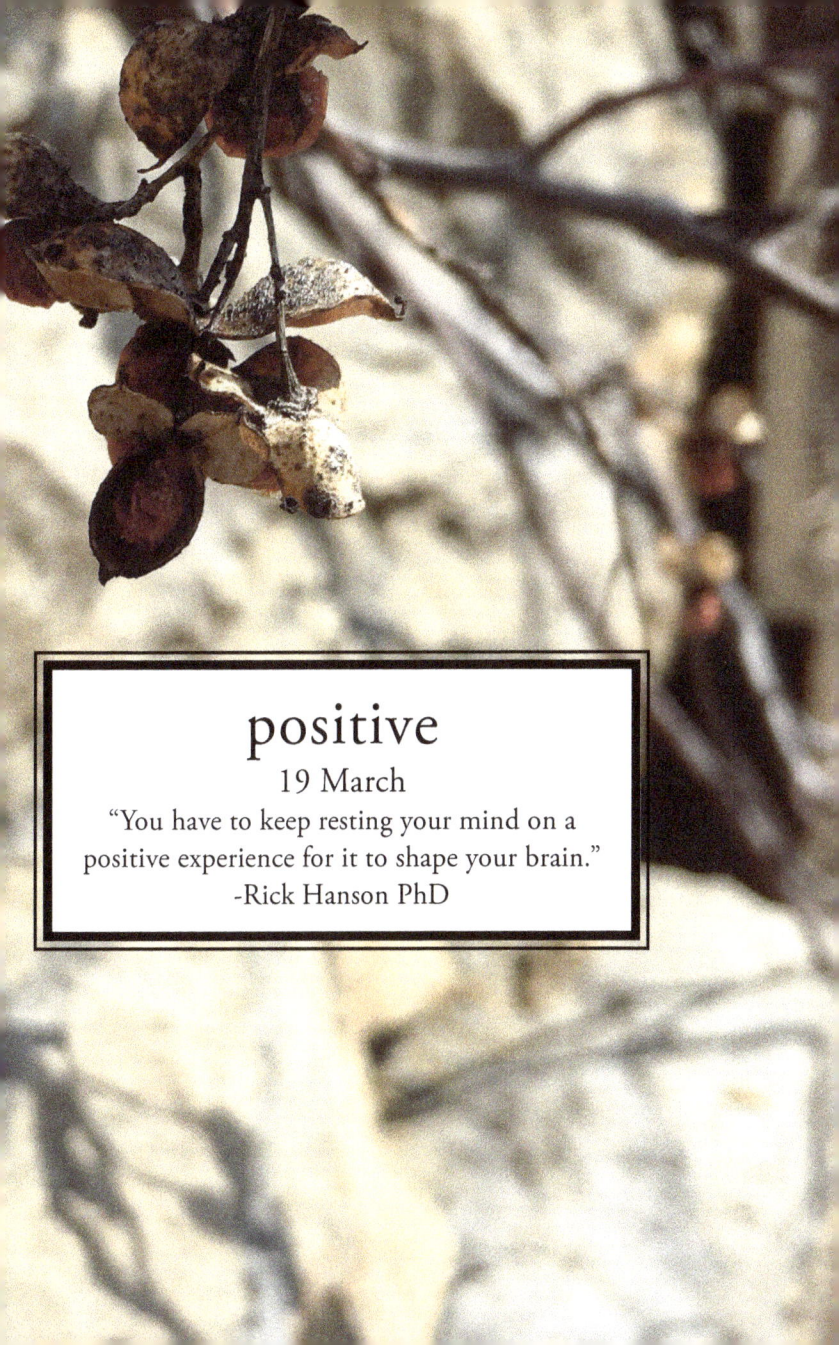

positive
19 March
"You have to keep resting your mind on a positive experience for it to shape your brain."
-Rick Hanson PhD

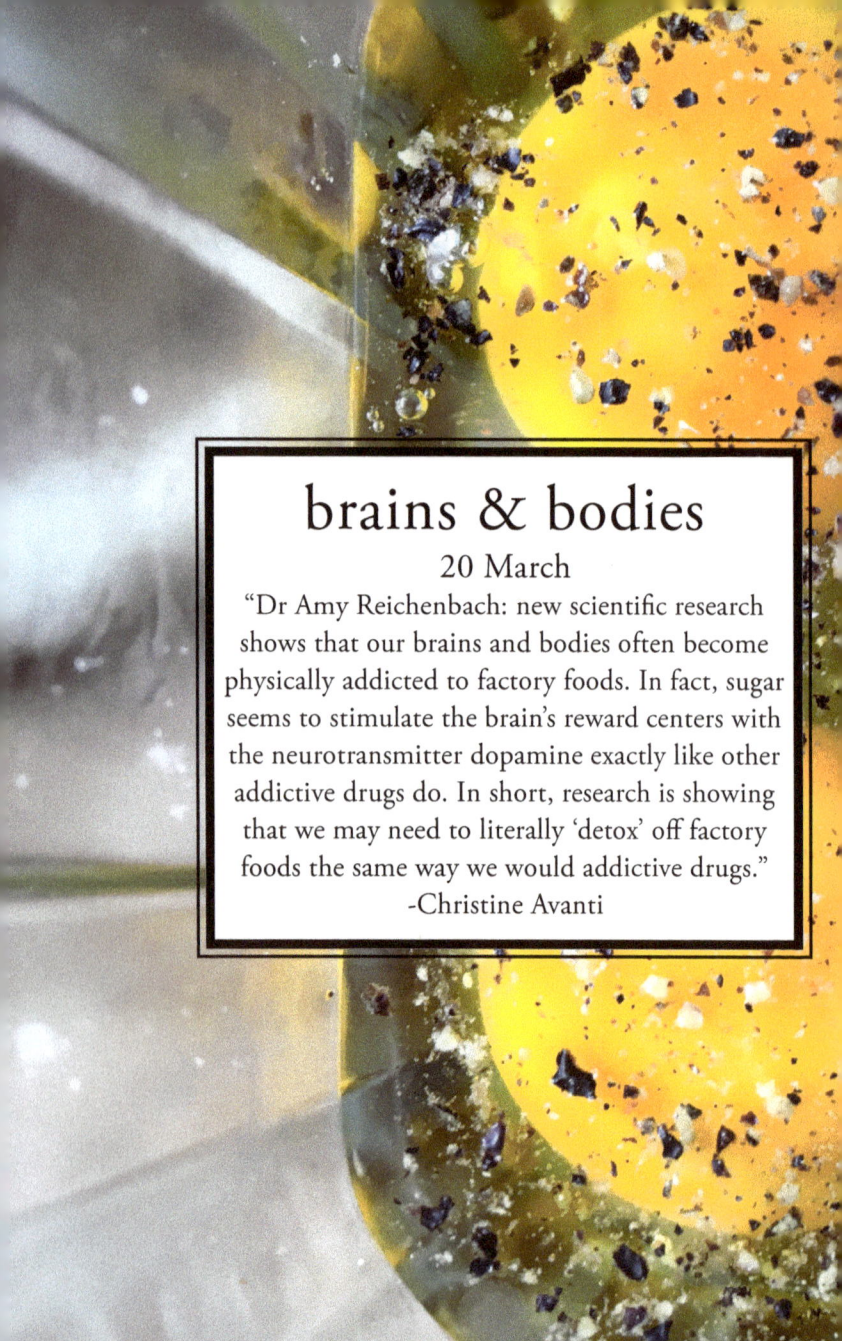

brains & bodies
20 March

"Dr Amy Reichenbach: new scientific research shows that our brains and bodies often become physically addicted to factory foods. In fact, sugar seems to stimulate the brain's reward centers with the neurotransmitter dopamine exactly like other addictive drugs do. In short, research is showing that we may need to literally 'detox' off factory foods the same way we would addictive drugs."
-Christine Avanti

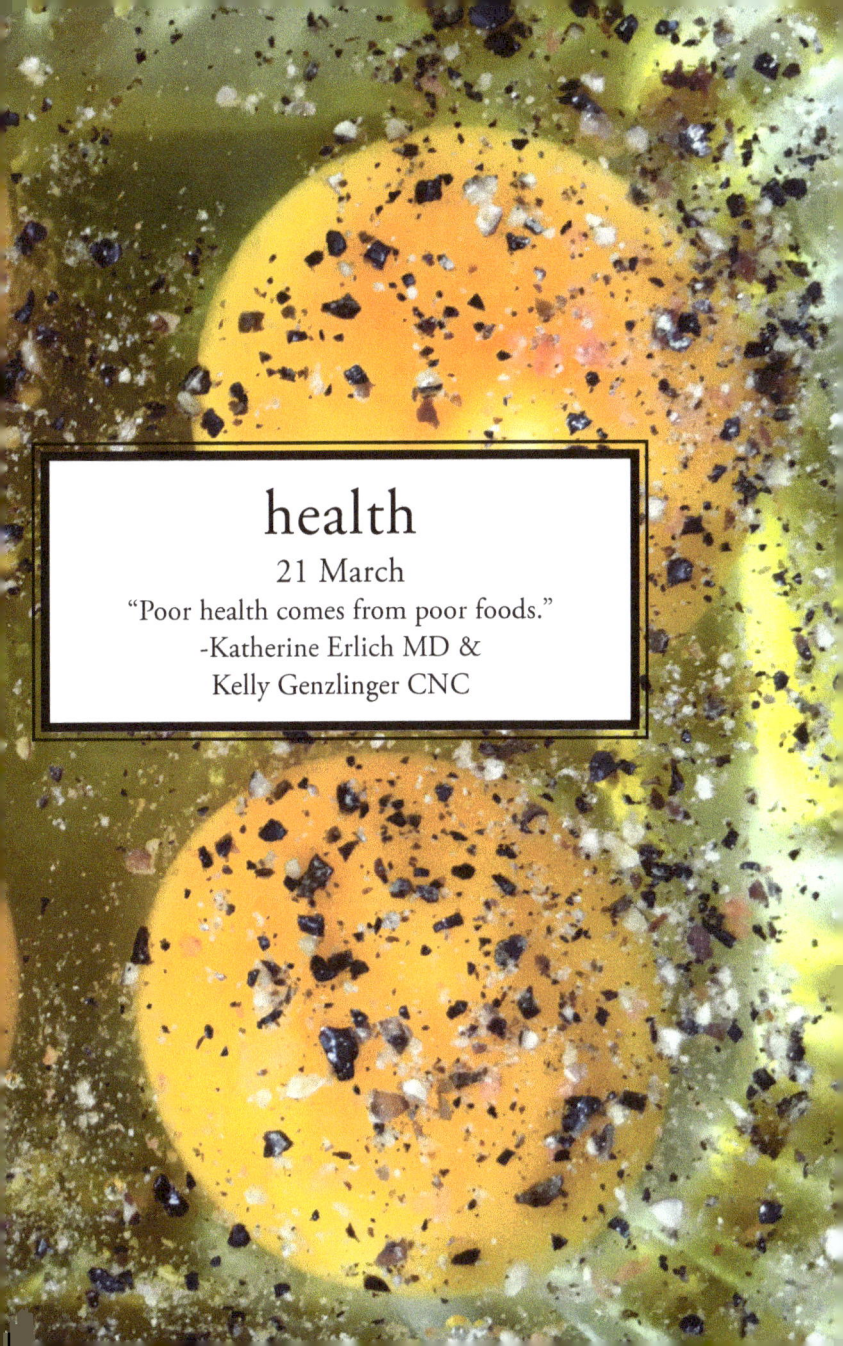

health

21 March
"Poor health comes from poor foods."
-Katherine Erlich MD &
Kelly Genzlinger CNC

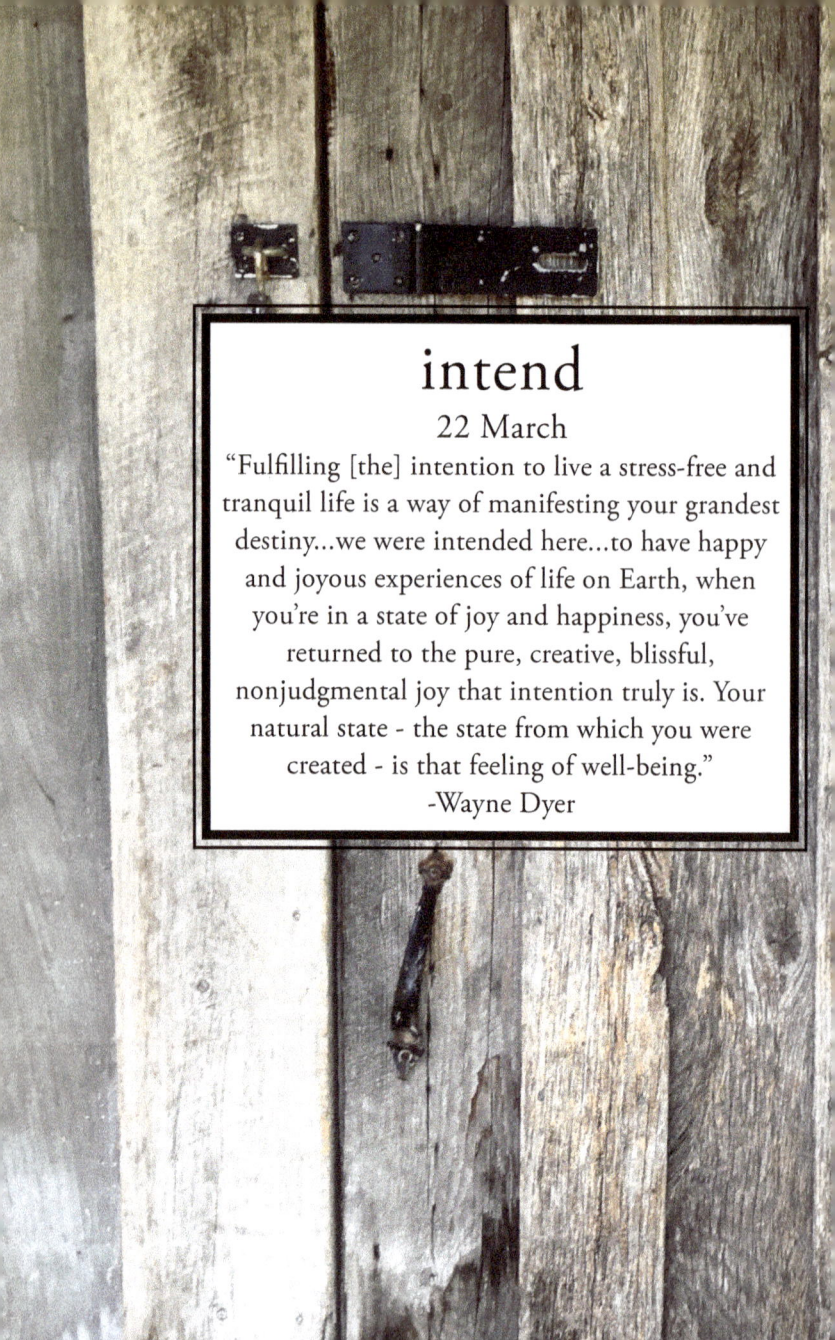

intend

22 March

"Fulfilling [the] intention to live a stress-free and tranquil life is a way of manifesting your grandest destiny...we were intended here...to have happy and joyous experiences of life on Earth, when you're in a state of joy and happiness, you've returned to the pure, creative, blissful, nonjudgmental joy that intention truly is. Your natural state - the state from which you were created - is that feeling of well-being."
-Wayne Dyer

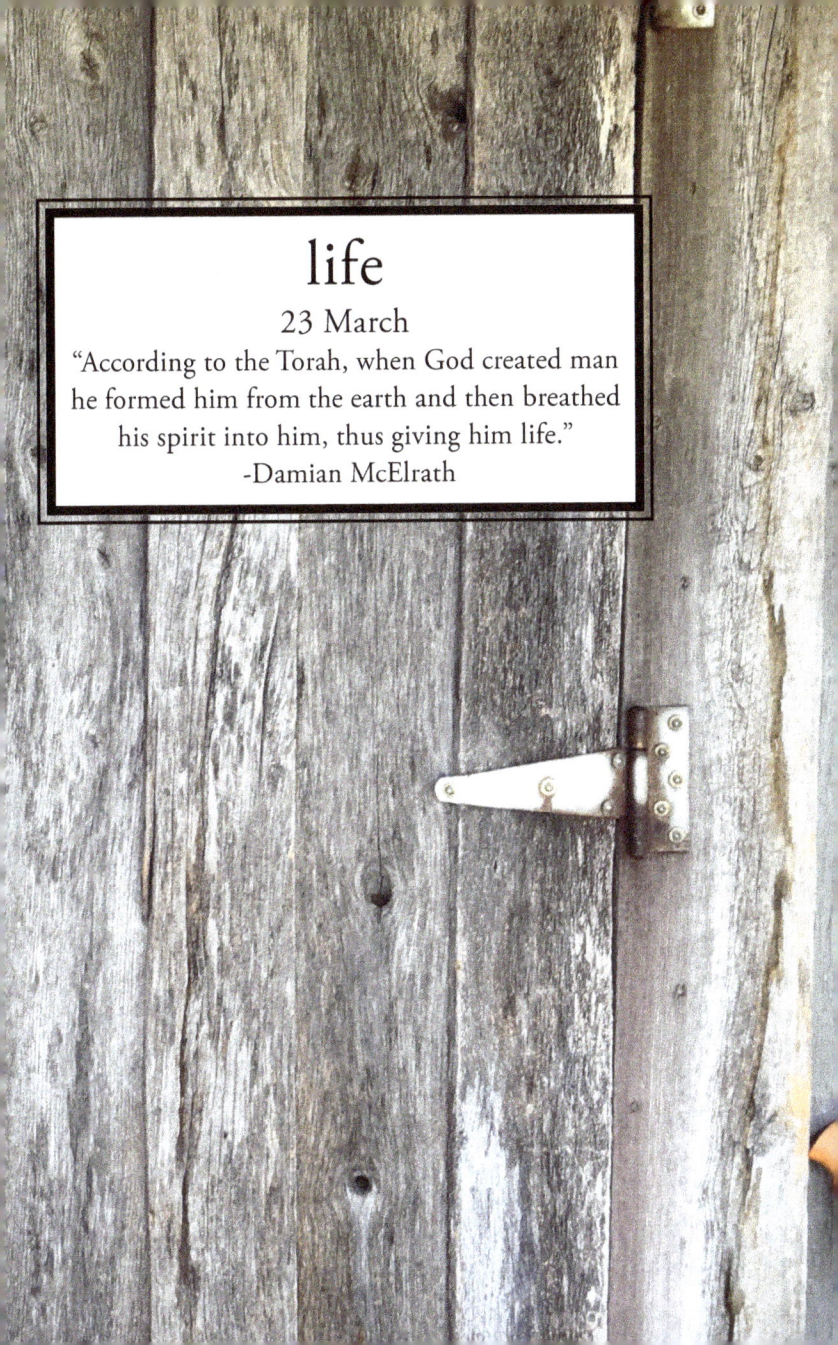

life

23 March

"According to the Torah, when God created man he formed him from the earth and then breathed his spirit into him, thus giving him life."
-Damian McElrath

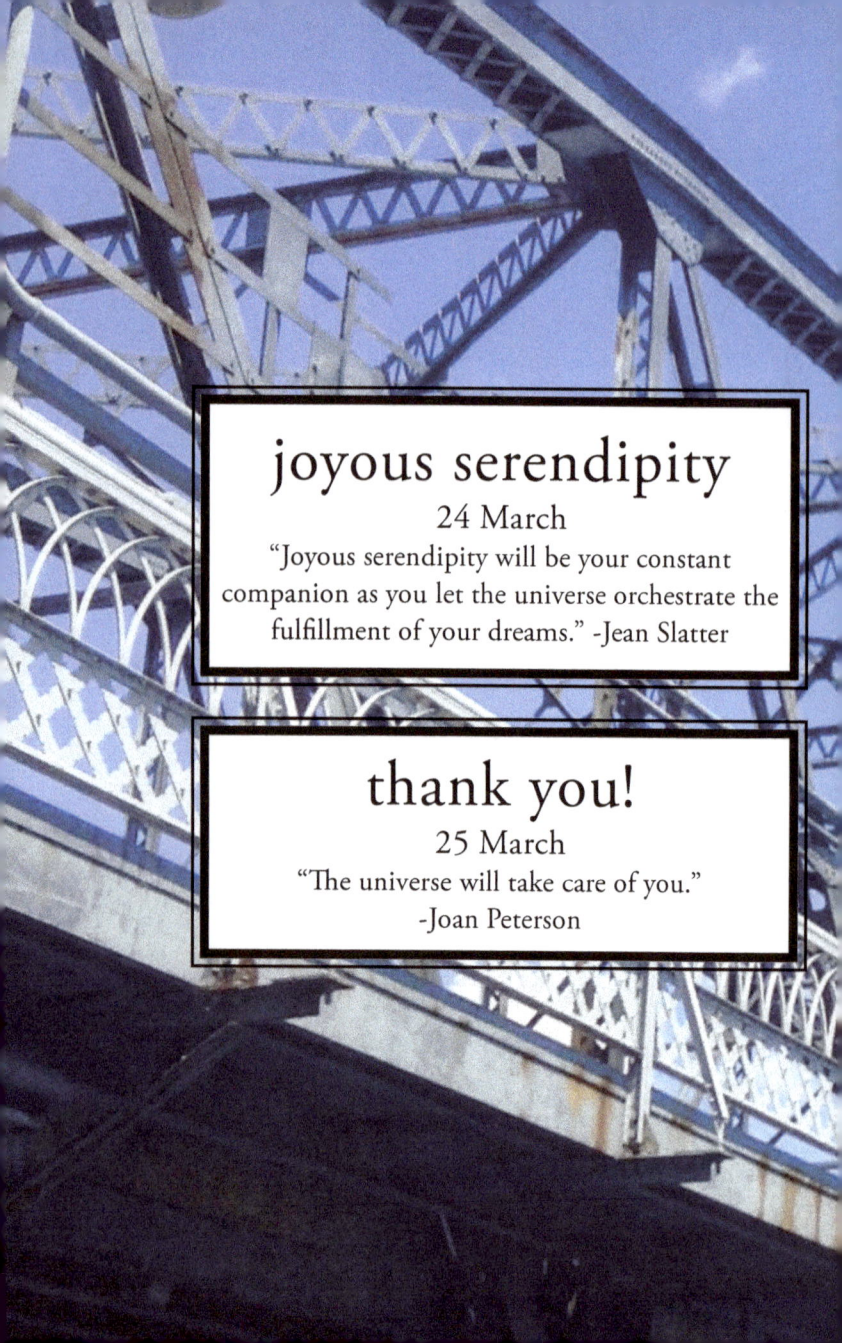

joyous serendipity
24 March
"Joyous serendipity will be your constant companion as you let the universe orchestrate the fulfillment of your dreams." -Jean Slatter

thank you!
25 March
"The universe will take care of you."
-Joan Peterson

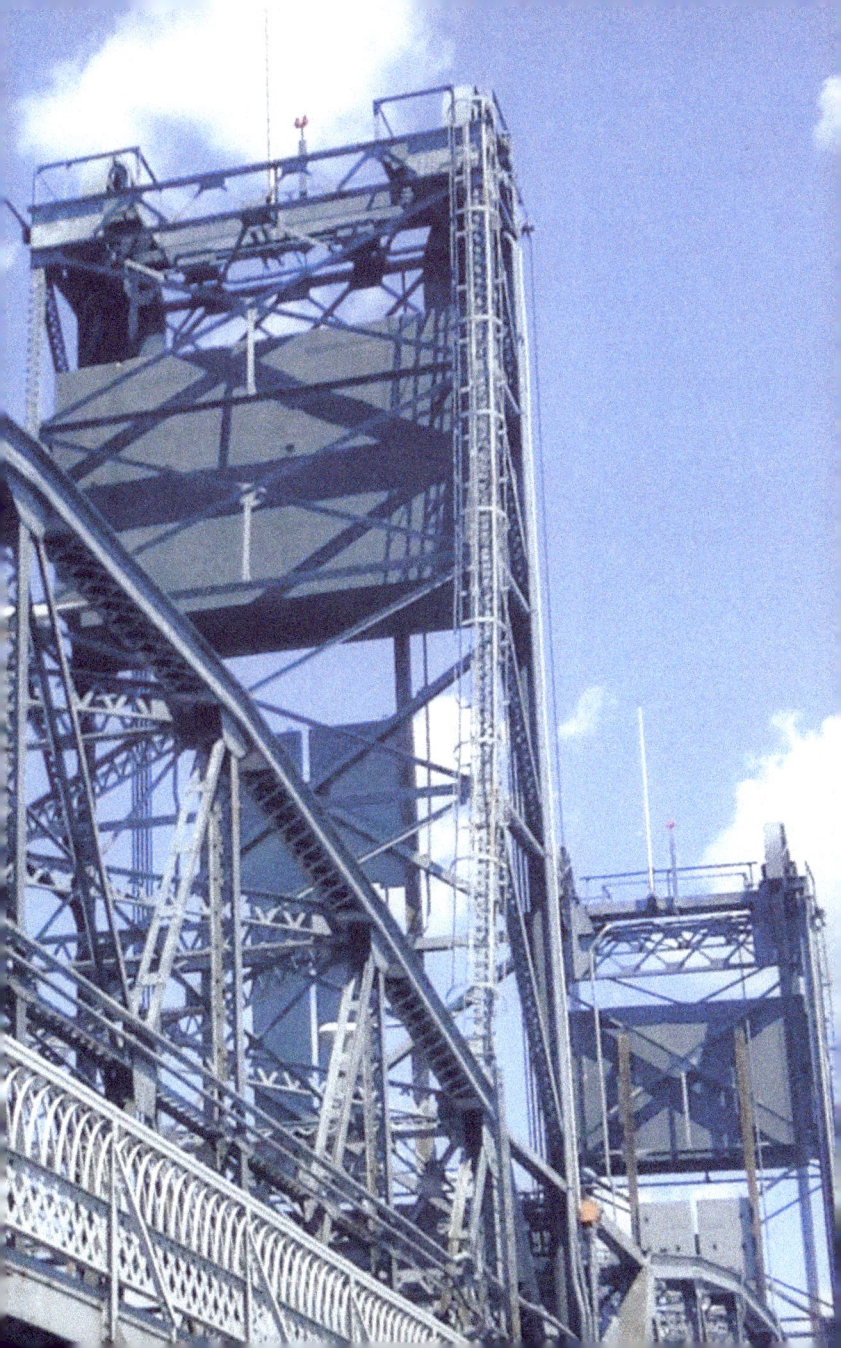

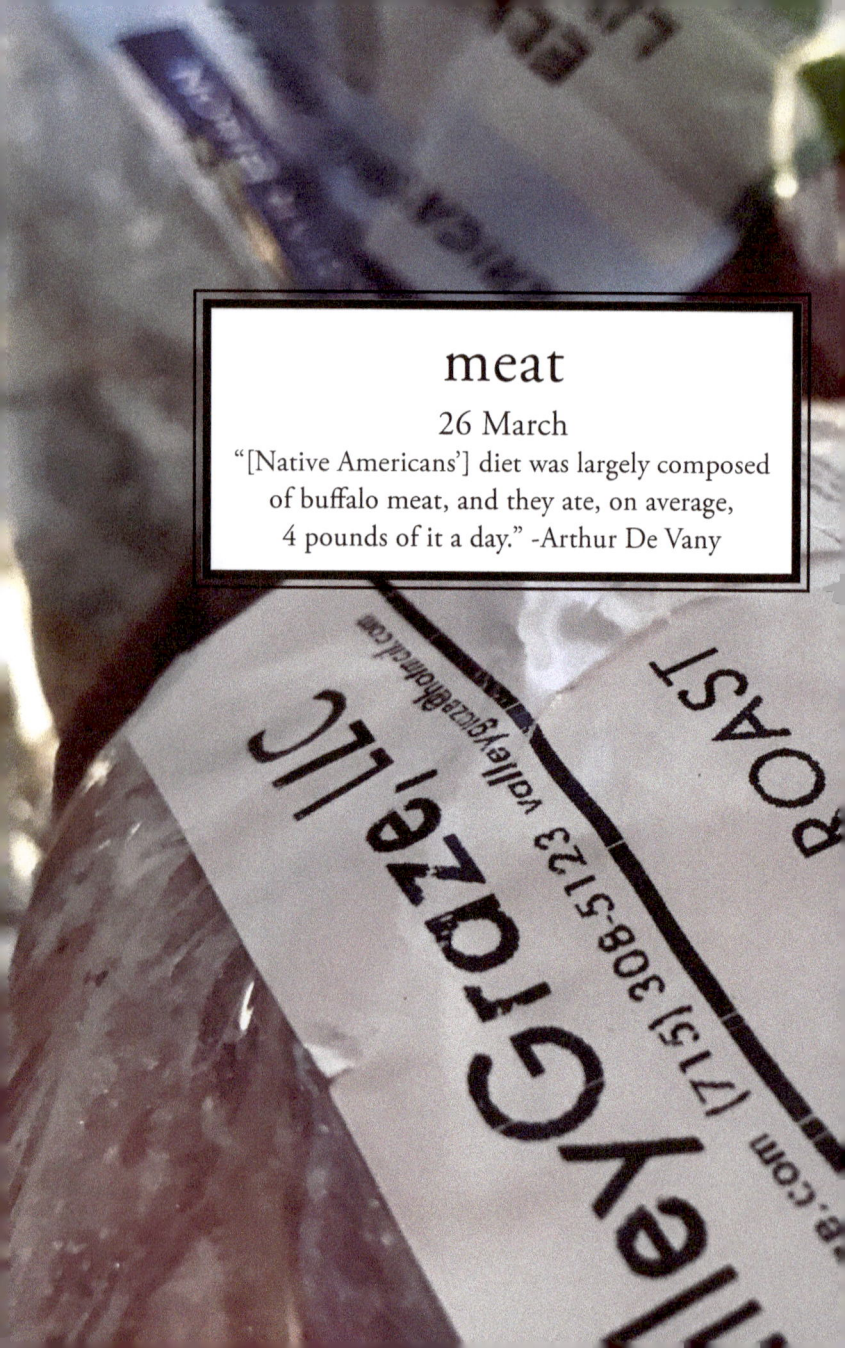

meat

26 March

"[Native Americans'] diet was largely composed of buffalo meat, and they ate, on average, 4 pounds of it a day." -Arthur De Vany

history, science & nature

27 March

"History, science and nature all lead us back to grass-fed beef despite the fact that there has been some adaptation by human beings over the last several hundred thousand years, we are still 'cavemen' from a nutritional standpoint. The optimal nutrition present during that period when the human gut and immune systems evolved consisted of fruits, vegetables and wild game for the most part. The meat in this wild game was very similar to that which can be acquired through pasture-feeding of modern livestock. Most research suggests that our ancestors consumed more lean, pasture-fed animal protein than contemporary man."

-Christopher M. Foley MD

perfect joy

28 March

"Perfect joy means total joy, and everything you desire is included in that." -James Twyman

ananda

29 March

ananda: perfect, divine joy;
supreme, eternal bliss;
one of the highest states of being

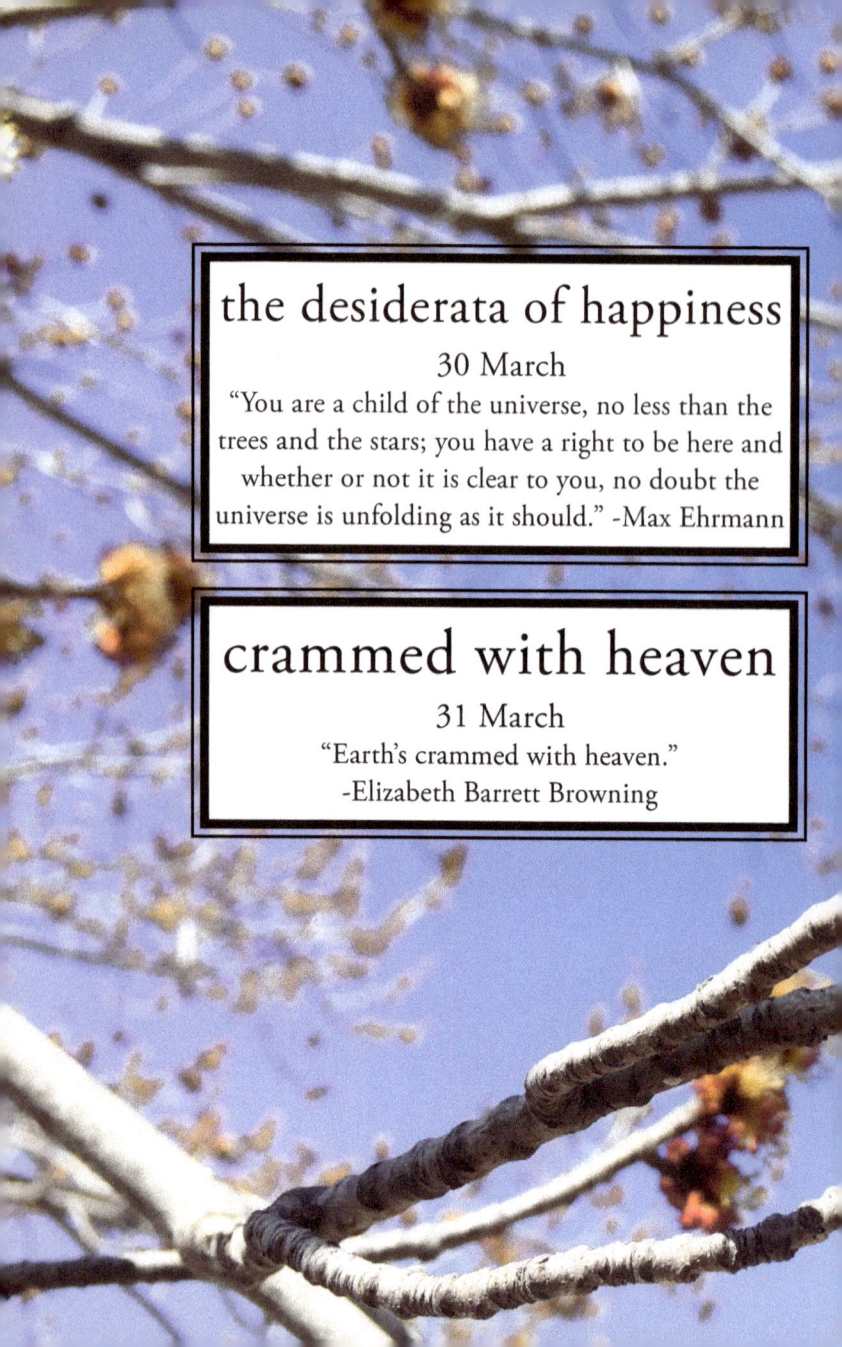

the desiderata of happiness
30 March
"You are a child of the universe, no less than the trees and the stars; you have a right to be here and whether or not it is clear to you, no doubt the universe is unfolding as it should." -Max Ehrmann

crammed with heaven
31 March
"Earth's crammed with heaven."
-Elizabeth Barrett Browning

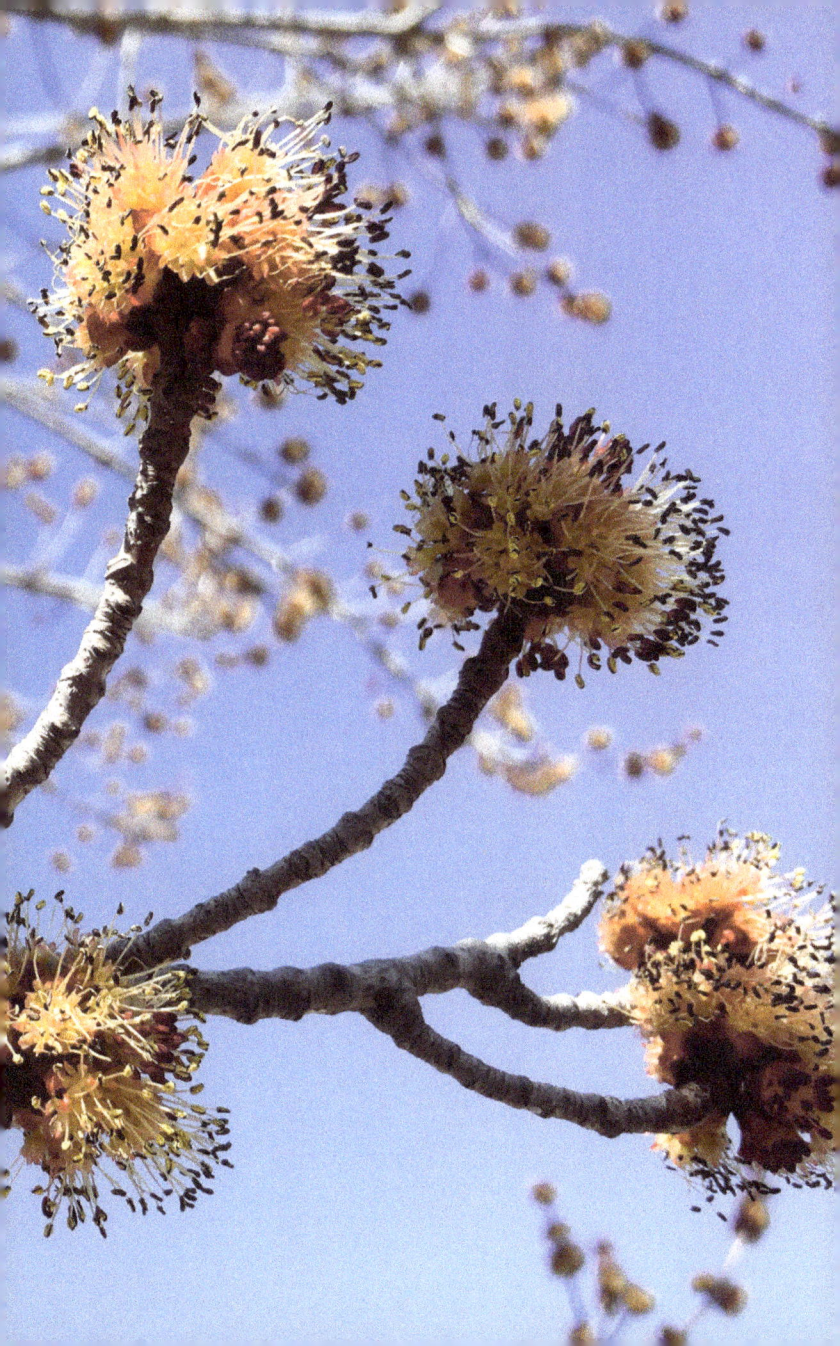

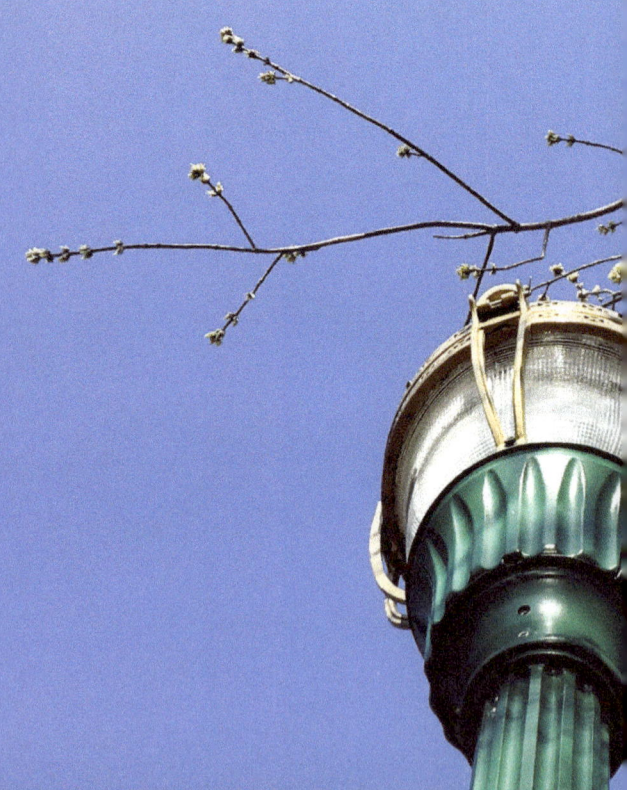

completeness
1 April
"I live in completeness. All of us do, though we may not realize it. I don't know anything; I don't have to figure anything out...I exist as a don't-know mind. This leaves nothing but peace and joy." -Byron Katie

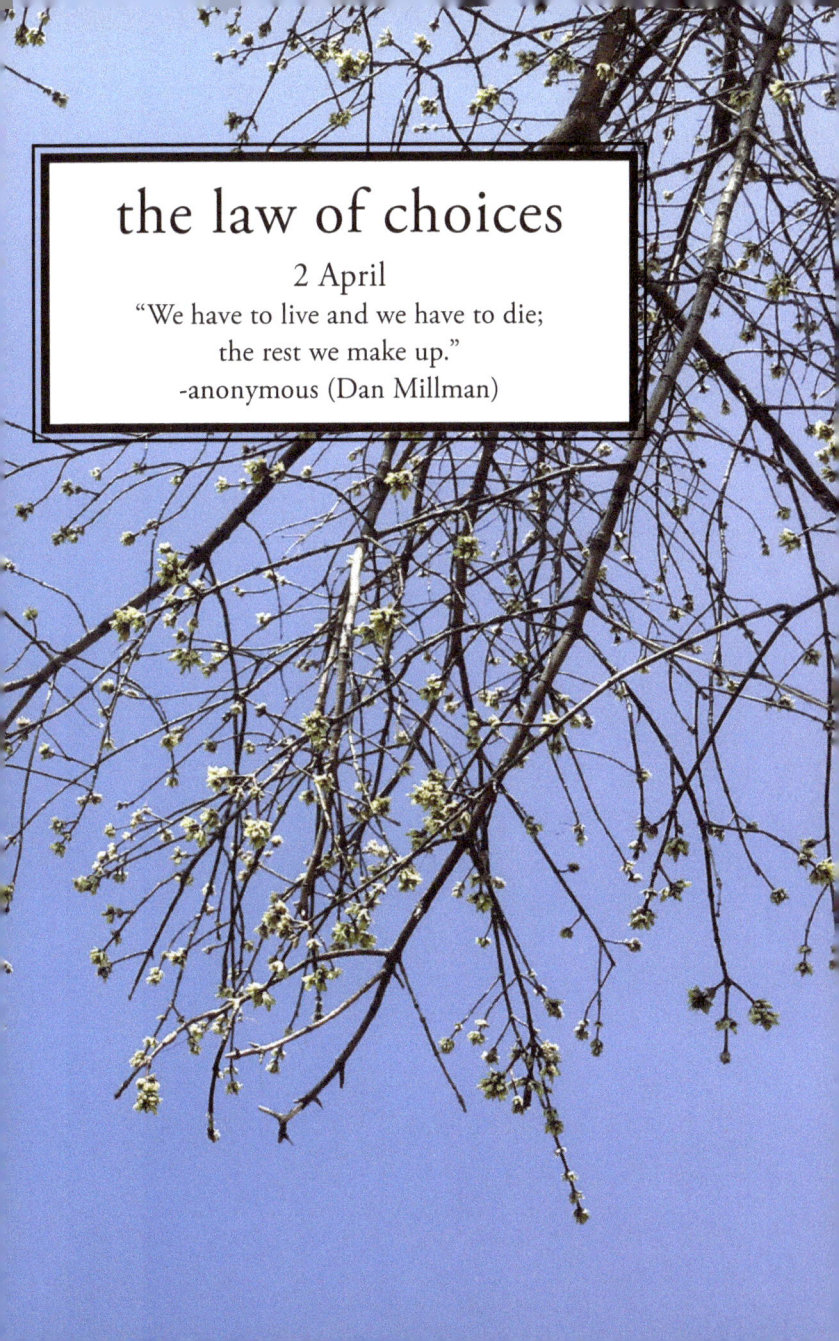

the law of choices

2 April

"We have to live and we have to die;
the rest we make up."
-anonymous (Dan Millman)

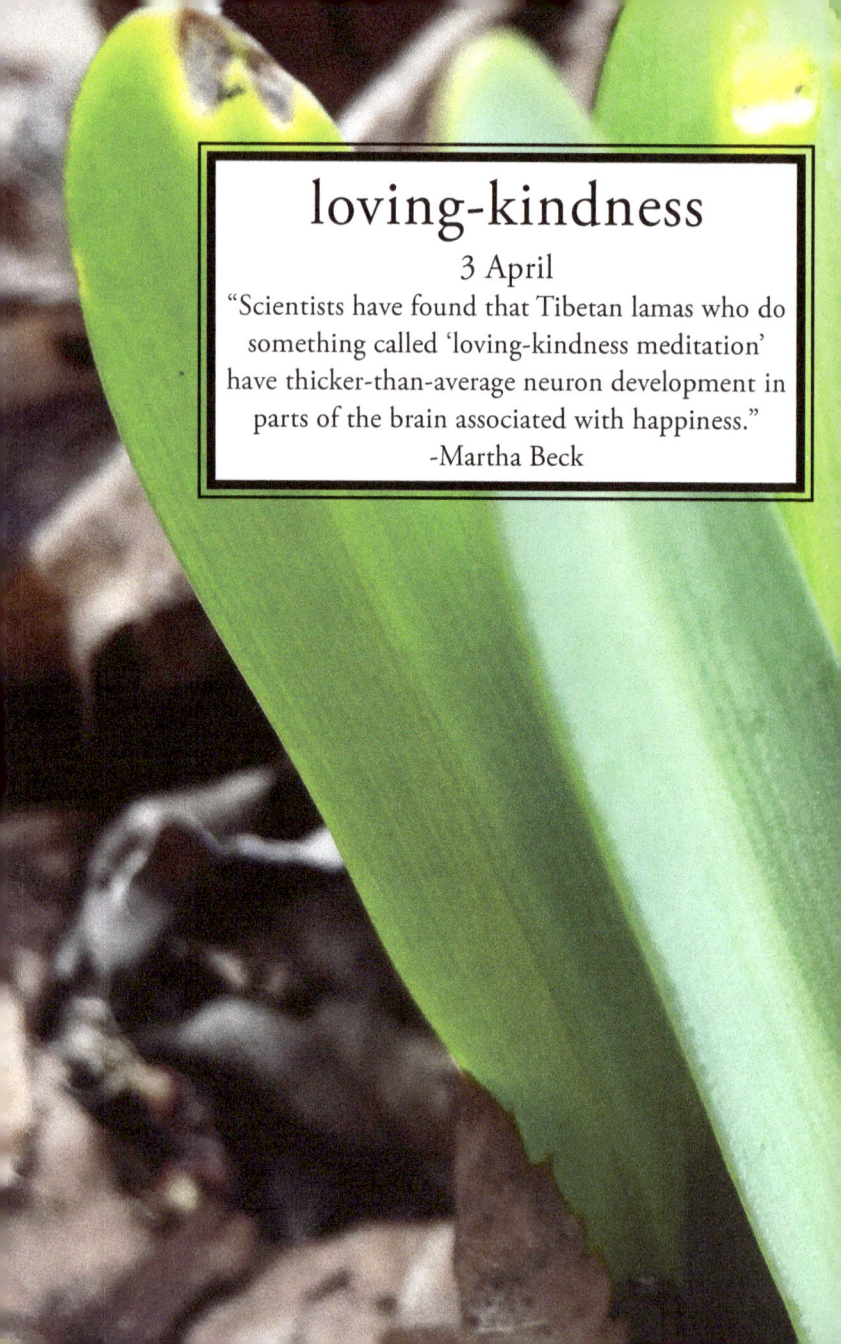

loving-kindness
3 April
"Scientists have found that Tibetan lamas who do something called 'loving-kindness meditation' have thicker-than-average neuron development in parts of the brain associated with happiness."
-Martha Beck

love "infused with love"

4 April
Steps & blinks & heartbeats & inhales & exhales
ALL "infused with love"!
(Thich Nhat Hanh)

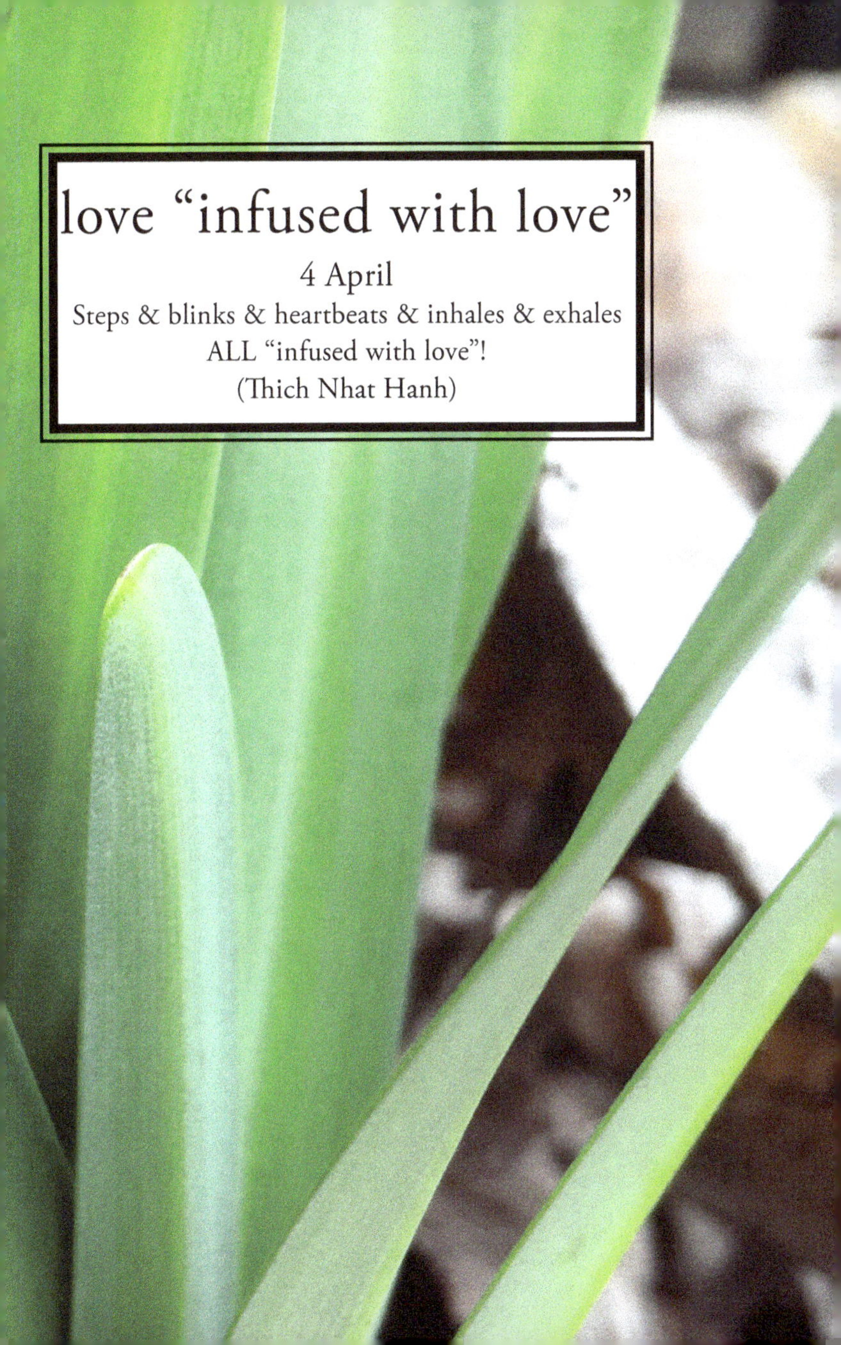

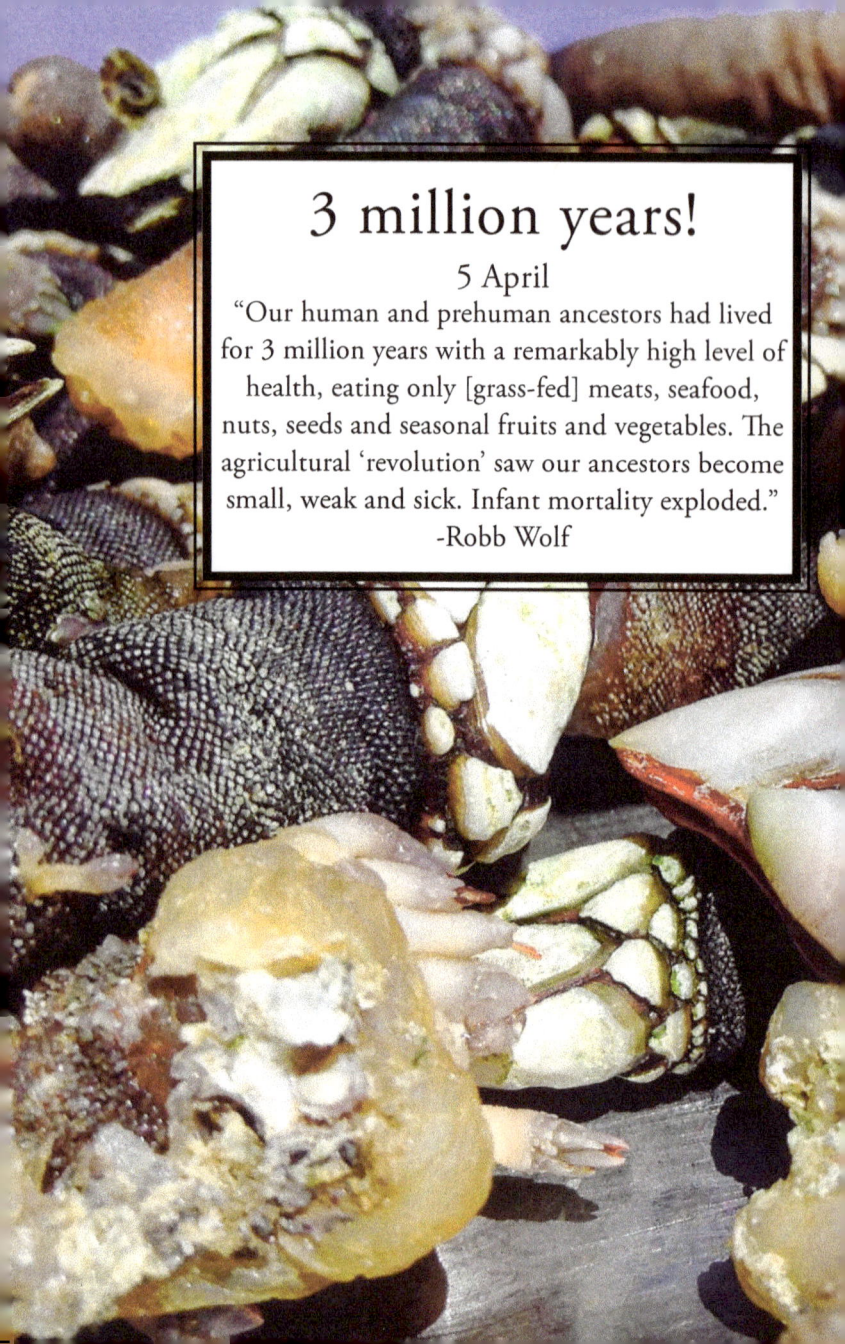

3 million years!
5 April

"Our human and prehuman ancestors had lived for 3 million years with a remarkably high level of health, eating only [grass-fed] meats, seafood, nuts, seeds and seasonal fruits and vegetables. The agricultural 'revolution' saw our ancestors become small, weak and sick. Infant mortality exploded."
-Robb Wolf

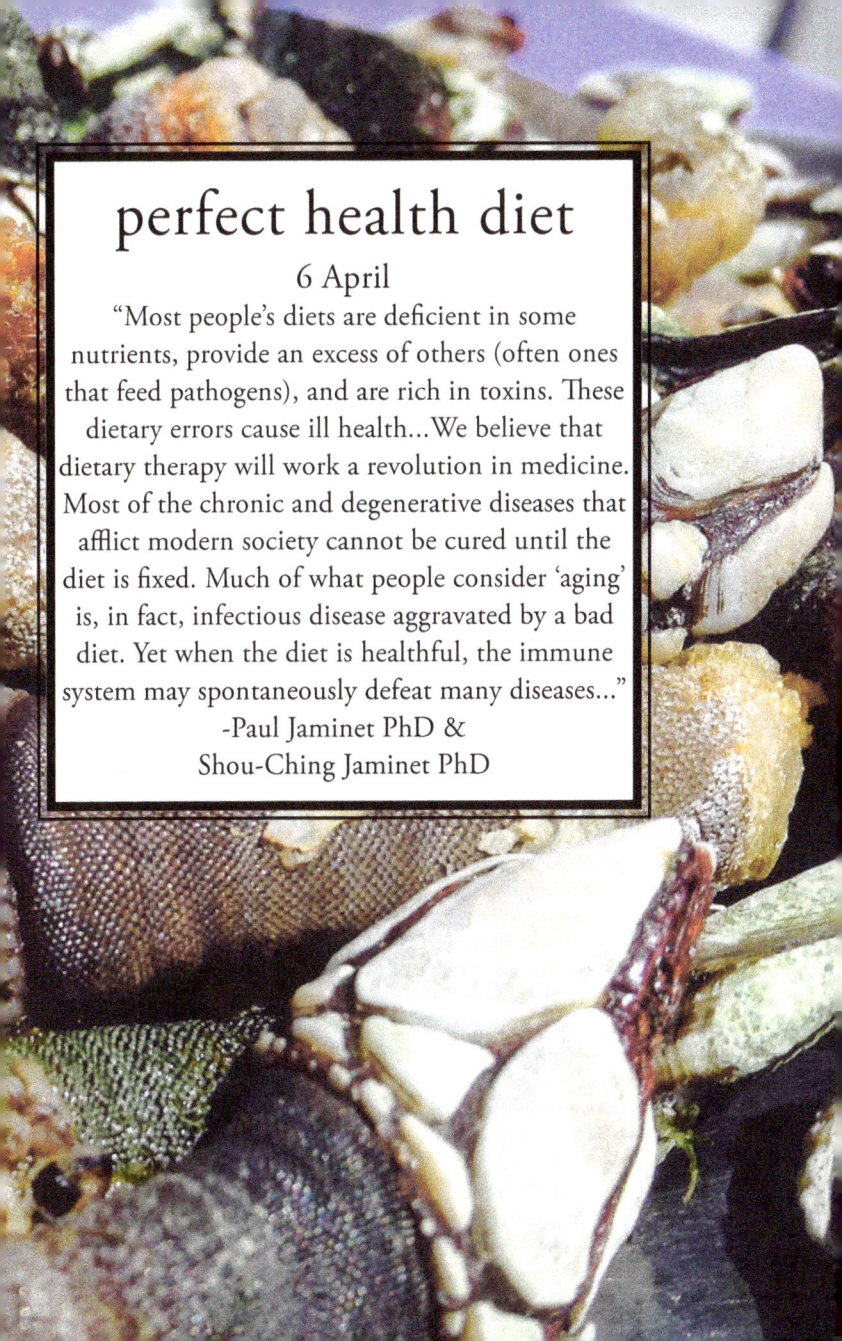

perfect health diet

6 April

"Most people's diets are deficient in some nutrients, provide an excess of others (often ones that feed pathogens), and are rich in toxins. These dietary errors cause ill health...We believe that dietary therapy will work a revolution in medicine. Most of the chronic and degenerative diseases that afflict modern society cannot be cured until the diet is fixed. Much of what people consider 'aging' is, in fact, infectious disease aggravated by a bad diet. Yet when the diet is healthful, the immune system may spontaneously defeat many diseases..."

-Paul Jaminet PhD &
Shou-Ching Jaminet PhD

happiness

7 April

"Happiness is the natural state for someone who knows that there's nothing to know and that we already have everything we need, right here, now."
-Byron Katie

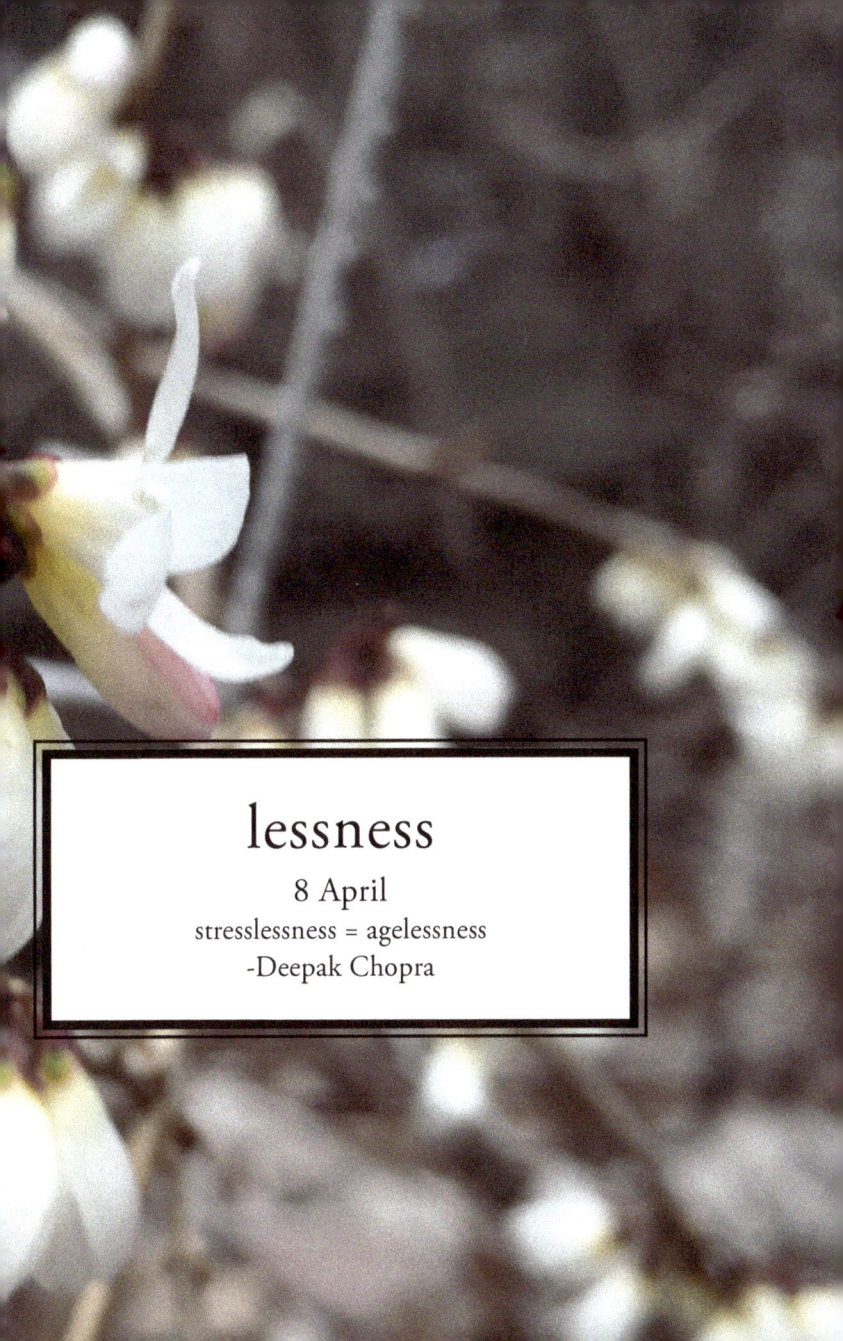

lessness

8 April

stresslessness = agelessness

-Deepak Chopra

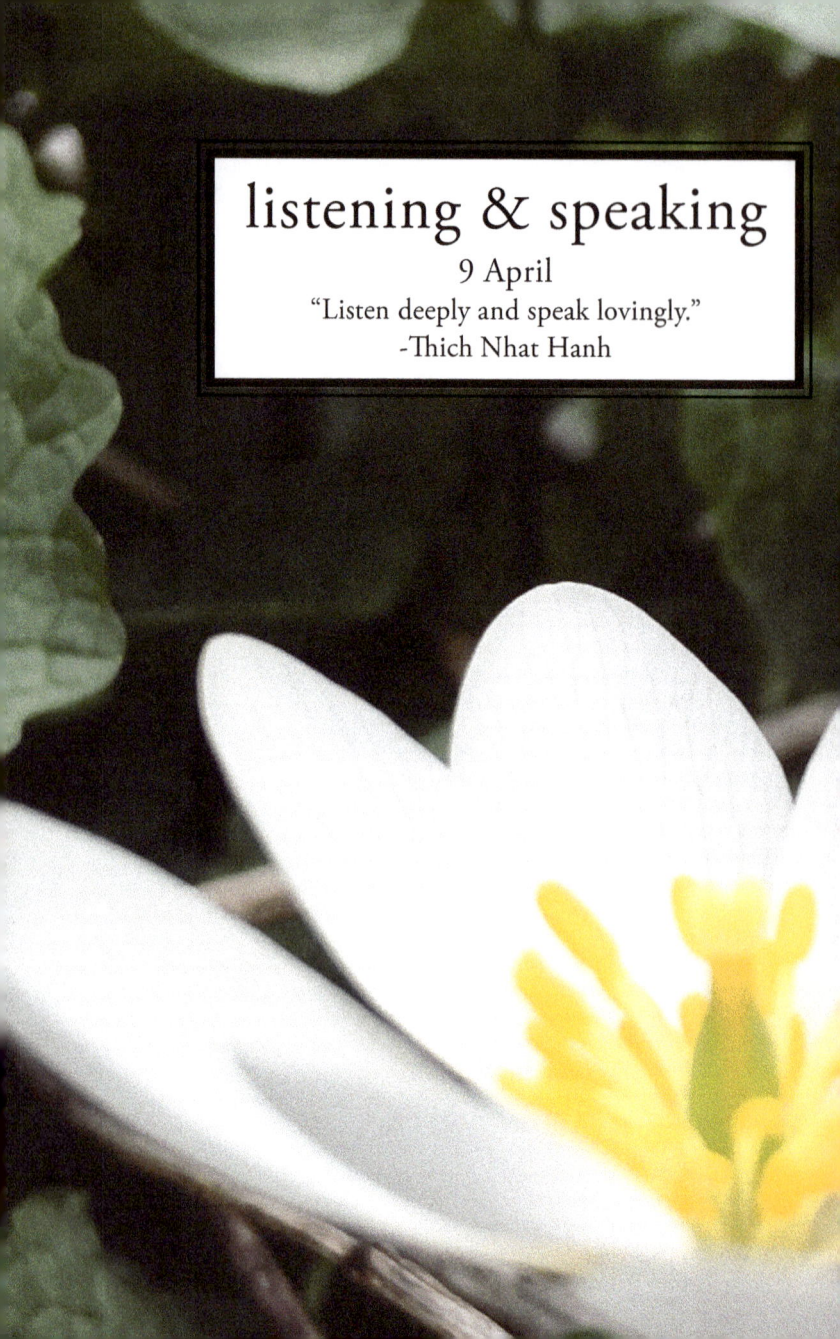

listening & speaking
9 April
"Listen deeply and speak lovingly."
-Thich Nhat Hanh

yay

10 April
"Jogging is a useless exercise."
-Arthur De Vany PhD

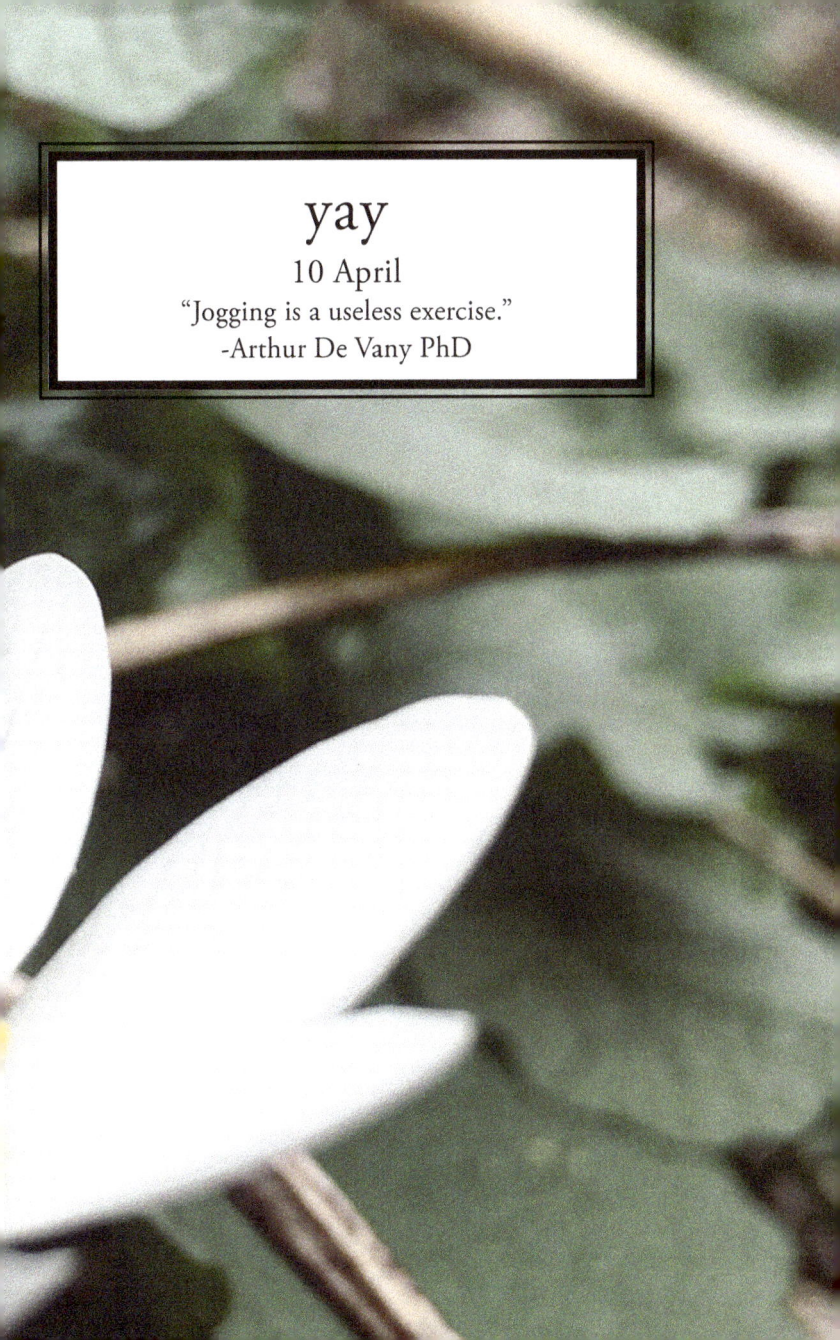

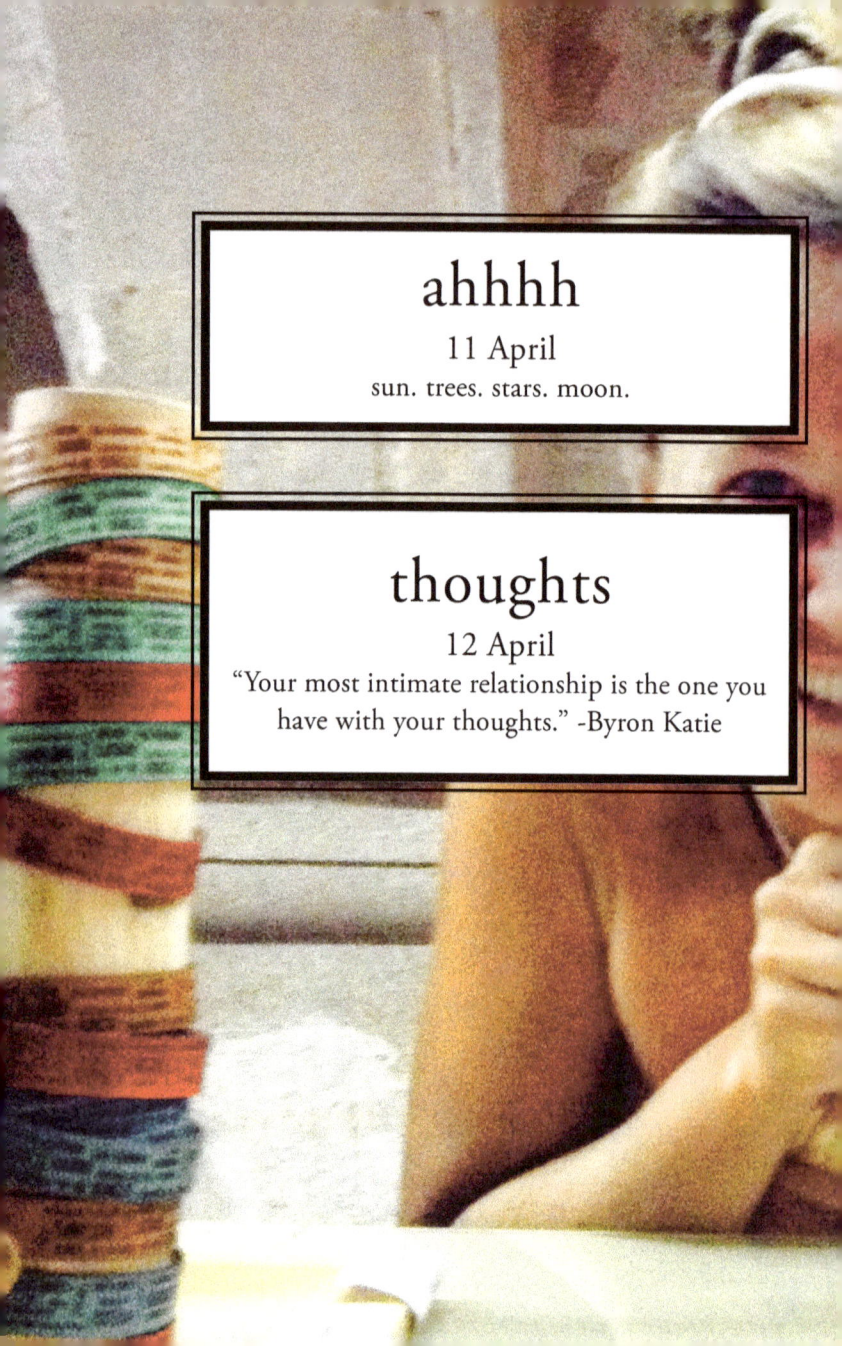

ahhhh
11 April
sun. trees. stars. moon.

thoughts
12 April
"Your most intimate relationship is the one you have with your thoughts." -Byron Katie

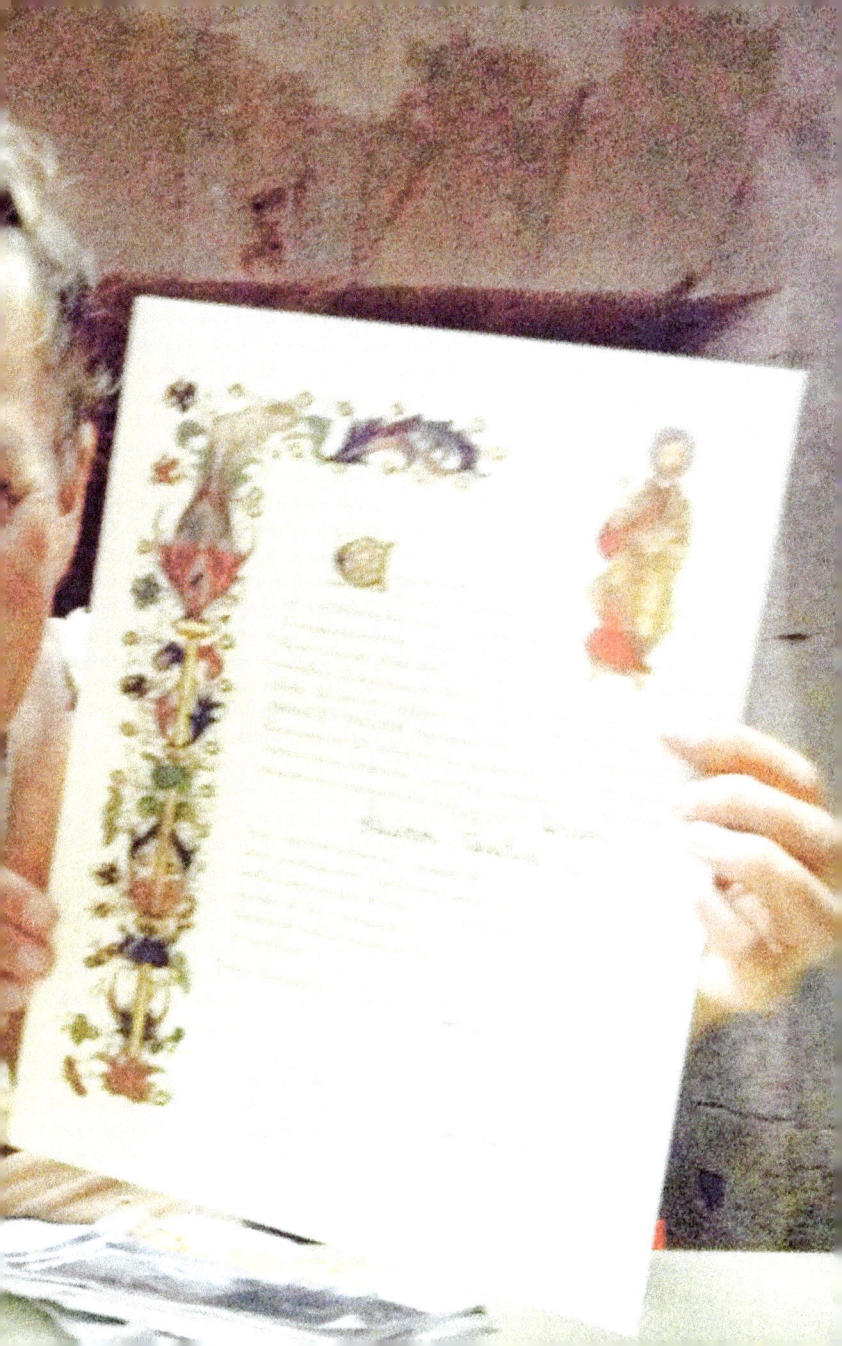

bewilderment

13 April

"Sell your cleverness and buy bewilderment."
-Rumi

10 years younger

14 April

"By cutting down on the toxins entering your body from poor food and drink choices and by reducing the amount of sugar in your diet, you'll see a dramatic difference. If you eat organic, free range [grass-fed] meats, you don't have to worry about cutting the fat away and you can eat red meats. In no time, you'll have more energy, your cholesterol levels are likely to normalize, and you'll be far more interested in getting the exercise you need…you'll look and feel at least ten years younger!" -Paul Chek

nt Love, I

blessings with

spiritual trek.

her always.

amply

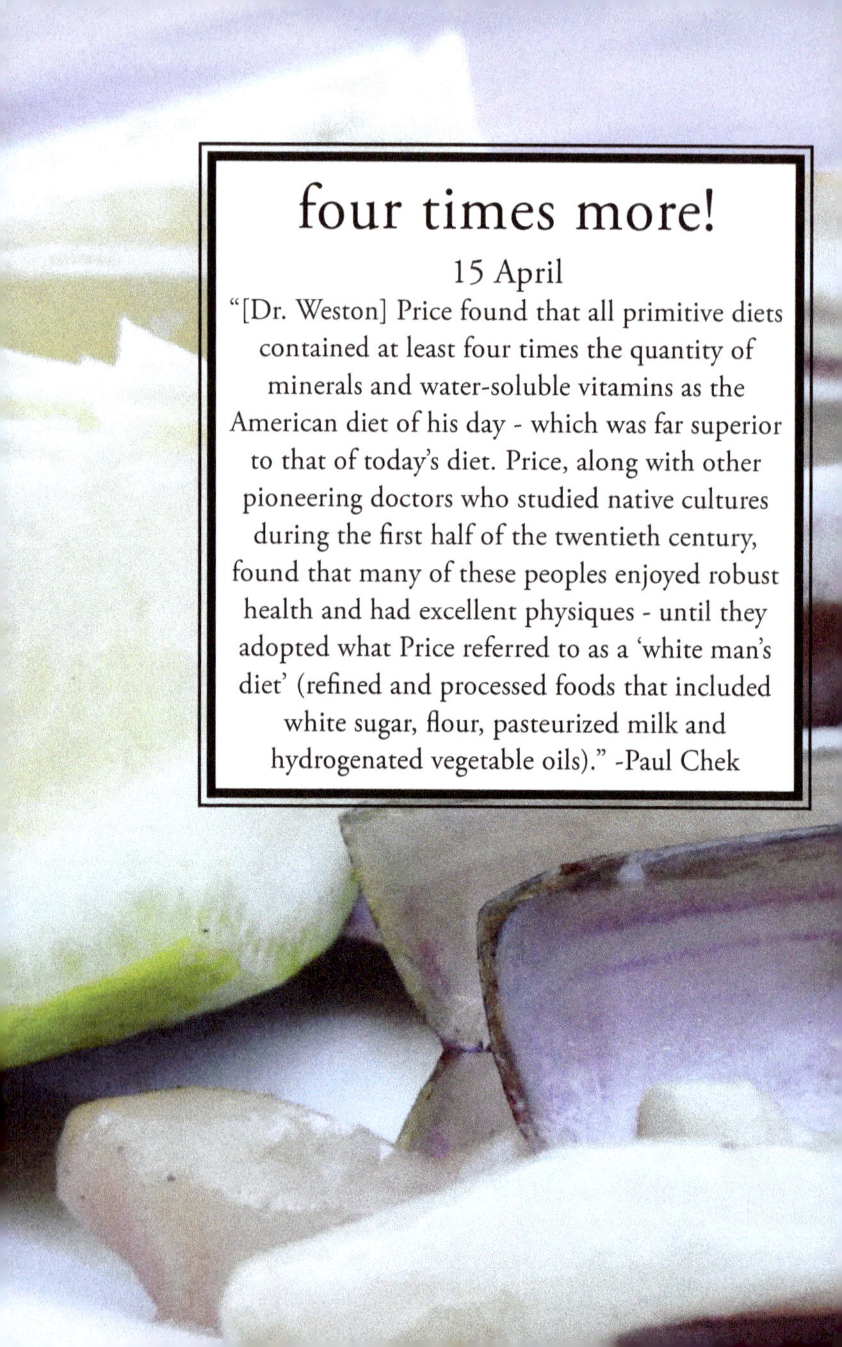

four times more!

15 April

"[Dr. Weston] Price found that all primitive diets contained at least four times the quantity of minerals and water-soluble vitamins as the American diet of his day - which was far superior to that of today's diet. Price, along with other pioneering doctors who studied native cultures during the first half of the twentieth century, found that many of these peoples enjoyed robust health and had excellent physiques - until they adopted what Price referred to as a 'white man's diet' (refined and processed foods that included white sugar, flour, pasteurized milk and hydrogenated vegetable oils)." -Paul Chek

evolutionary concepts
16 April

"They [our ancestors] also consumed much larger amounts of fruits and vegetables, had higher potassium and calcium content in the diet, and rarely depended on sodium-rich foods or grains. The extent to which modern diets can recapture these evolutionary concepts may guide us away from any number of chronic inflammatory diseases, insulin resistant diabetes, and obesity. One basic fundamental of this so-called 'paleo-nutrition' is the consumption of pasture-fed meats instead of grain-fed meat."

-Christopher M. Foley MD

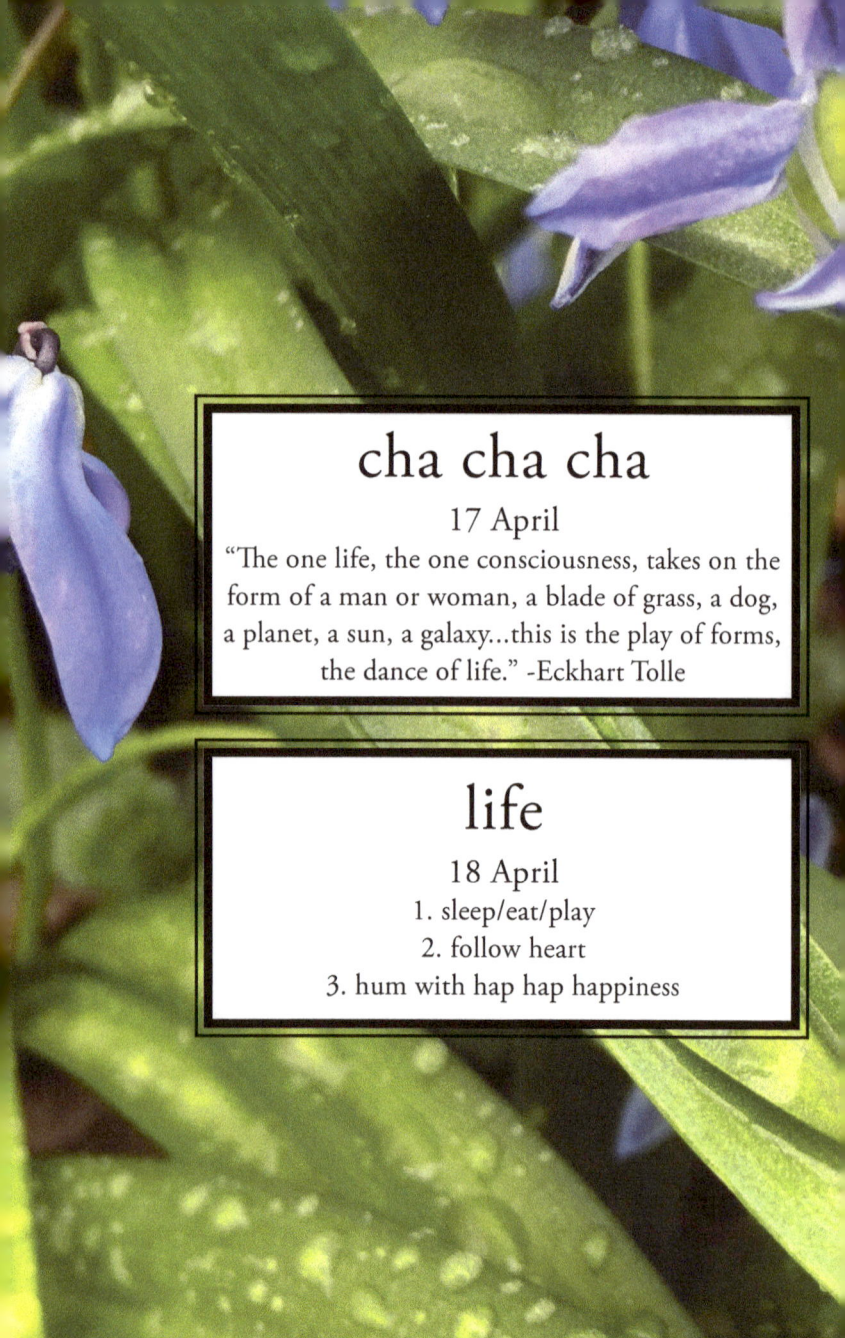

cha cha cha

17 April

"The one life, the one consciousness, takes on the form of a man or woman, a blade of grass, a dog, a planet, a sun, a galaxy...this is the play of forms, the dance of life." -Eckhart Tolle

life

18 April
1. sleep/eat/play
2. follow heart
3. hum with hap hap happiness

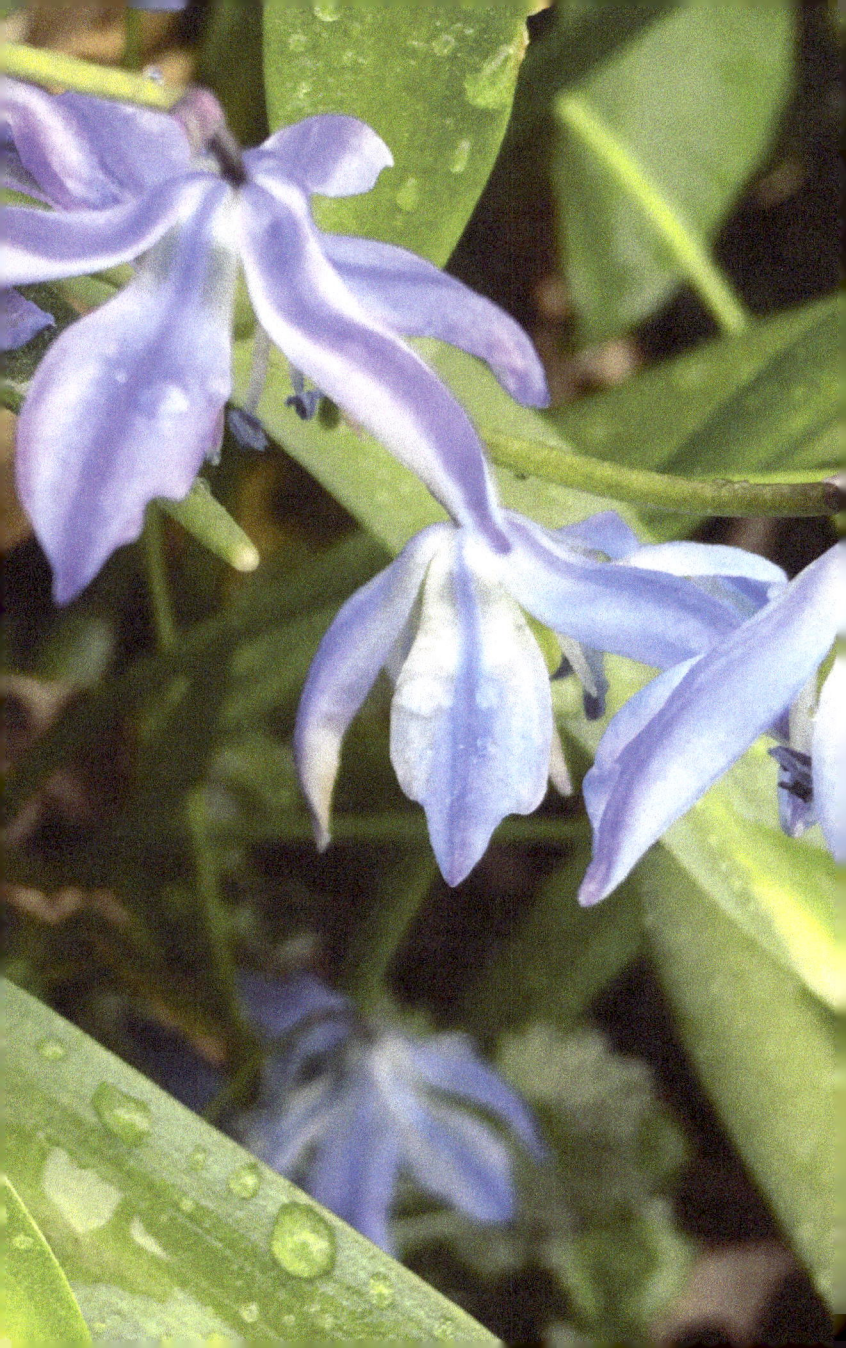

known

19 April
"If you begin to look upon everything as alive, it will come closer and want to be known."
-unknown

all one

20 April
"The plants and we are one. The molecule heme, that structures the faction of our blood called hemoglobin, is the same molecule that structures the blood of plants - chlorophyll. We really are all one." -TS Wiley with Bent Formby PhD

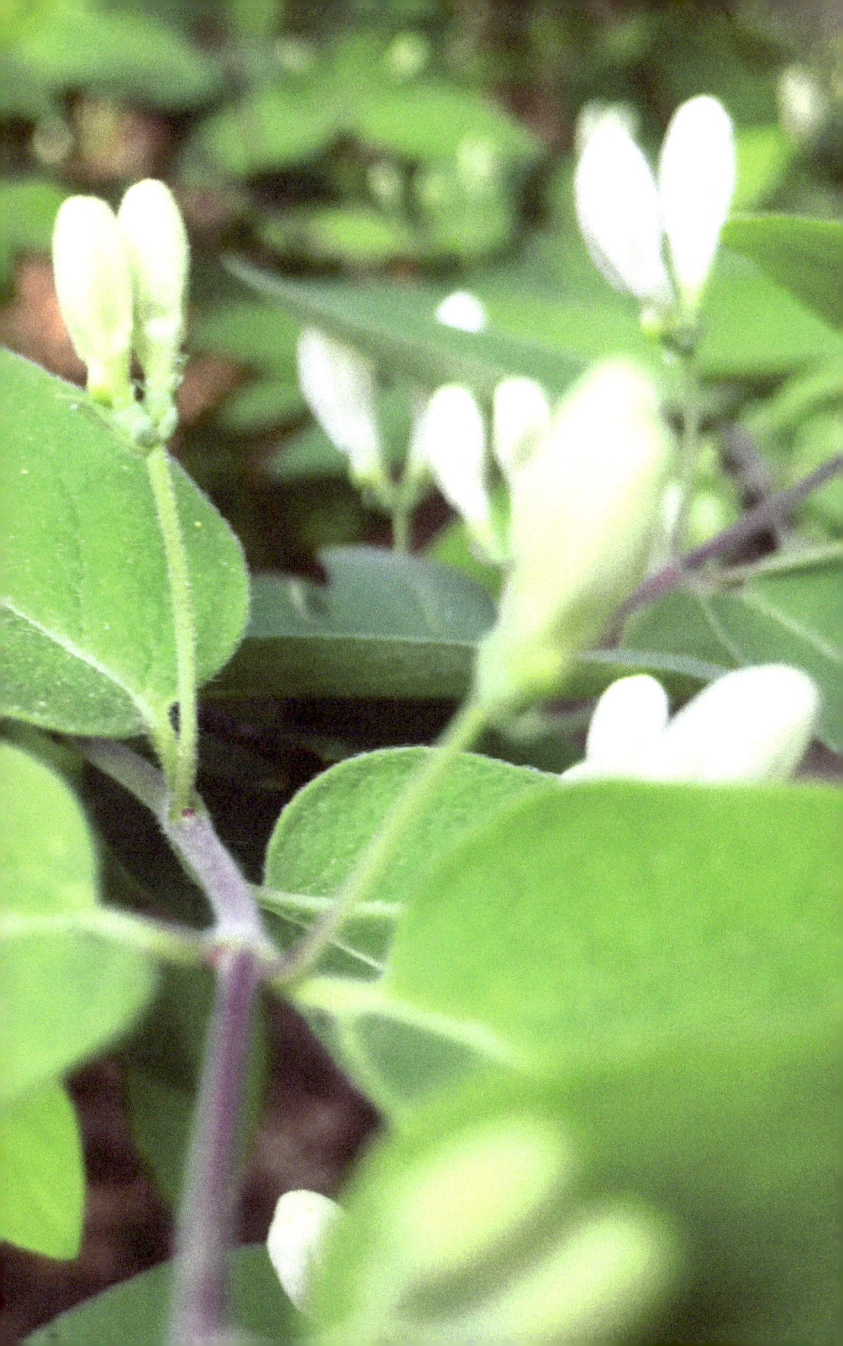

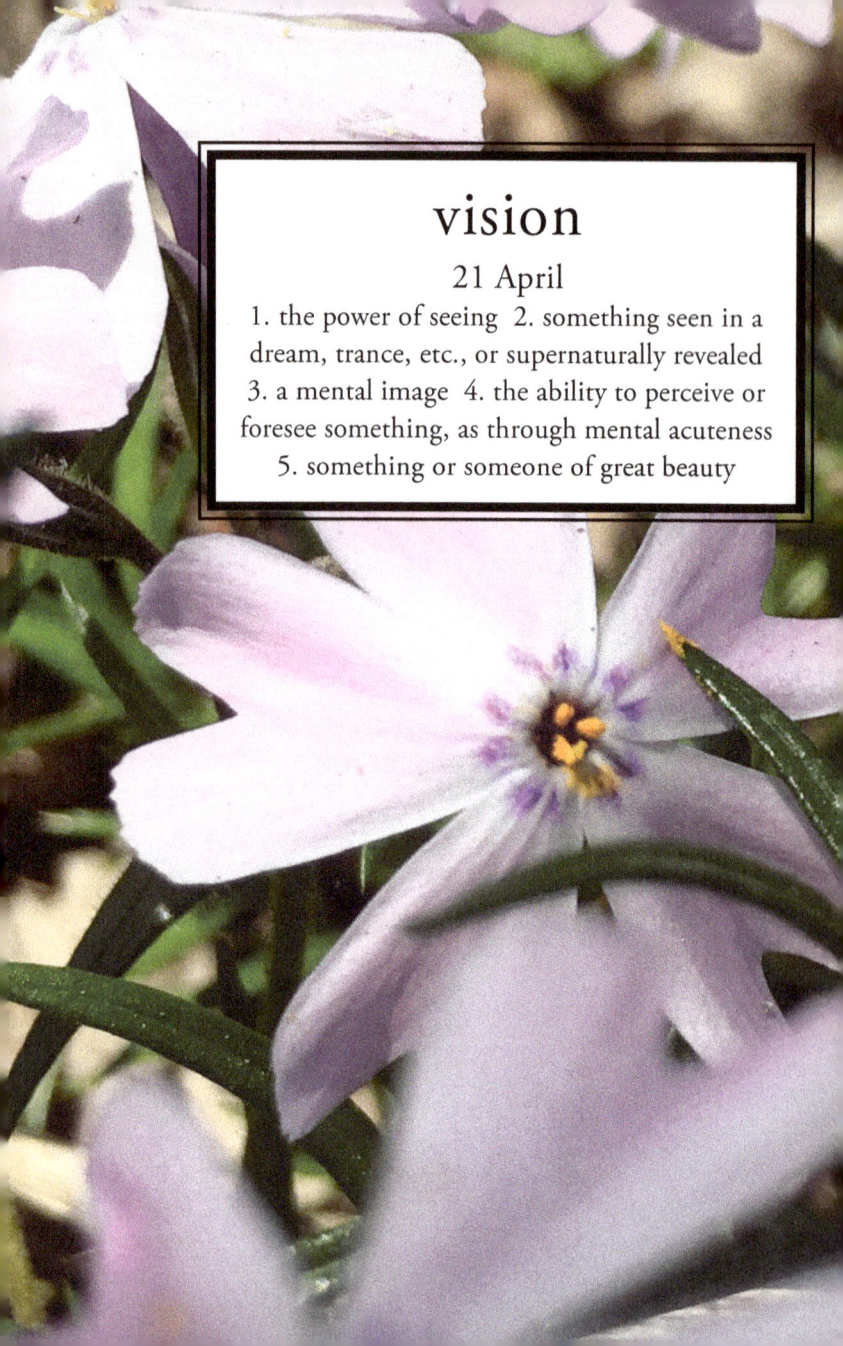

vision
21 April
1. the power of seeing 2. something seen in a dream, trance, etc., or supernaturally revealed 3. a mental image 4. the ability to perceive or foresee something, as through mental acuteness 5. something or someone of great beauty

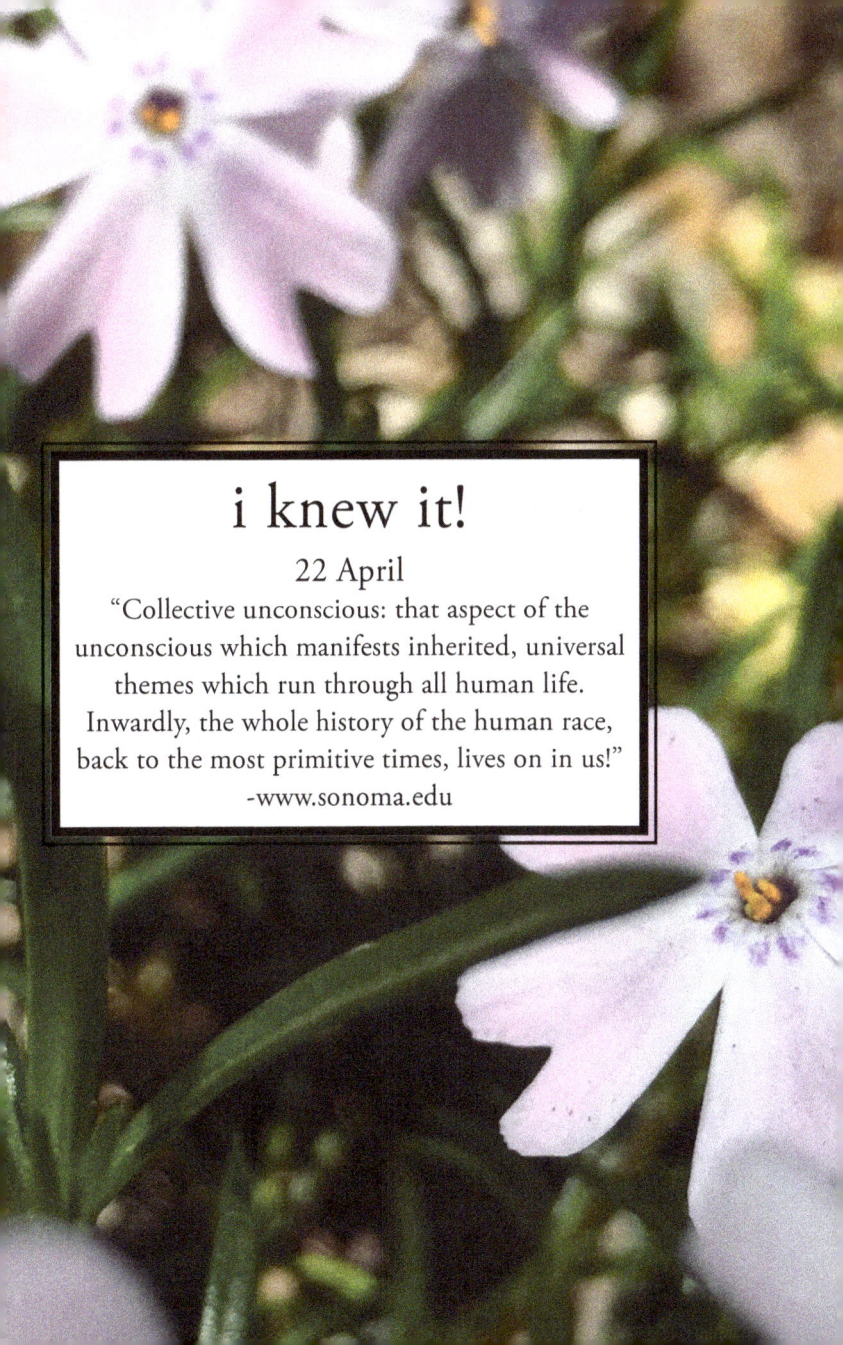

i knew it!

22 April

"Collective unconscious: that aspect of the unconscious which manifests inherited, universal themes which run through all human life. Inwardly, the whole history of the human race, back to the most primitive times, lives on in us!"
-www.sonoma.edu

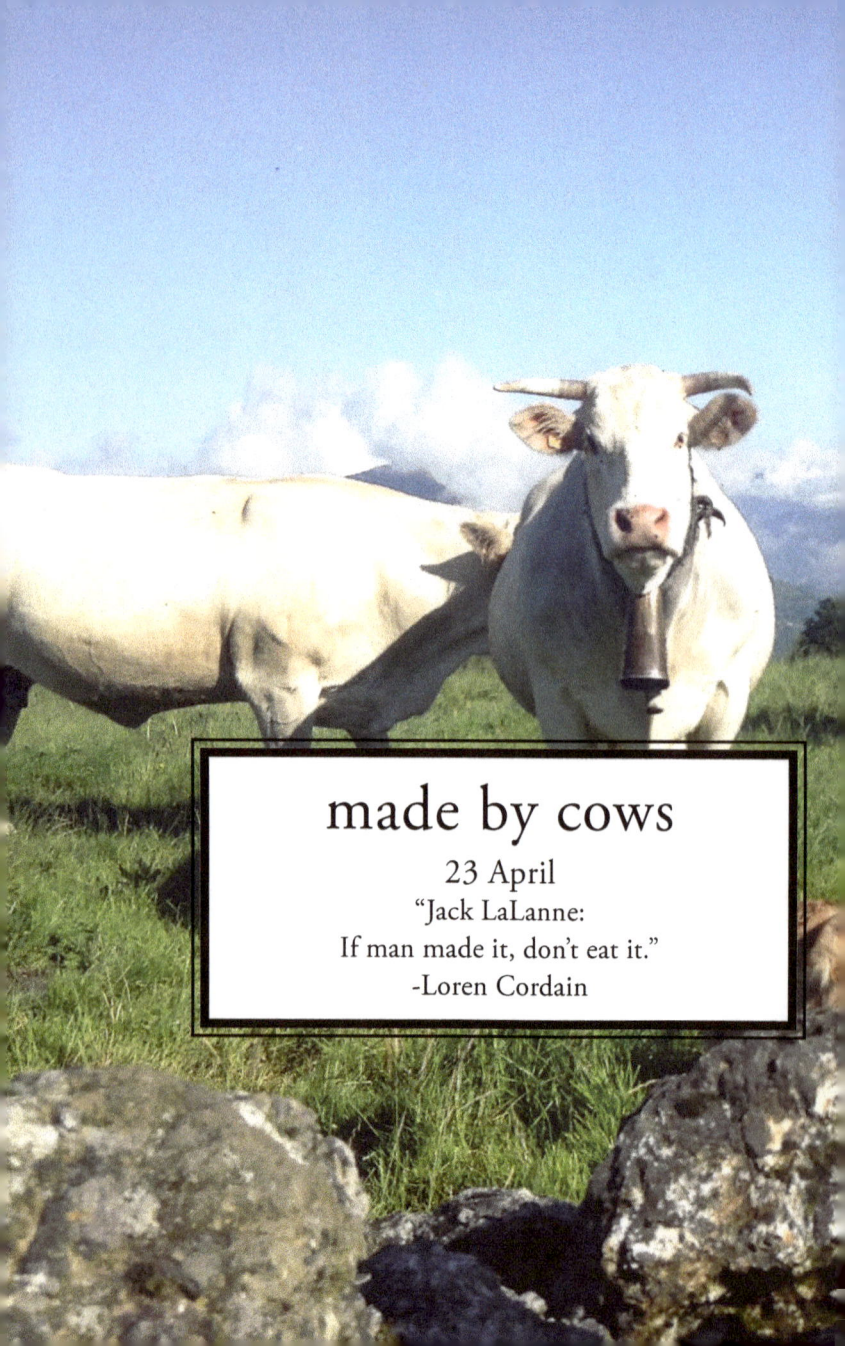

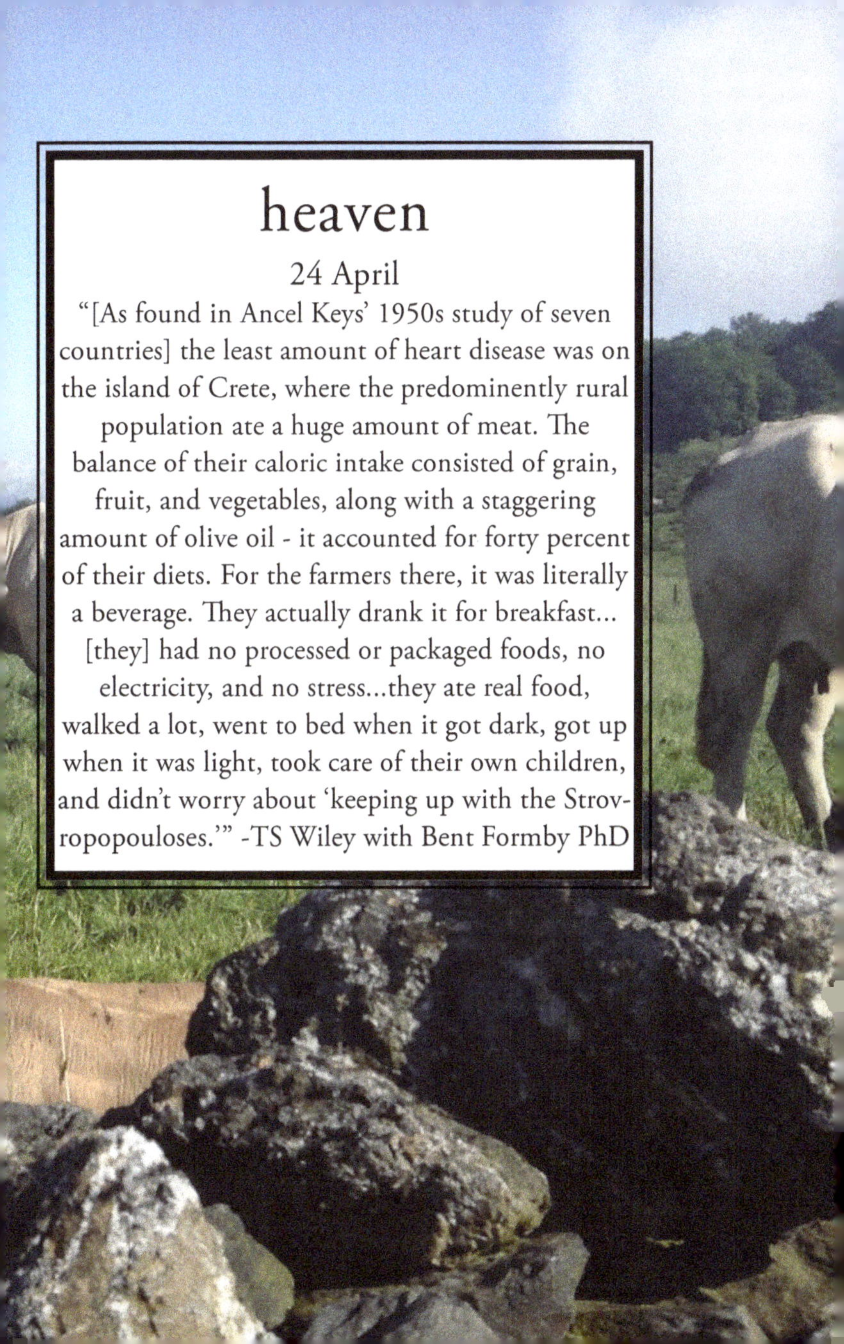

heaven

24 April

"[As found in Ancel Keys' 1950s study of seven countries] the least amount of heart disease was on the island of Crete, where the predominently rural population ate a huge amount of meat. The balance of their caloric intake consisted of grain, fruit, and vegetables, along with a staggering amount of olive oil - it accounted for forty percent of their diets. For the farmers there, it was literally a beverage. They actually drank it for breakfast... [they] had no processed or packaged foods, no electricity, and no stress...they ate real food, walked a lot, went to bed when it got dark, got up when it was light, took care of their own children, and didn't worry about 'keeping up with the Strovropopouloses.'" -TS Wiley with Bent Formby PhD

mystery

25 April

"For [Carl] Jung life was a great mystery. We know and understand very little of it. He never hesitated to say, 'I don't know.' Always admitted when he came to the end of his understanding."
-www.sonoma.edu

attentive

26 April
"The present moment is filled with joy and happiness. If you are attentive, you will see it."
-Thich Nhat Hanh

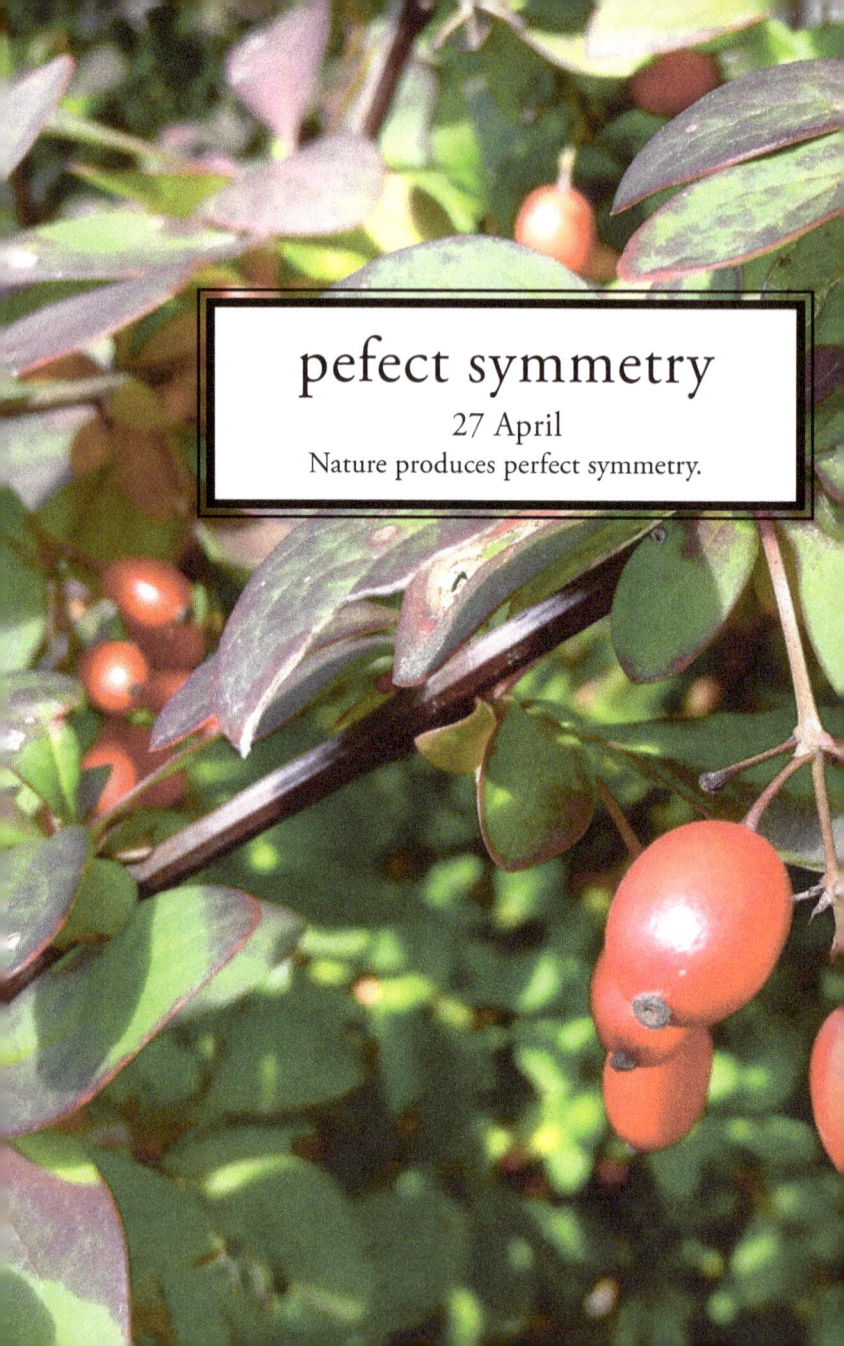

pefect symmetry
27 April
Nature produces perfect symmetry.

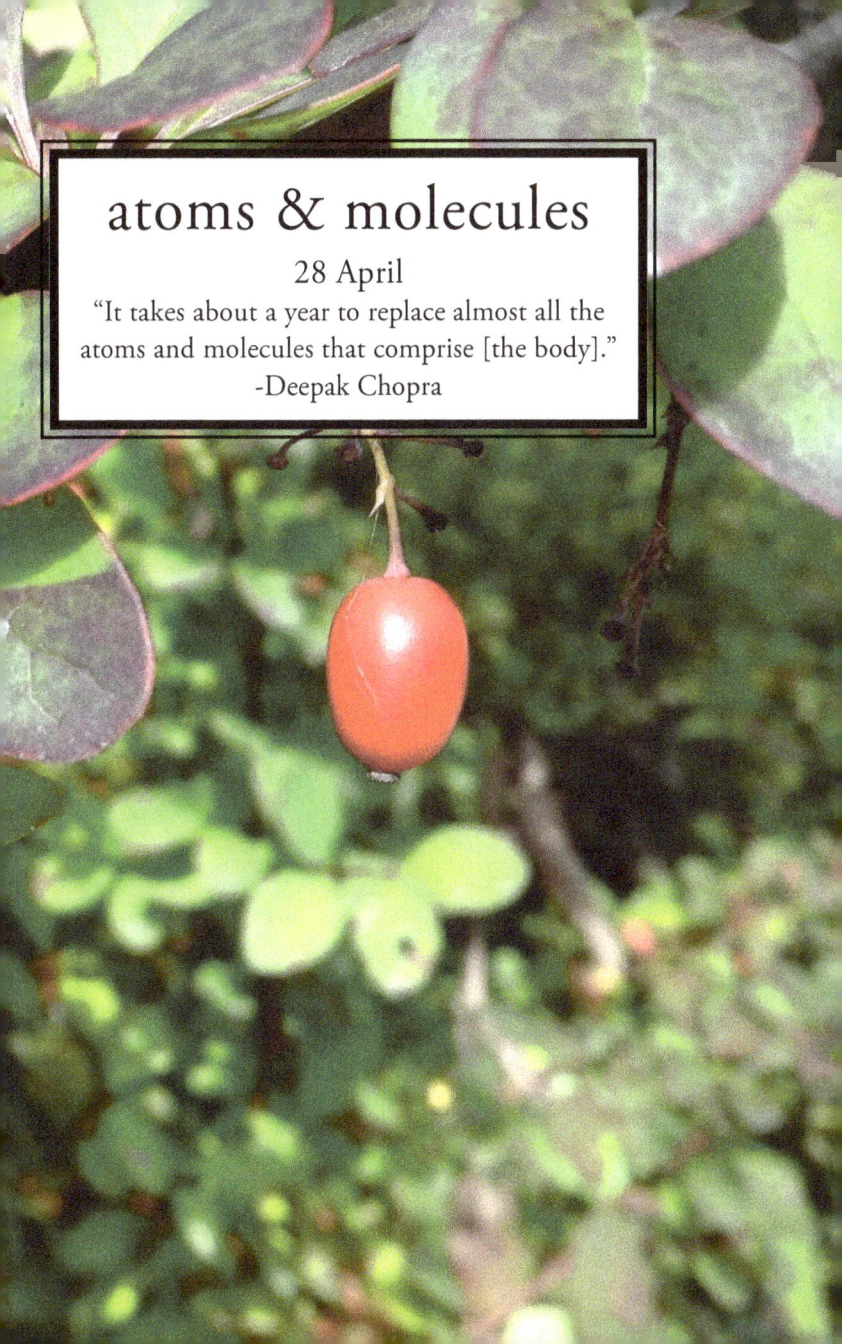

atoms & molecules

28 April

"It takes about a year to replace almost all the atoms and molecules that comprise [the body]."
-Deepak Chopra

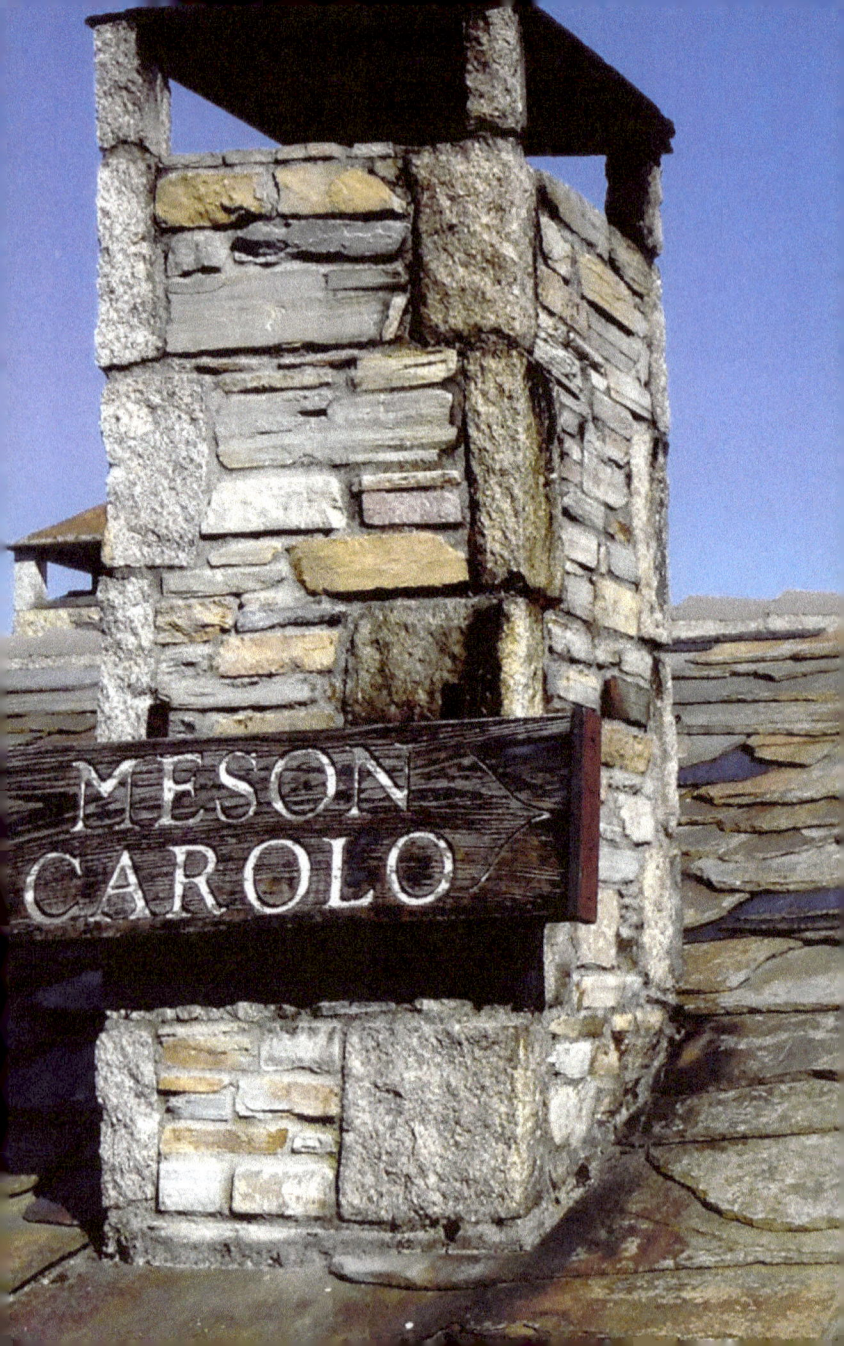

optimal performance
29 April
"Dr Leila Denmark was the world's oldest active pediatrician when she retired at the age of 103; she recently died at age 114...At her 100th birthday she refused cake because it had sugar in it, and at her 103rd birthday party, when she again refused cake, she explained that she hadn't eaten any food made with sugar for seventy years."
-Paul Jaminet PhD &
Shou-Ching Jaminet PhD

MonTuesWedThursFriSatSun
30 April
cooking eating sleeping b e i n g

lush grasses & pretty cows
1 May

"Food is like a language, an unbroken information stream that connects every cell in your body to an aspect of the natural world...If you eat a properly cooked steak from an open-range, grass-fed cow, then you are receiving information not only about the health of that cow's body, but about the health of the grasses from which it ate, and the soil from which those grasses grew. If you want to know whether or not a steak, or a fish, or a carrot is good for you, ask yourself what portions of the natural world it represents, and whether or not the bulk of that information remains intact. This requires traveling backwards down the food chain, step by step, until you reach the ground or the sea."

-Catherine Shanahan MD & Luke Shanahan

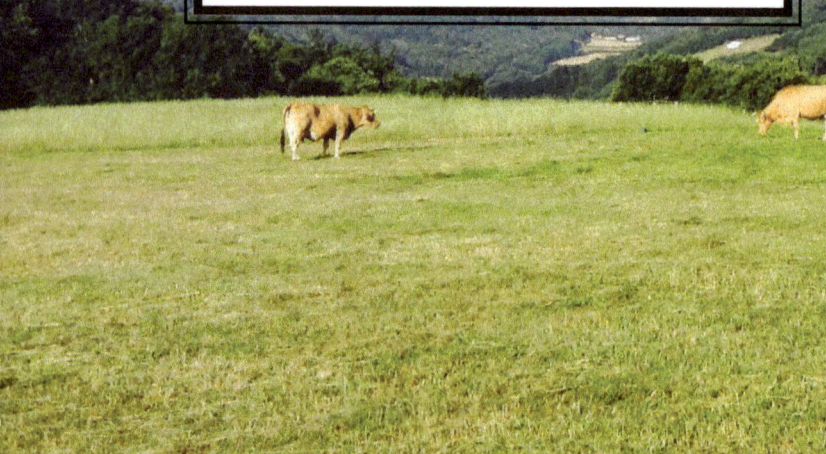

ahhhhh

2 May

"4 reasons why you should make [grass-fed] protein a major part of your diet: 1. It can't be overeaten. 2. It raises your metabolism, causing you to burn more calories. 3. It satisfies your appetite, causing you to feel less hungry between meals. 4. It improves insulin sensitivity."
-Loren Cordain

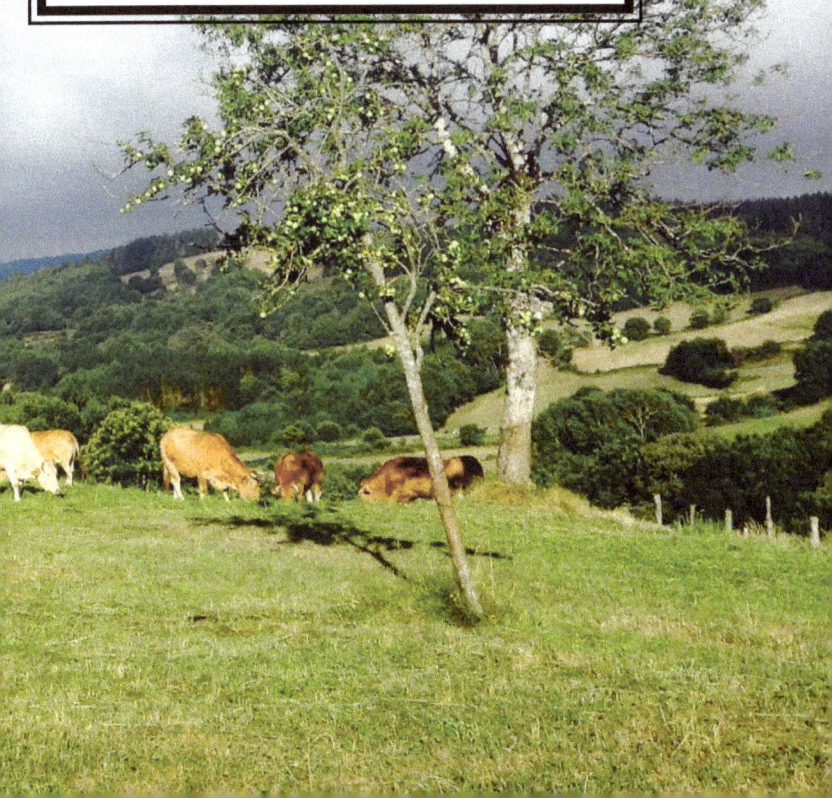

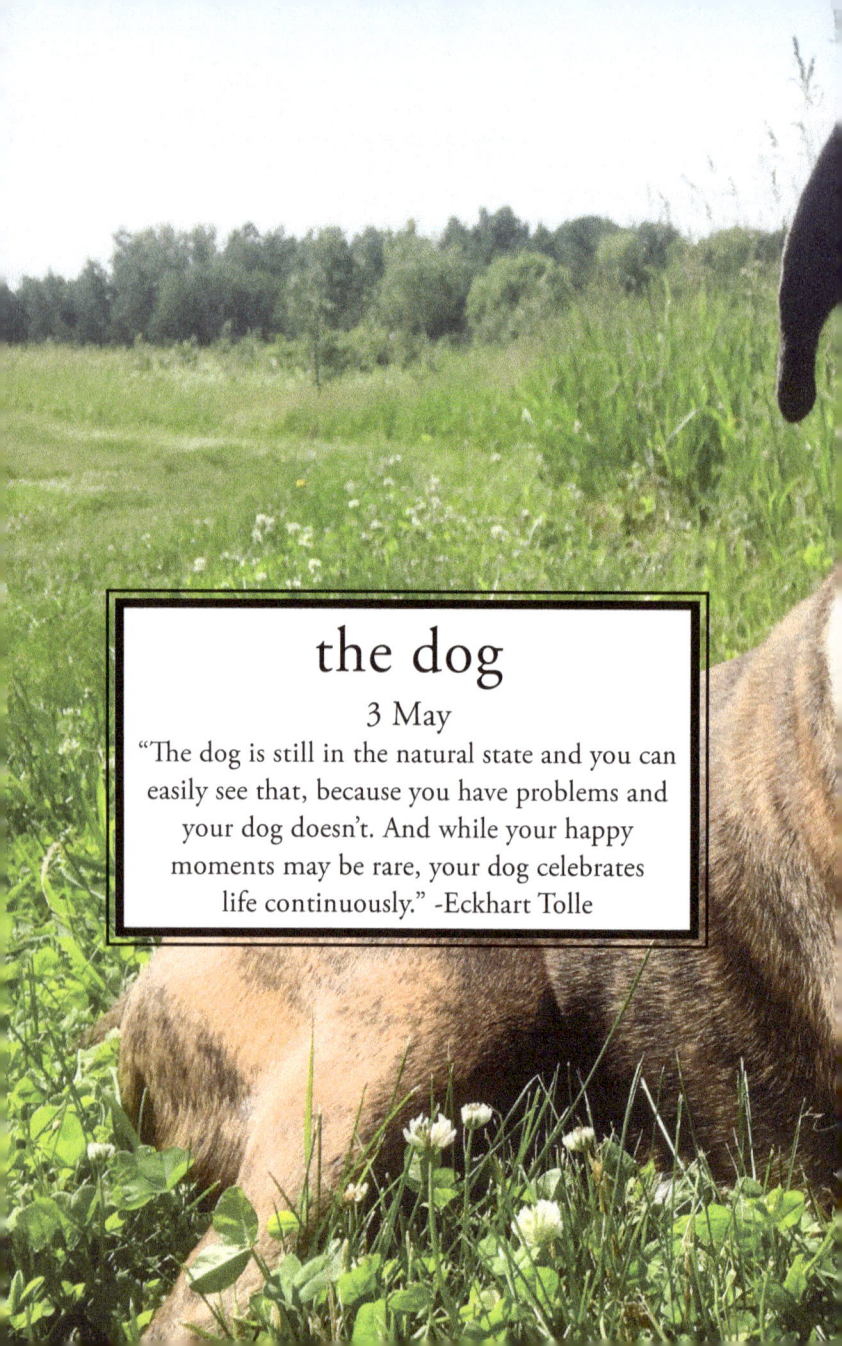

the dog

3 May

"The dog is still in the natural state and you can easily see that, because you have problems and your dog doesn't. And while your happy moments may be rare, your dog celebrates life continuously." -Eckhart Tolle

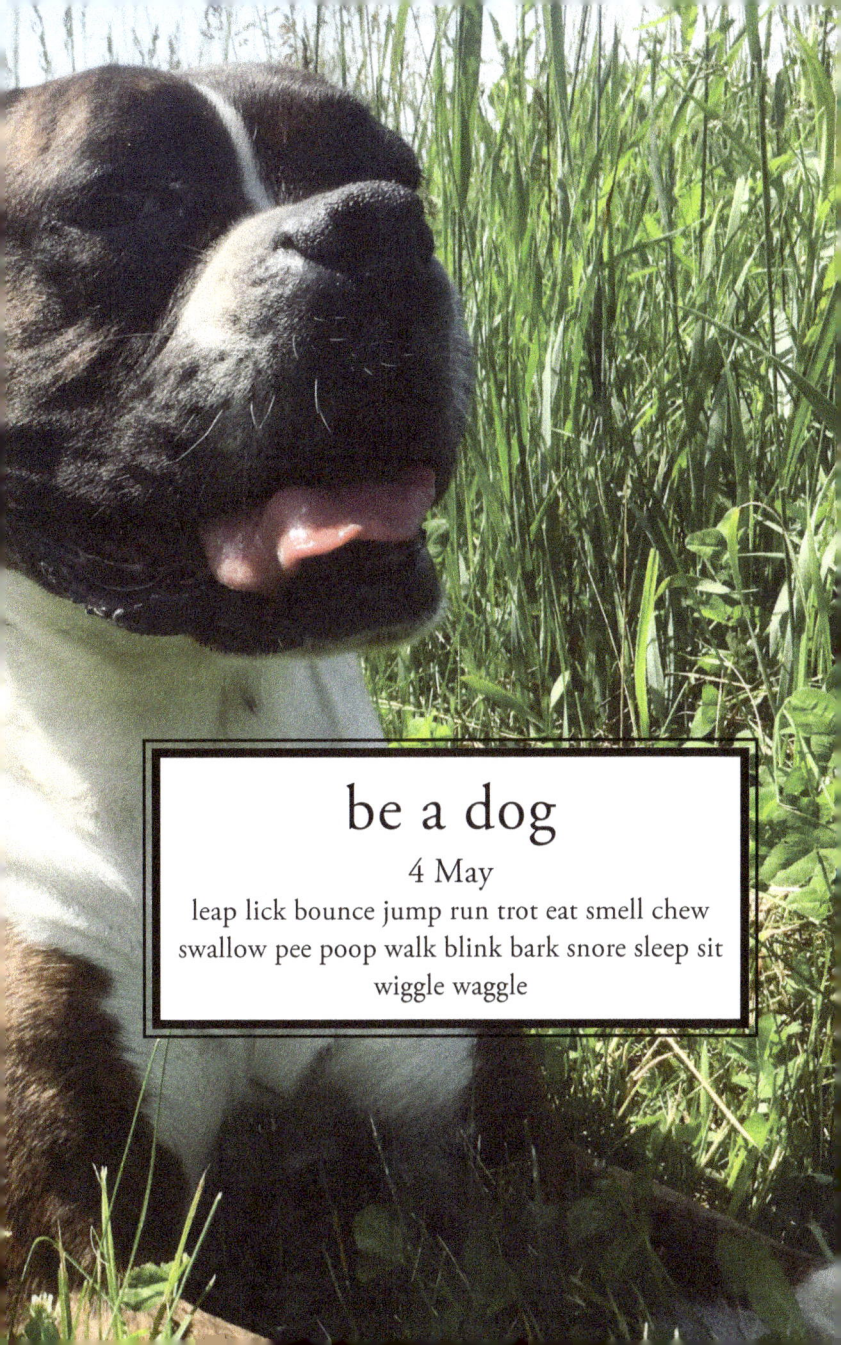

be a dog

4 May

leap lick bounce jump run trot eat smell chew swallow pee poop walk blink bark snore sleep sit wiggle waggle

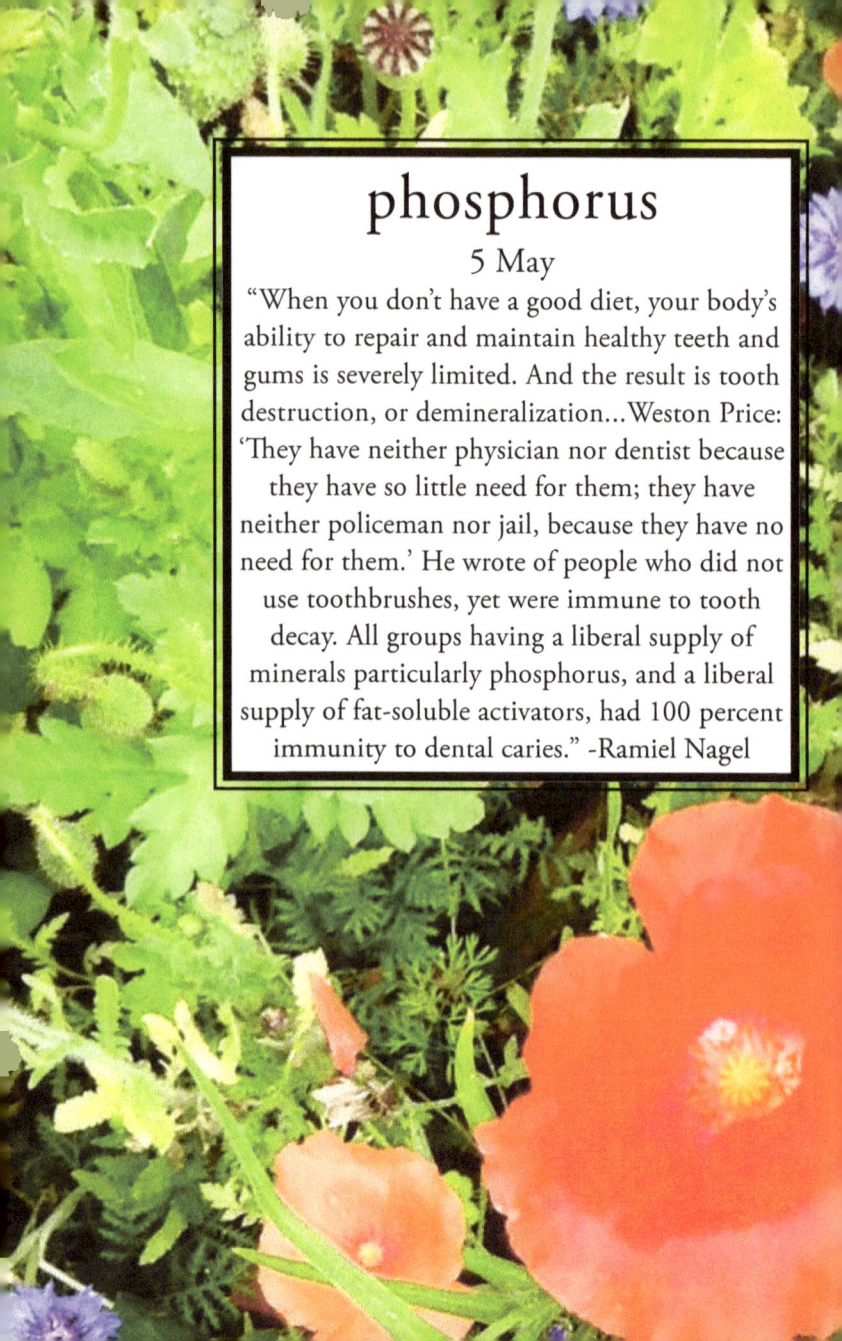

phosphorus
5 May

"When you don't have a good diet, your body's ability to repair and maintain healthy teeth and gums is severely limited. And the result is tooth destruction, or demineralization...Weston Price: 'They have neither physician nor dentist because they have so little need for them; they have neither policeman nor jail, because they have no need for them.' He wrote of people who did not use toothbrushes, yet were immune to tooth decay. All groups having a liberal supply of minerals particularly phosphorus, and a liberal supply of fat-soluble activators, had 100 percent immunity to dental caries." -Ramiel Nagel

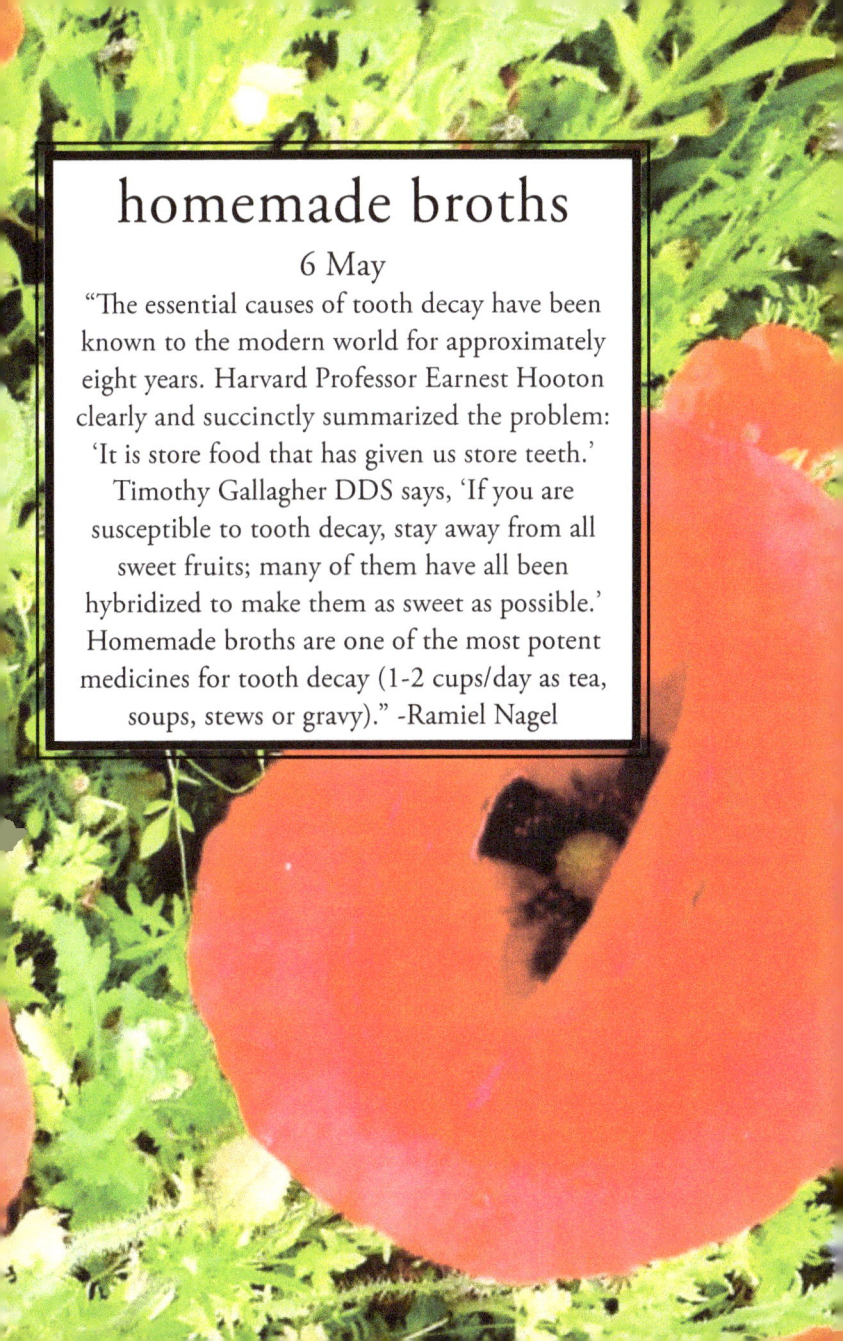

homemade broths

6 May

"The essential causes of tooth decay have been known to the modern world for approximately eight years. Harvard Professor Earnest Hooton clearly and succinctly summarized the problem: 'It is store food that has given us store teeth.' Timothy Gallagher DDS says, 'If you are susceptible to tooth decay, stay away from all sweet fruits; many of them have all been hybridized to make them as sweet as possible.' Homemade broths are one of the most potent medicines for tooth decay (1-2 cups/day as tea, soups, stews or gravy)." -Ramiel Nagel

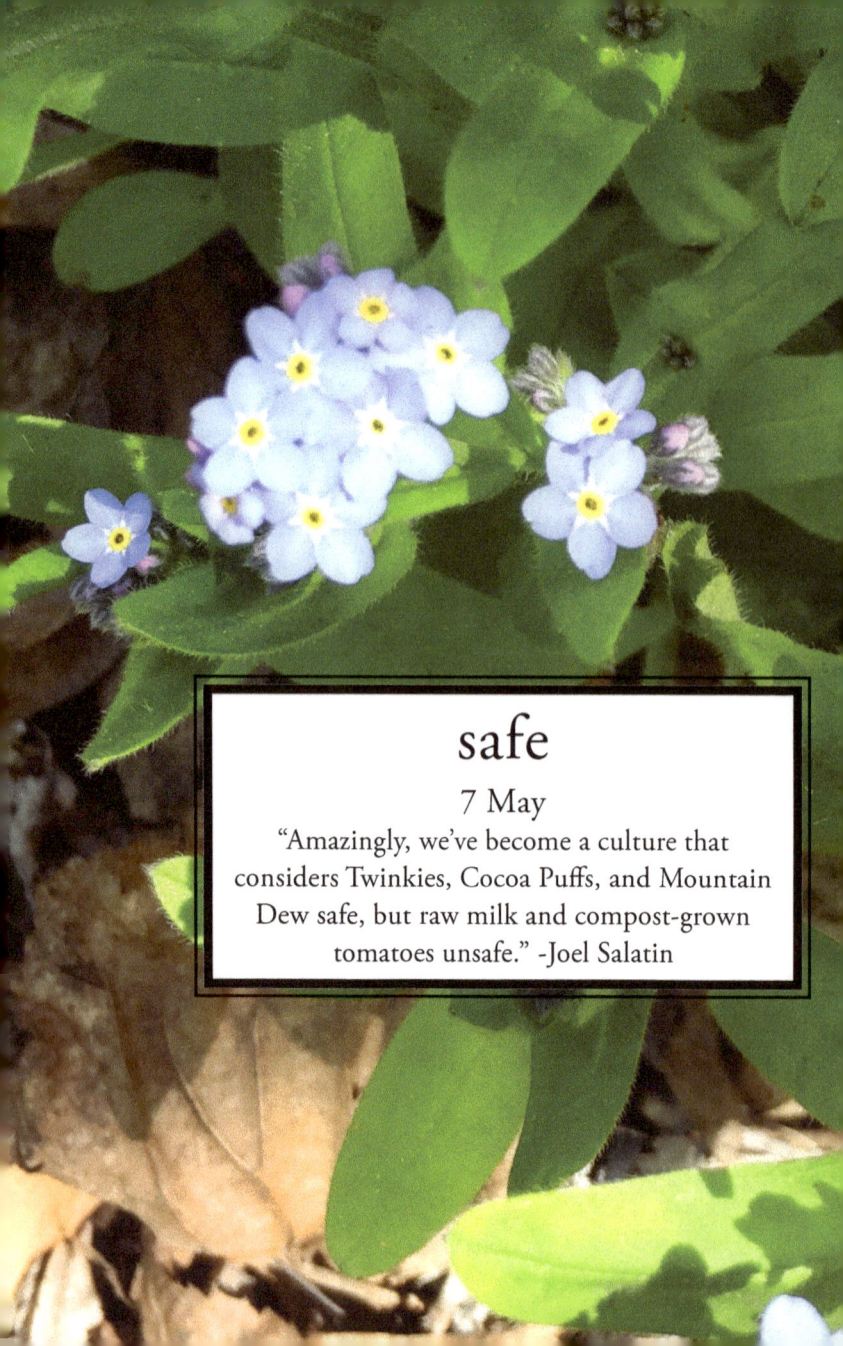

safe

7 May

"Amazingly, we've become a culture that considers Twinkies, Cocoa Puffs, and Mountain Dew safe, but raw milk and compost-grown tomatoes unsafe." -Joel Salatin

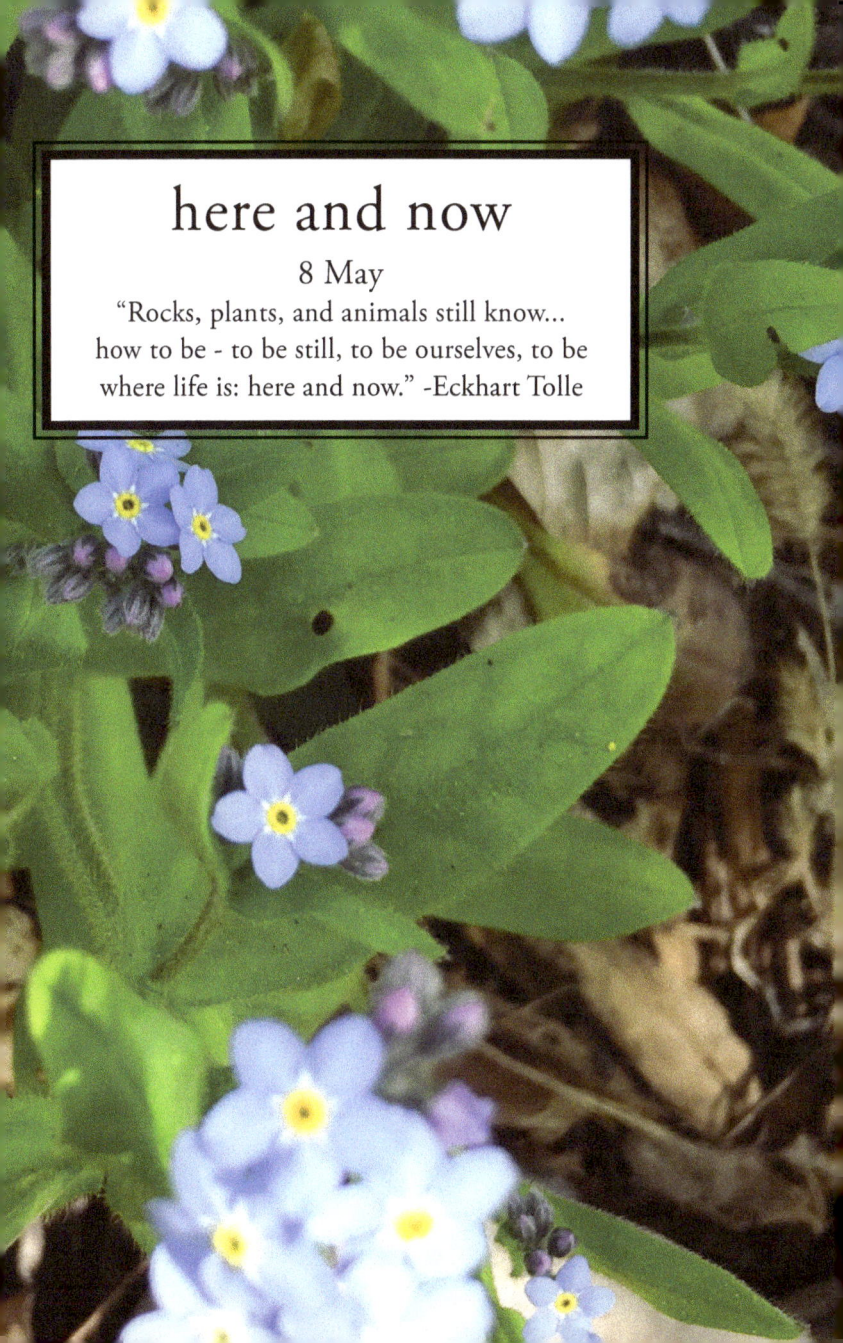

here and now

8 May

"Rocks, plants, and animals still know... how to be - to be still, to be ourselves, to be where life is: here and now." -Eckhart Tolle

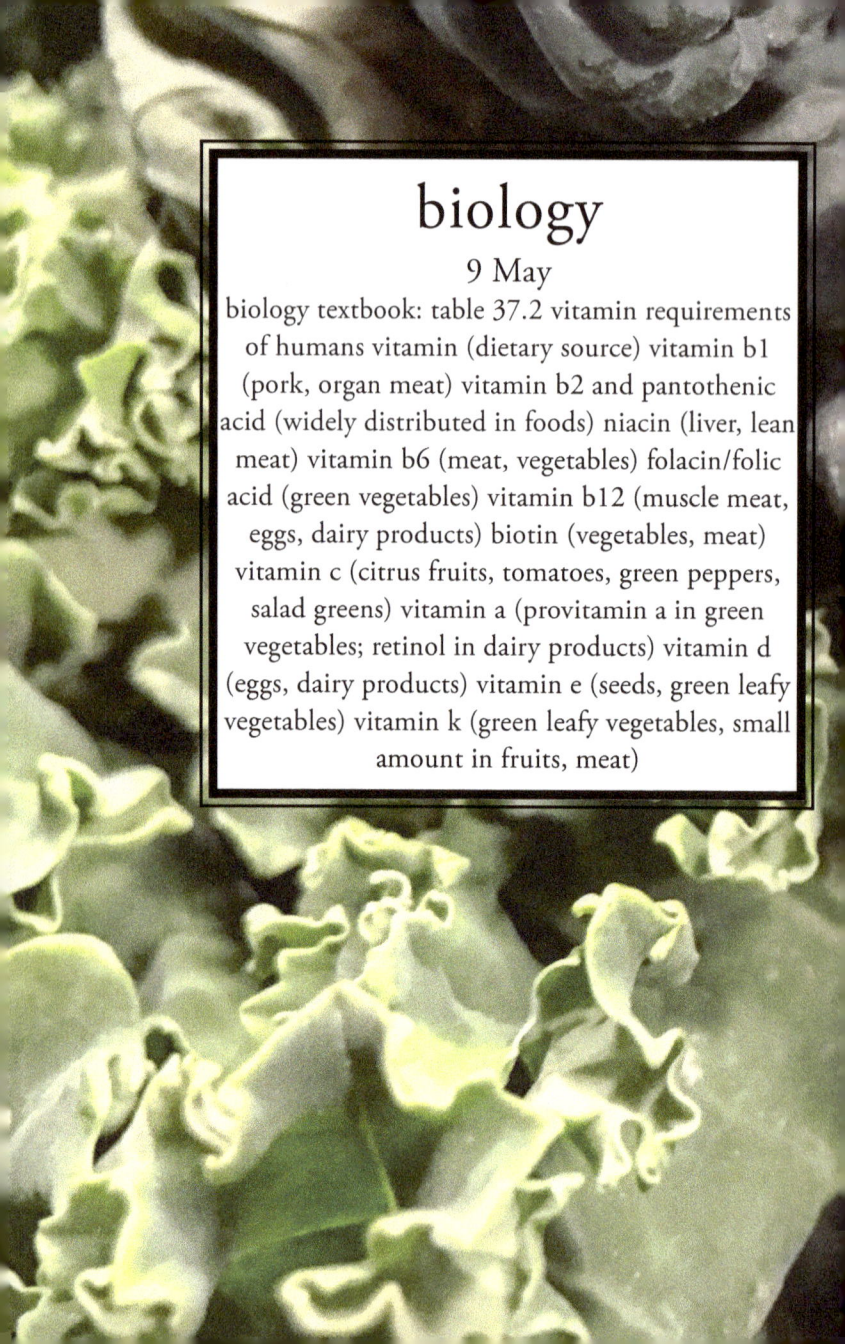

biology

9 May

biology textbook: table 37.2 vitamin requirements of humans vitamin (dietary source) vitamin b1 (pork, organ meat) vitamin b2 and pantothenic acid (widely distributed in foods) niacin (liver, lean meat) vitamin b6 (meat, vegetables) folacin/folic acid (green vegetables) vitamin b12 (muscle meat, eggs, dairy products) biotin (vegetables, meat) vitamin c (citrus fruits, tomatoes, green peppers, salad greens) vitamin a (provitamin a in green vegetables; retinol in dairy products) vitamin d (eggs, dairy products) vitamin e (seeds, green leafy vegetables) vitamin k (green leafy vegetables, small amount in fruits, meat)

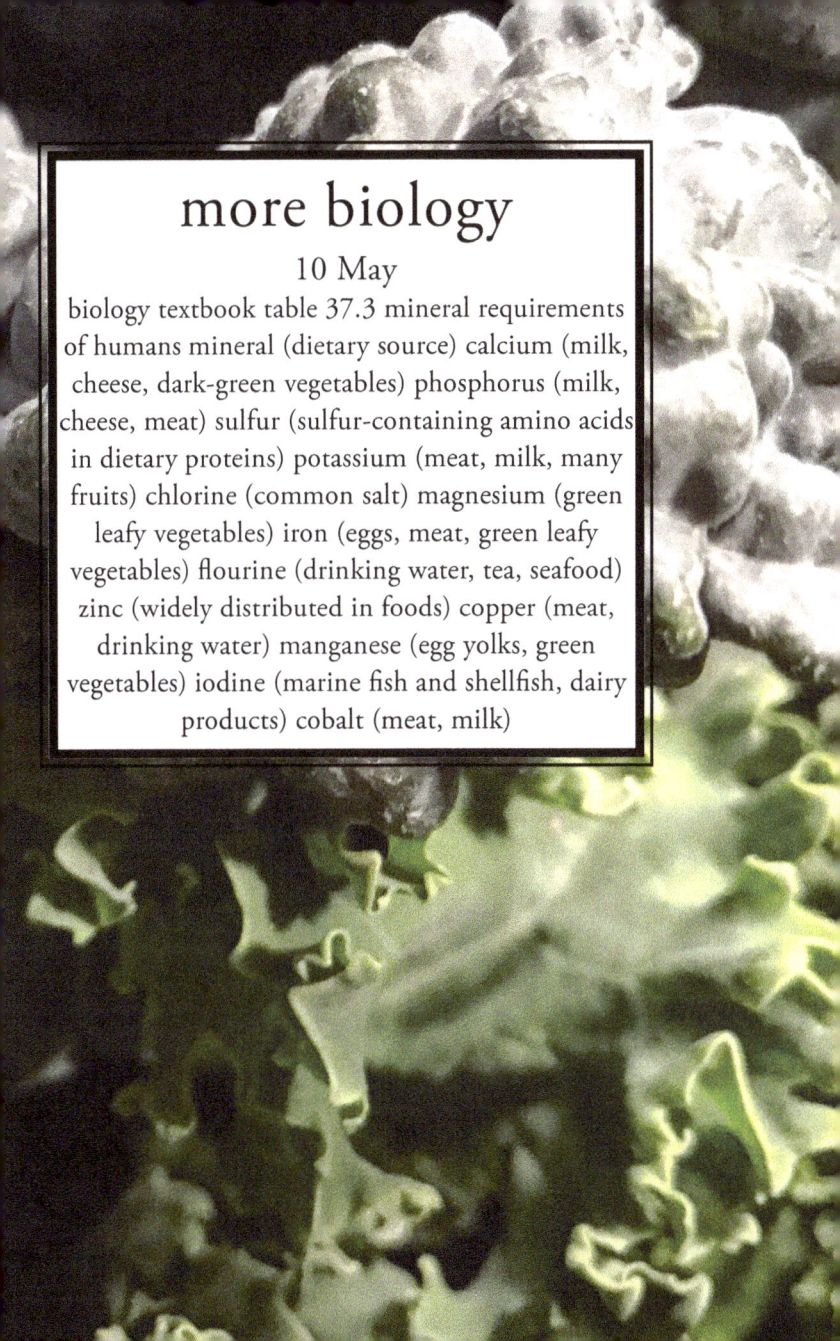

more biology
10 May

biology textbook table 37.3 mineral requirements of humans mineral (dietary source) calcium (milk, cheese, dark-green vegetables) phosphorus (milk, cheese, meat) sulfur (sulfur-containing amino acids in dietary proteins) potassium (meat, milk, many fruits) chlorine (common salt) magnesium (green leafy vegetables) iron (eggs, meat, green leafy vegetables) flourine (drinking water, tea, seafood) zinc (widely distributed in foods) copper (meat, drinking water) manganese (egg yolks, green vegetables) iodine (marine fish and shellfish, dairy products) cobalt (meat, milk)

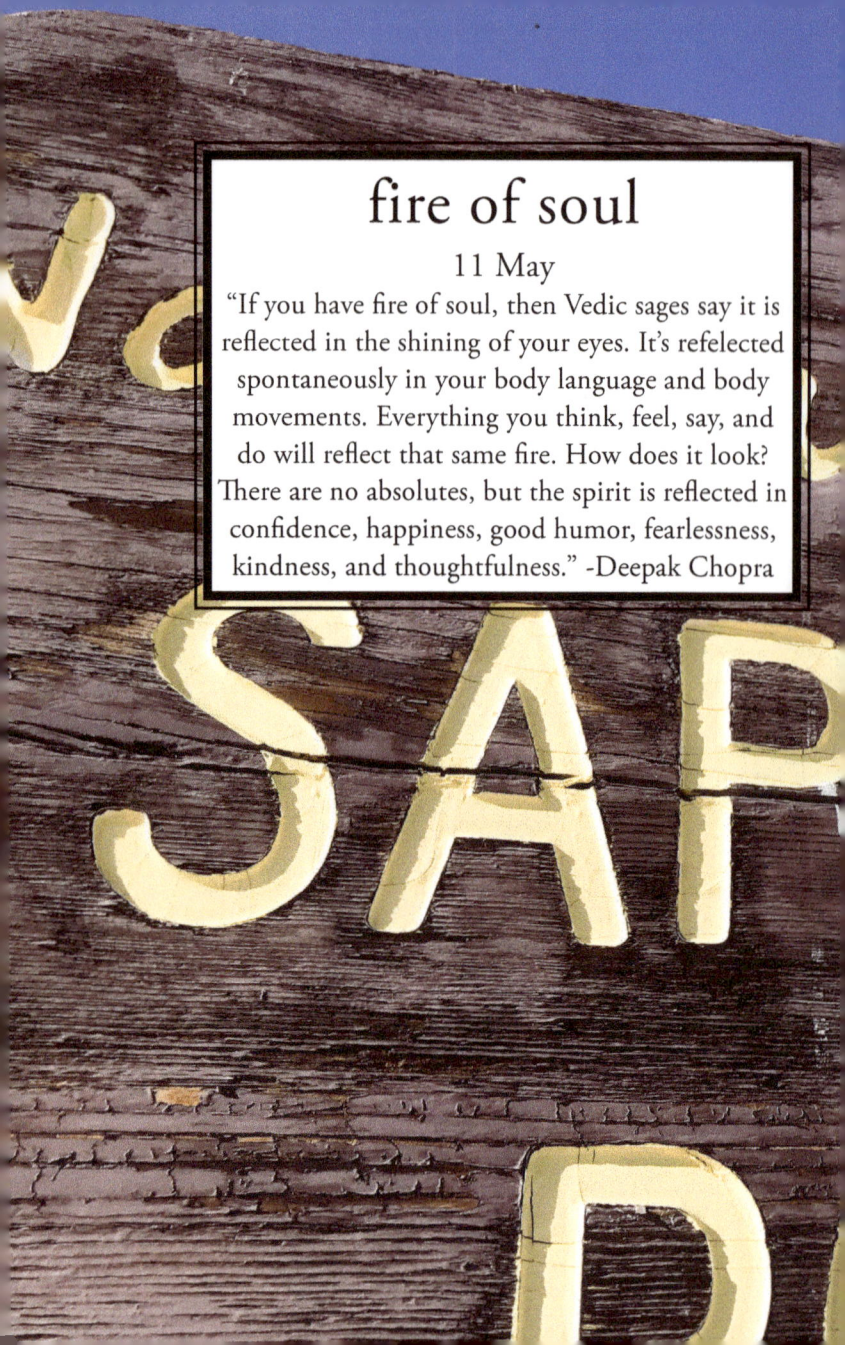

fire of soul

11 May

"If you have fire of soul, then Vedic sages say it is reflected in the shining of your eyes. It's refelcted spontaneously in your body language and body movements. Everything you think, feel, say, and do will reflect that same fire. How does it look? There are no absolutes, but the spirit is reflected in confidence, happiness, good humor, fearlessness, kindness, and thoughtfulness." -Deepak Chopra

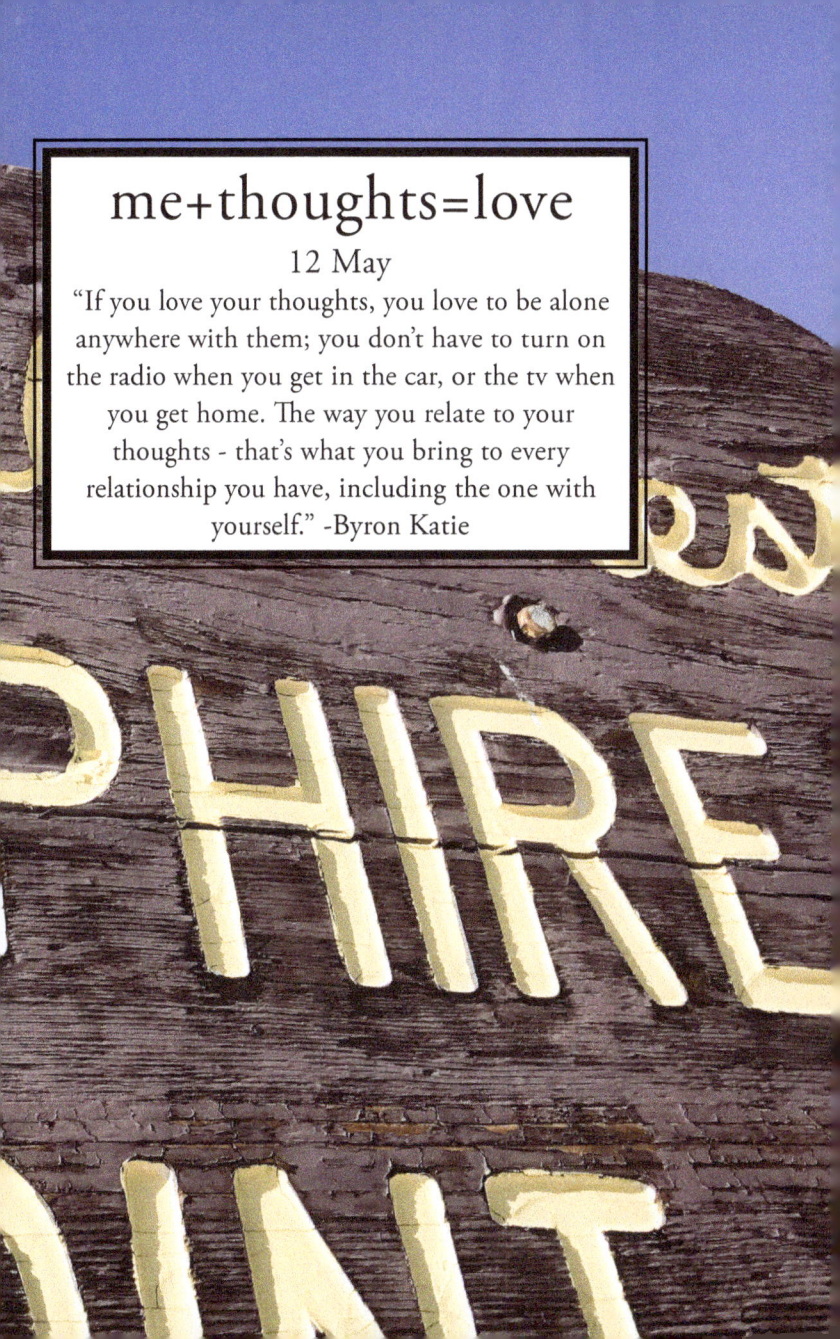

me+thoughts=love

12 May

"If you love your thoughts, you love to be alone anywhere with them; you don't have to turn on the radio when you get in the car, or the tv when you get home. The way you relate to your thoughts - that's what you bring to every relationship you have, including the one with yourself." -Byron Katie

living fully

13 May

"To live fully means lowering the risk for all disease and maximizing health at the cellular level. So many choices we make and things we encounter every day of our lives will impact our ability to live fully until we die. These include what we choose to eat and drink, where we sleep, what we put on our skin, and how we clean our homes." -Dr Myron Wentz & Dave Wentz

freedom

14 May
"Freedom is available at any time to anyone -and so is captivity." -Martha Beck

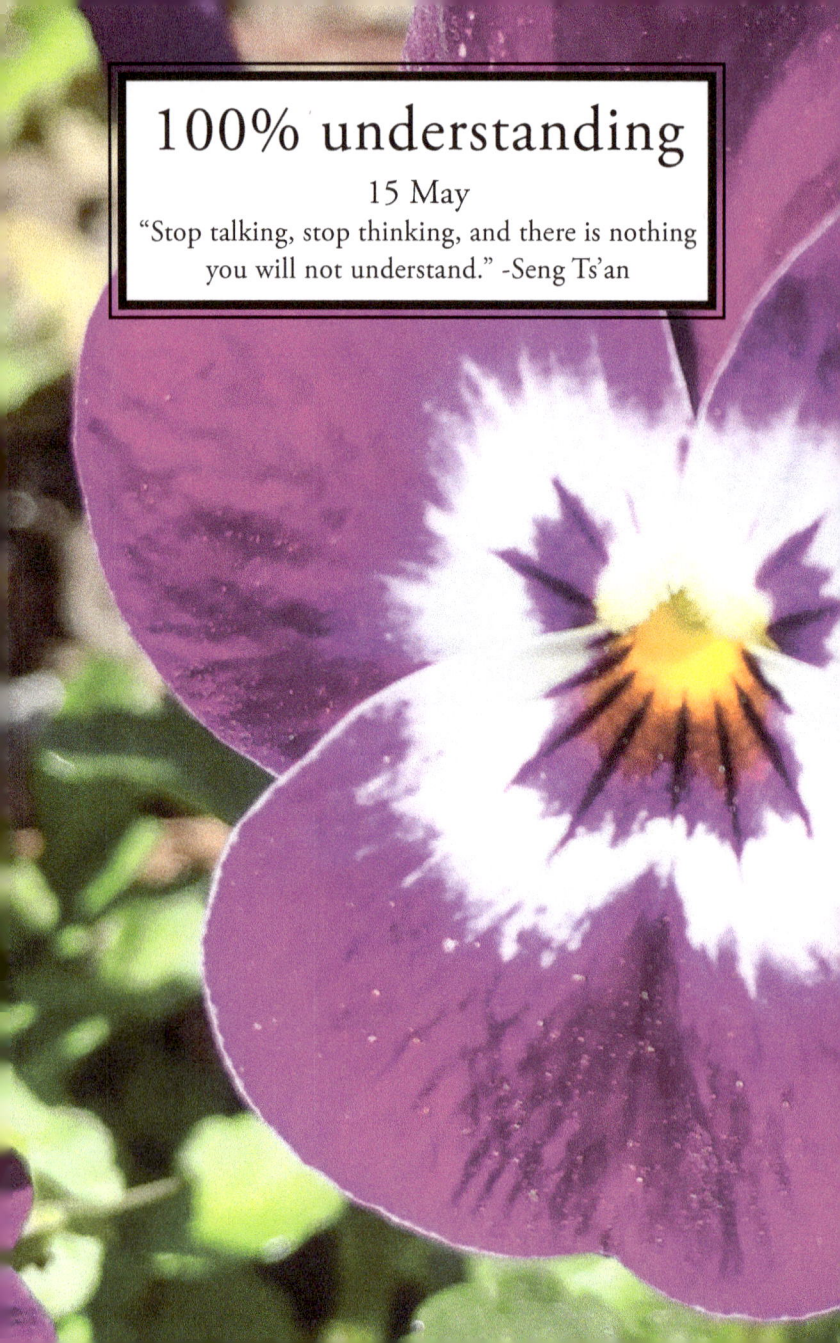

100% understanding

15 May
"Stop talking, stop thinking, and there is nothing you will not understand." -Seng Ts'an

blueprint
16 May

"I believe that God gives us our soul, our deepest identity, our True Self, our unique blueprint...We are given a span of years to discover it, to choose it, and to live our own destiny to the full. If we do not, our True Self will never be offered again, in our own unique form - which is perhaps why almost all religious traditions present the matter with utterly charged words like 'heaven' and 'hell.' Our soul's discovery is utterly crucial, momentous, and of pressing importance for each of us and for the world." -Richard Rohr

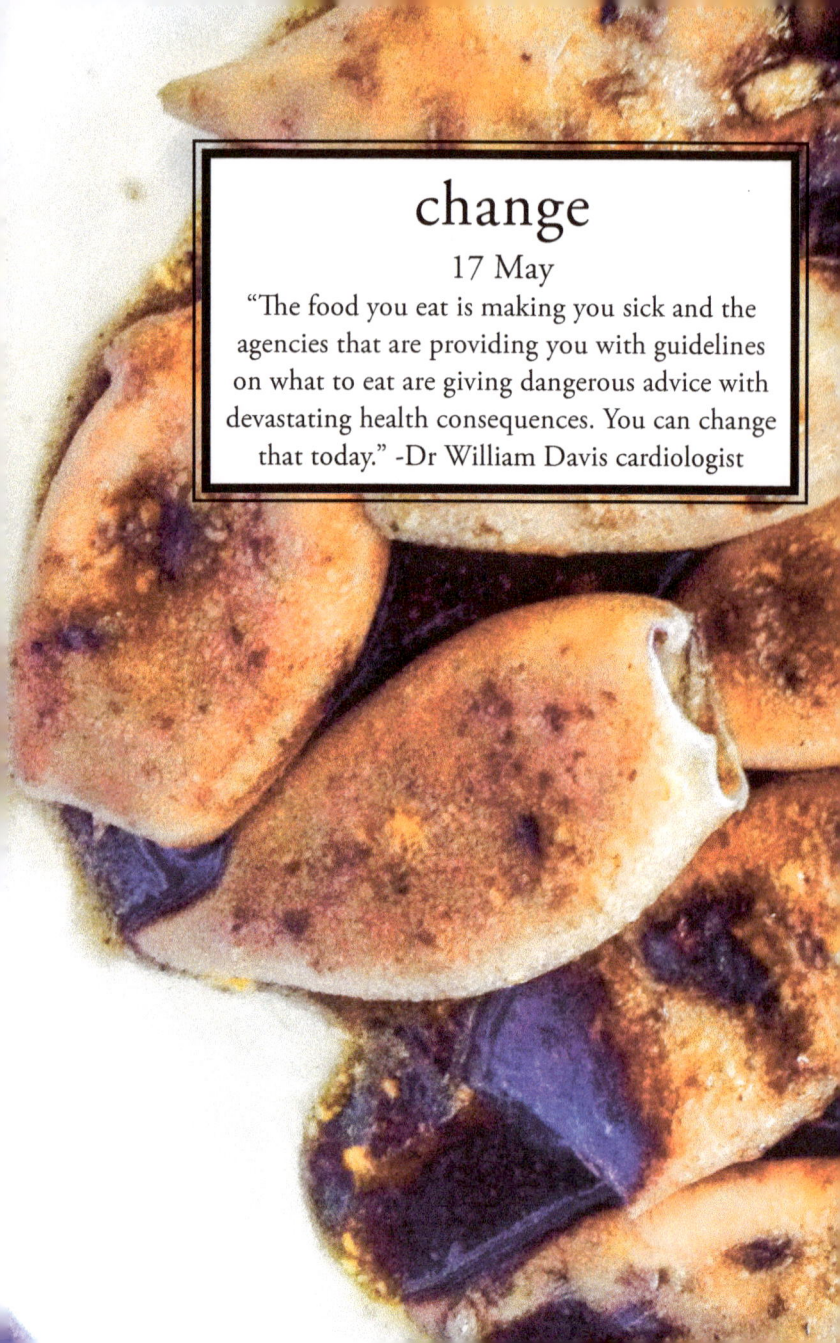

change
17 May
"The food you eat is making you sick and the agencies that are providing you with guidelines on what to eat are giving dangerous advice with devastating health consequences. You can change that today." -Dr William Davis cardiologist

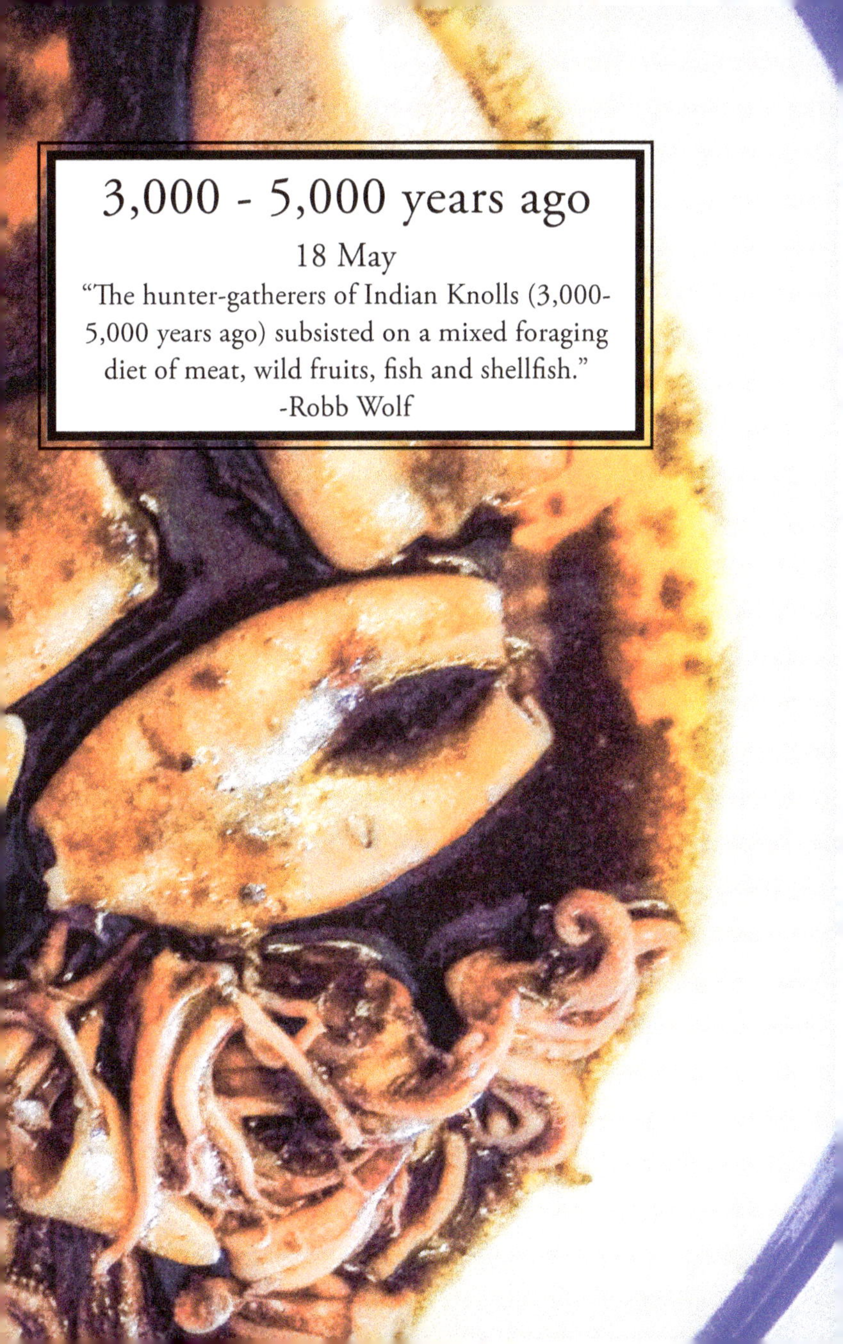

3,000 - 5,000 years ago
18 May
"The hunter-gatherers of Indian Knolls (3,000-5,000 years ago) subsisted on a mixed foraging diet of meat, wild fruits, fish and shellfish."
-Robb Wolf

birth

19 May
"When you are born, your work is placed in your heart." -Kahil Gibran

1. know thyself

20 May
"Knowing thyself is the first practice of love."
-unknown

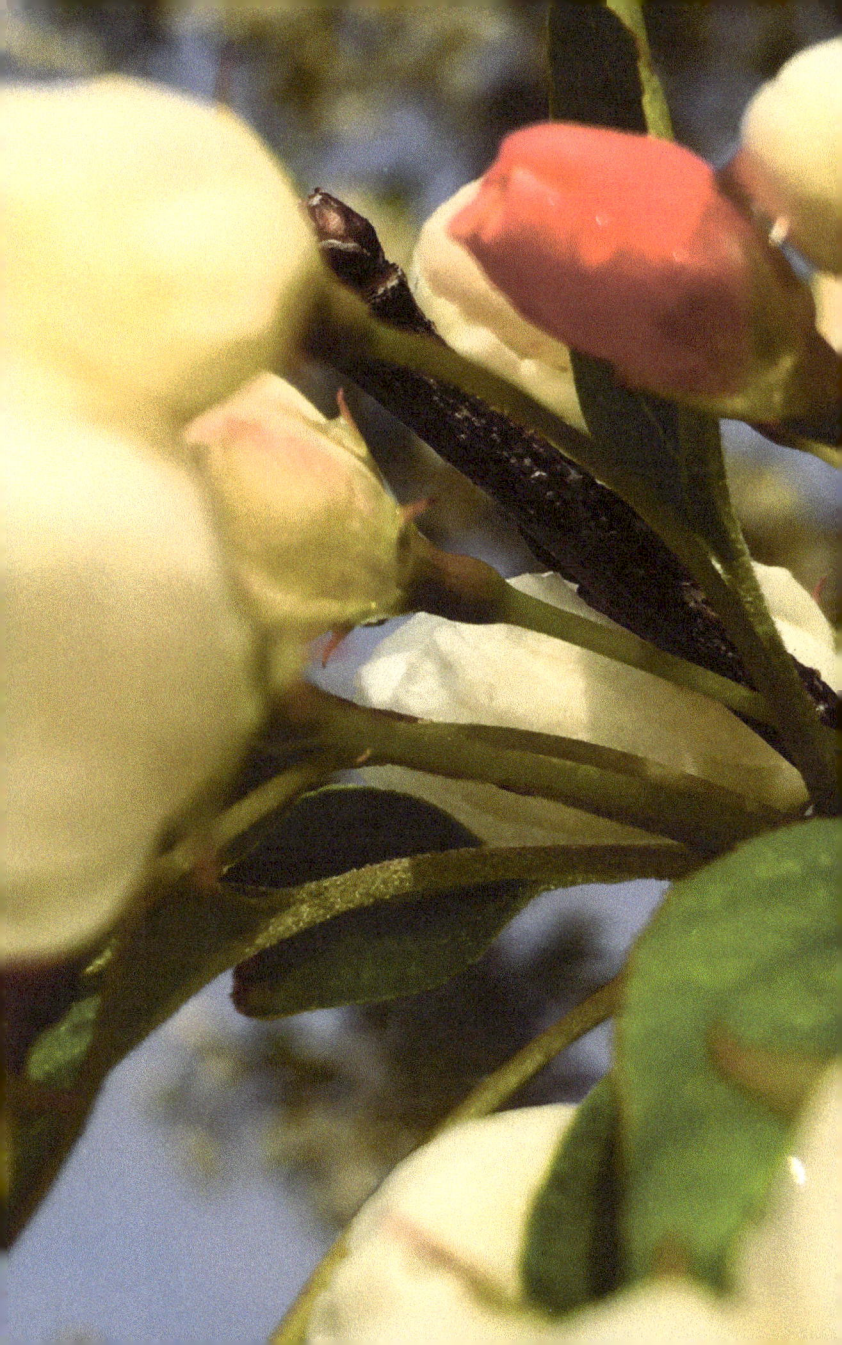

knowingness
21 May
just know

synchronicity
22 May
The meaningful coincidence of a
psychic and a physical state or event which have
no casual relationship to each other.

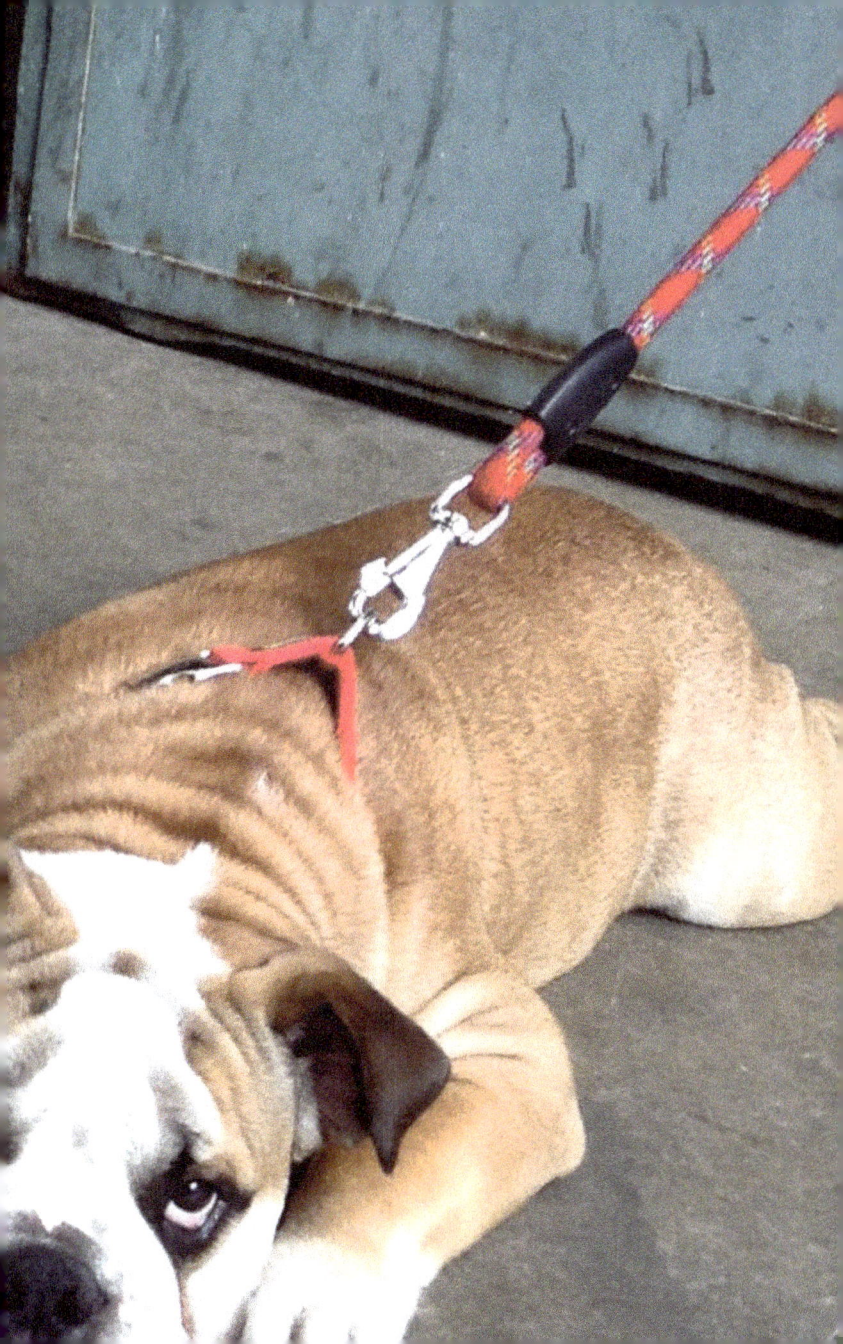

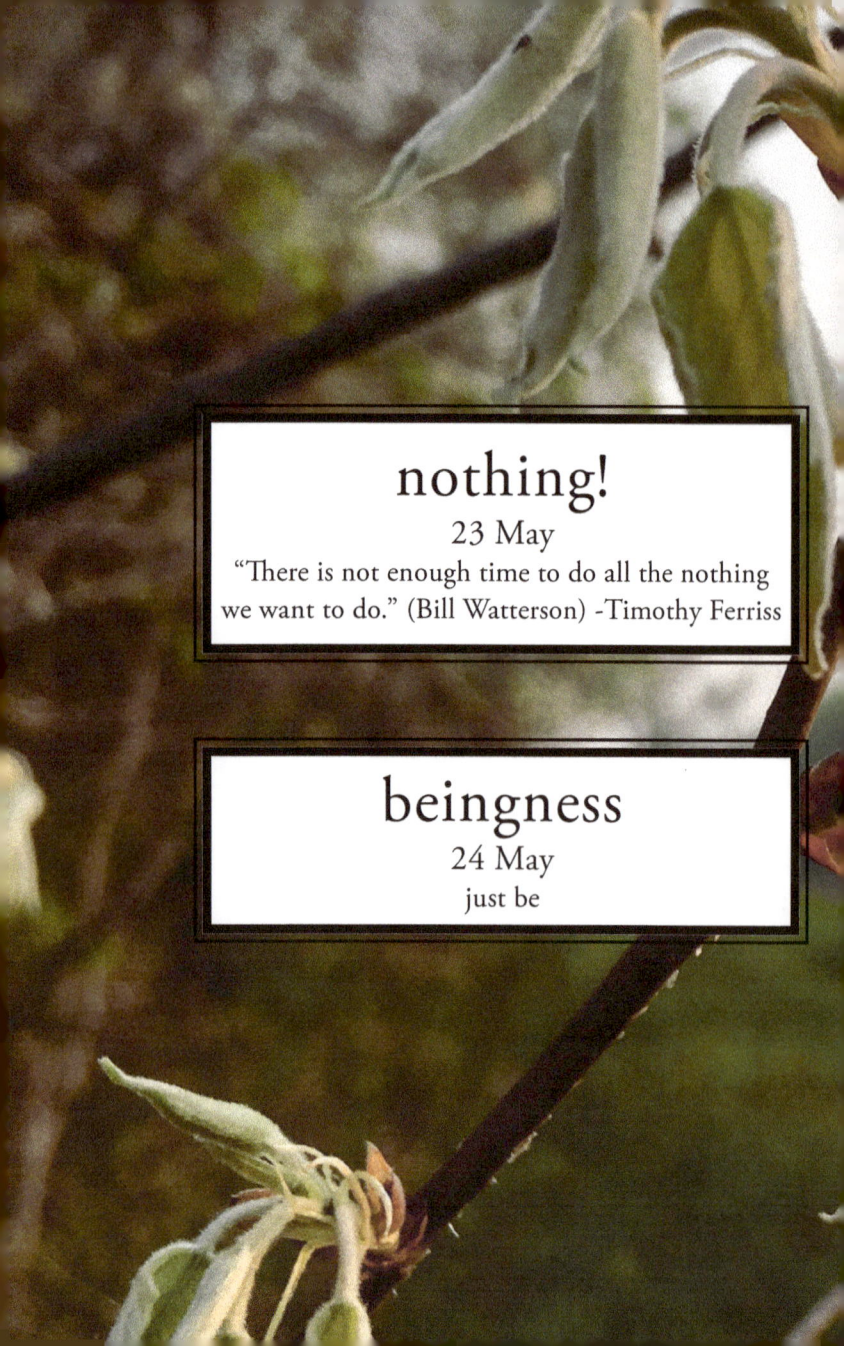

nothing!
23 May
"There is not enough time to do all the nothing we want to do." (Bill Watterson) -Timothy Ferriss

beingness
24 May
just be

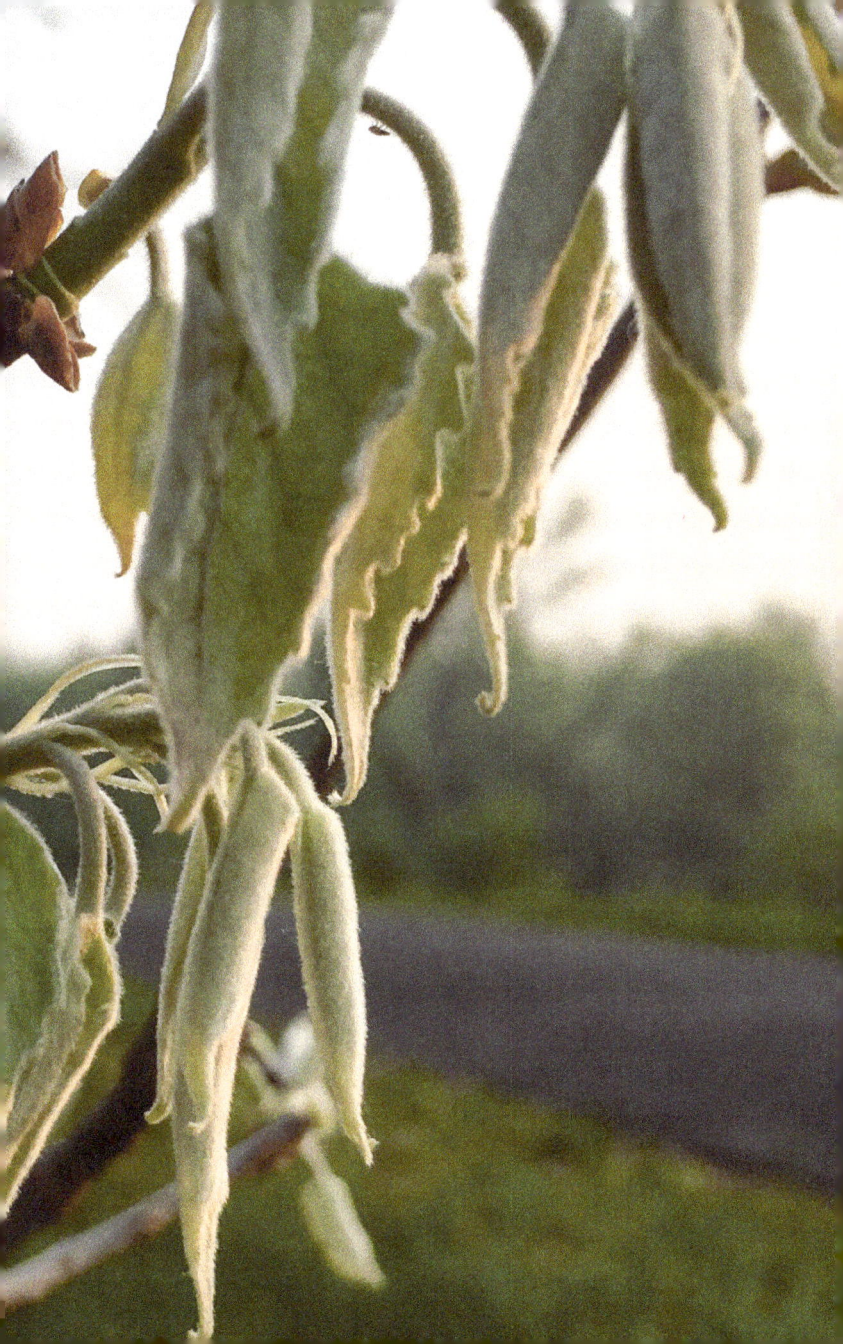

FAT

25 May

"Eat real fat. Fats become useless when they are accompanied by sugar, or when their chemical structure is changed. Chemical processes used in the packaging and processing of food can damage the structure of fat."
-TS Wiley with Bent Forby PhD

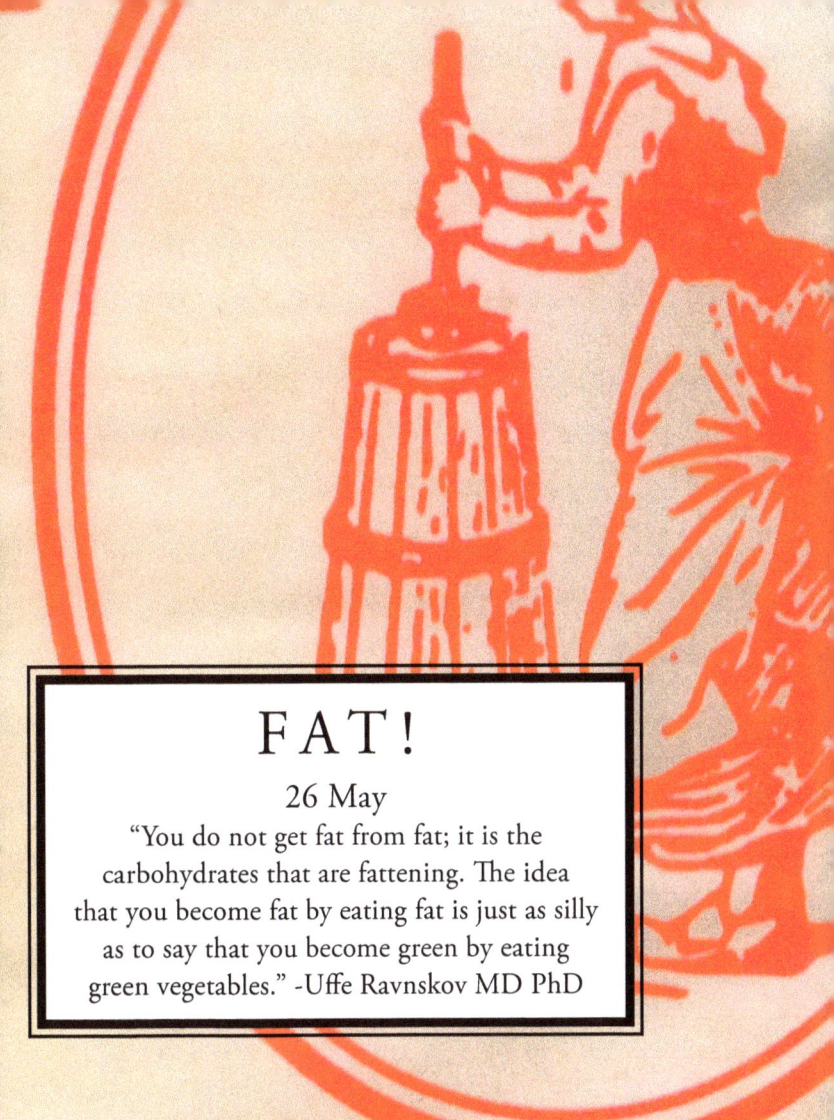

FAT!

26 May

"You do not get fat from fat; it is the carbohydrates that are fattening. The idea that you become fat by eating fat is just as silly as to say that you become green by eating green vegetables." -Uffe Ravnskov MD PhD

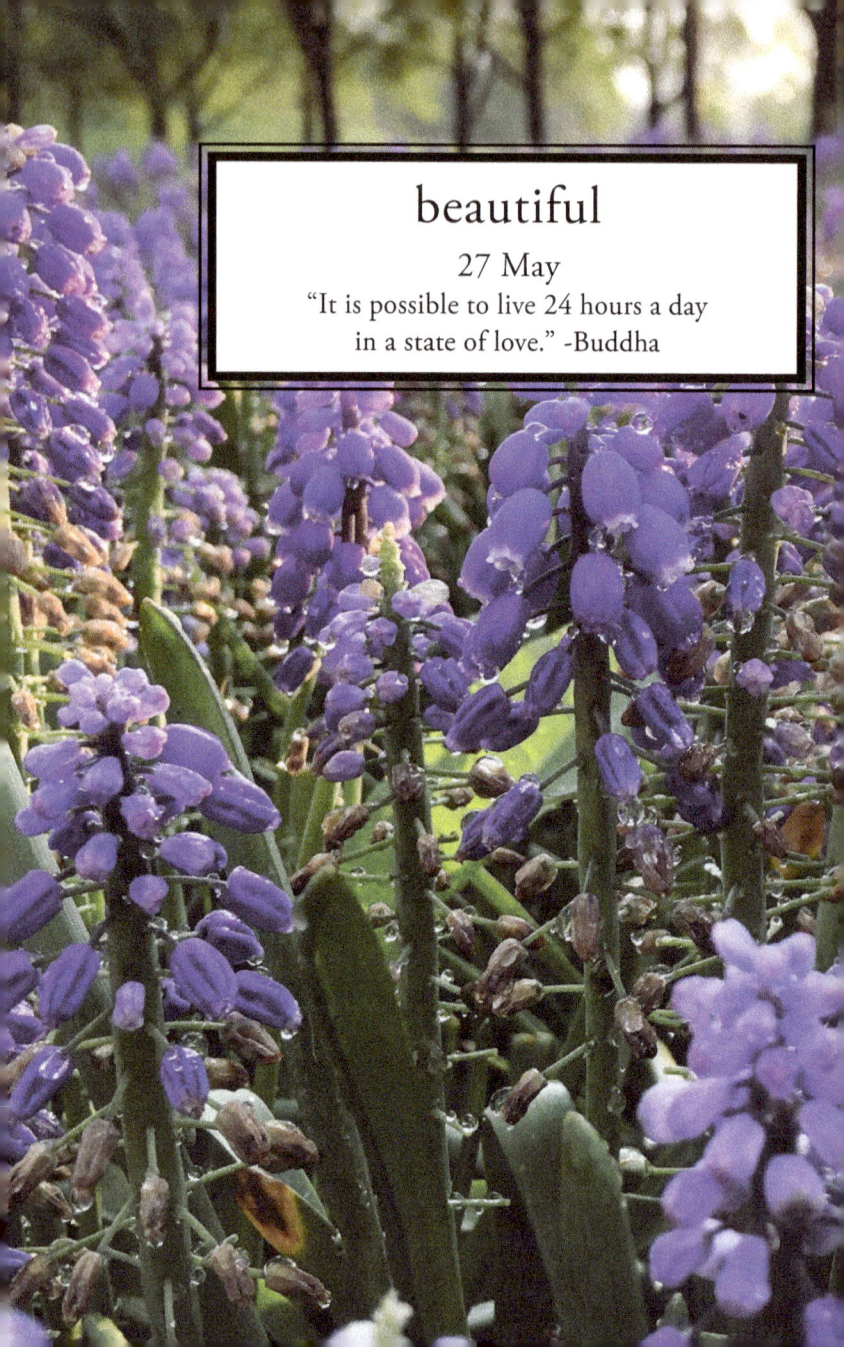

beautiful

27 May
"It is possible to live 24 hours a day in a state of love." -Buddha

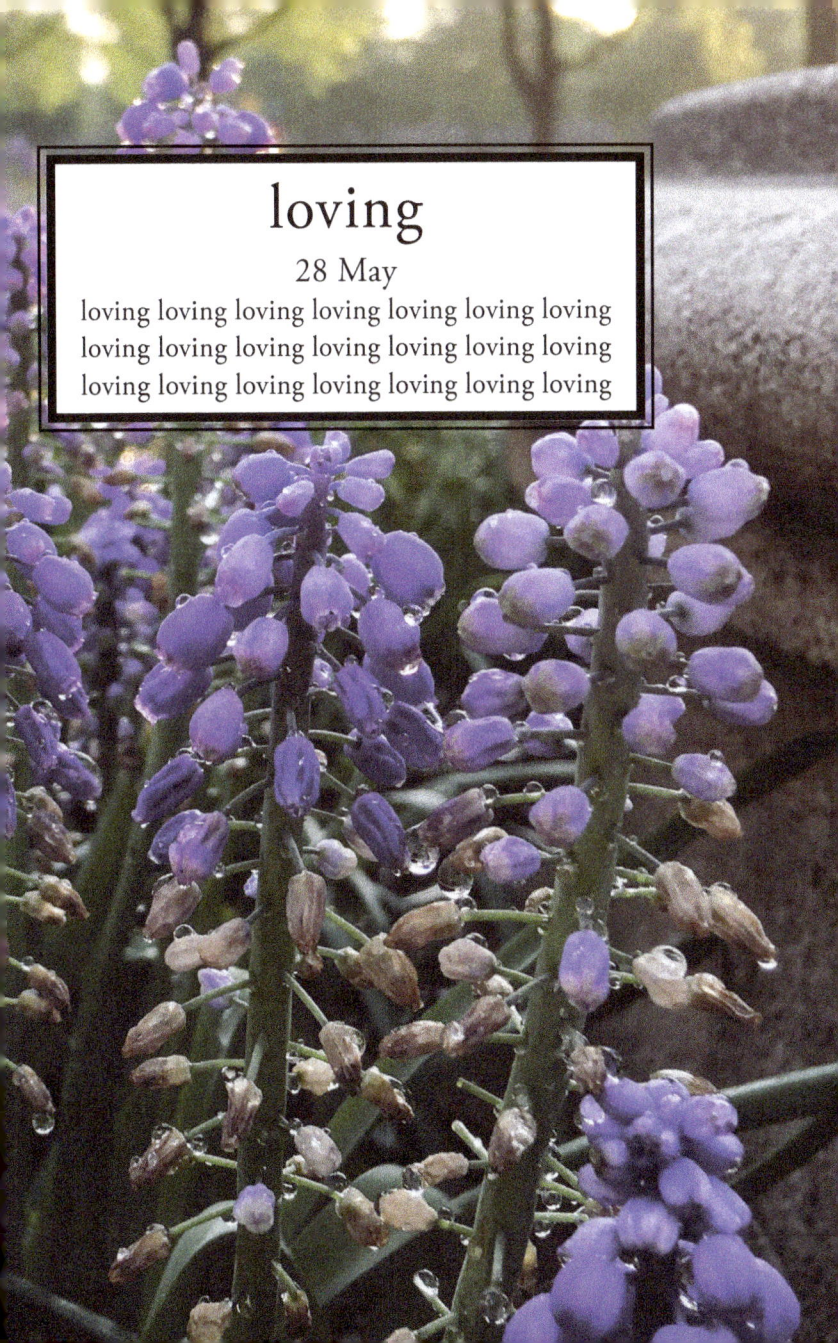

loving

28 May

loving loving loving loving loving loving loving
loving loving loving loving loving loving loving
loving loving loving loving loving loving loving

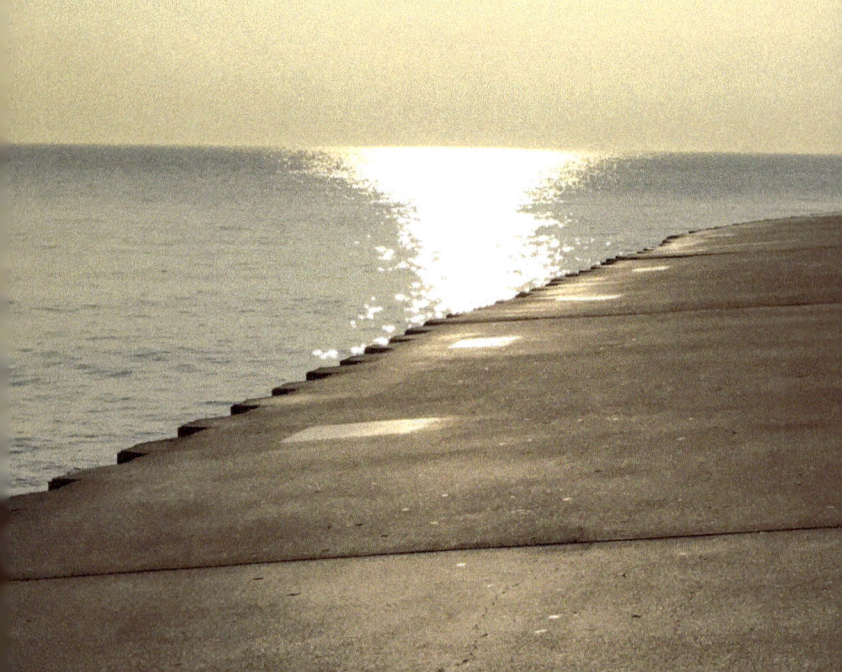

all things possible
29 May
"'All things are possible' leaves out nothing."
-Wayne Dyer

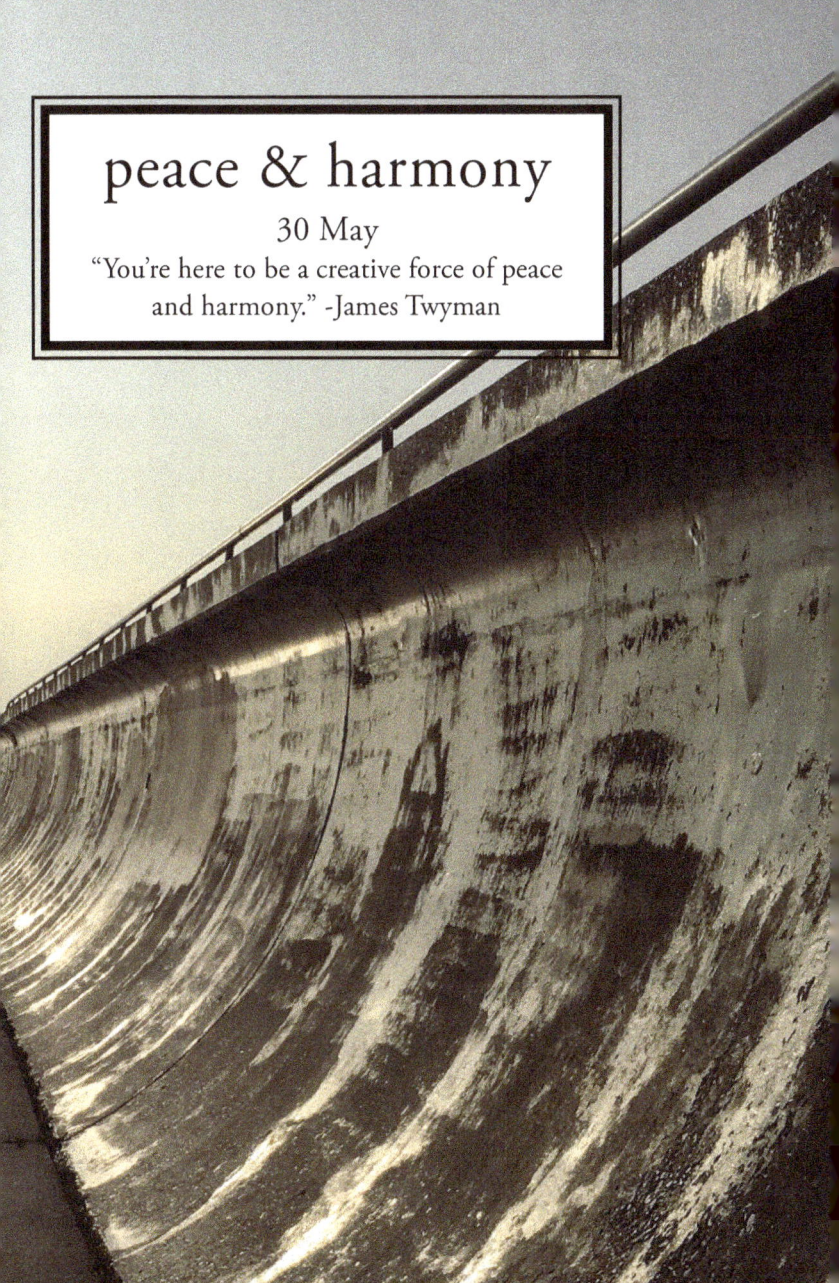

peace & harmony

30 May
"You're here to be a creative force of peace and harmony." -James Twyman

the l o v e

31 May
"Go where the love takes you every day."
-Martha Beck

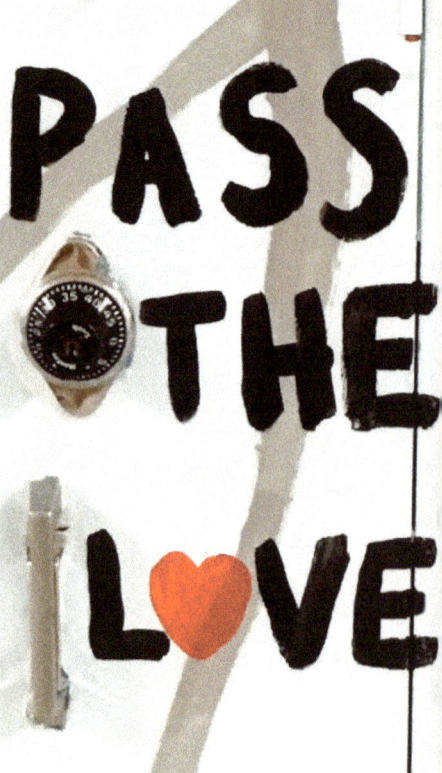

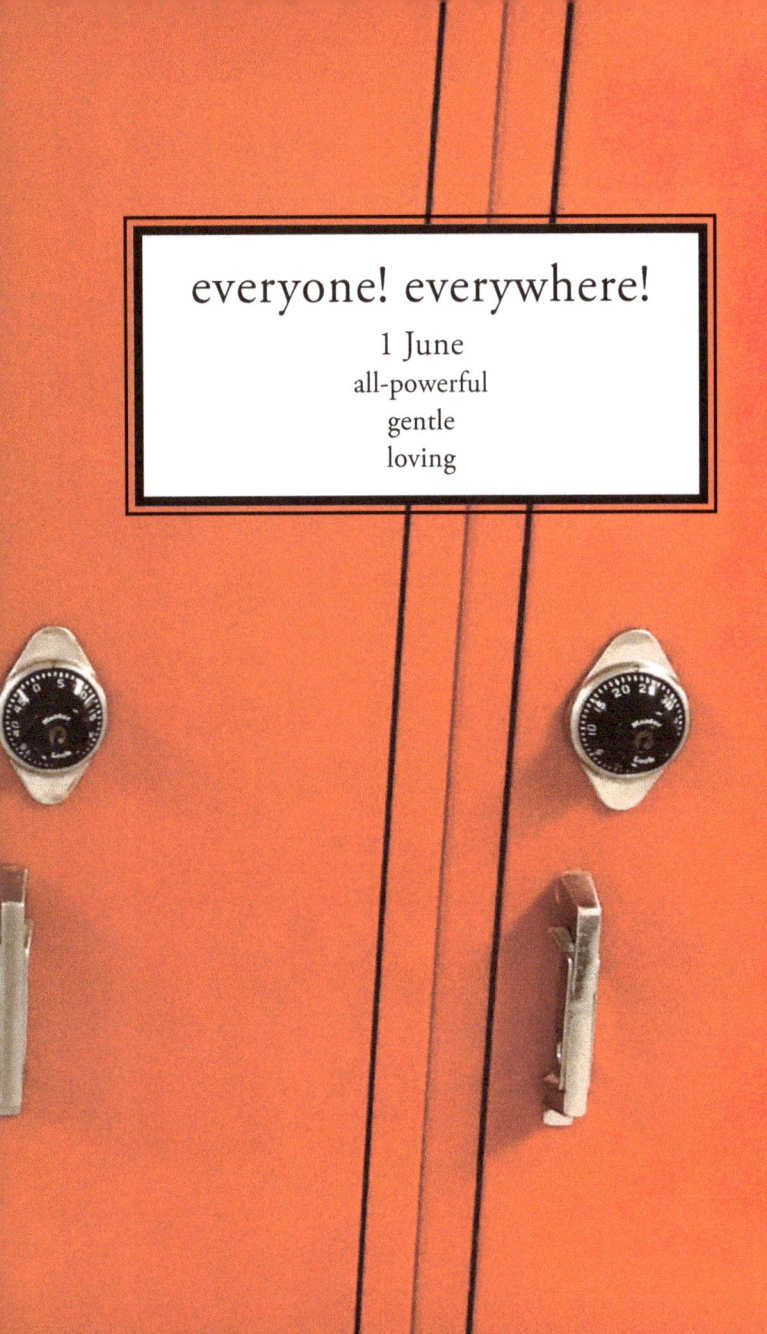

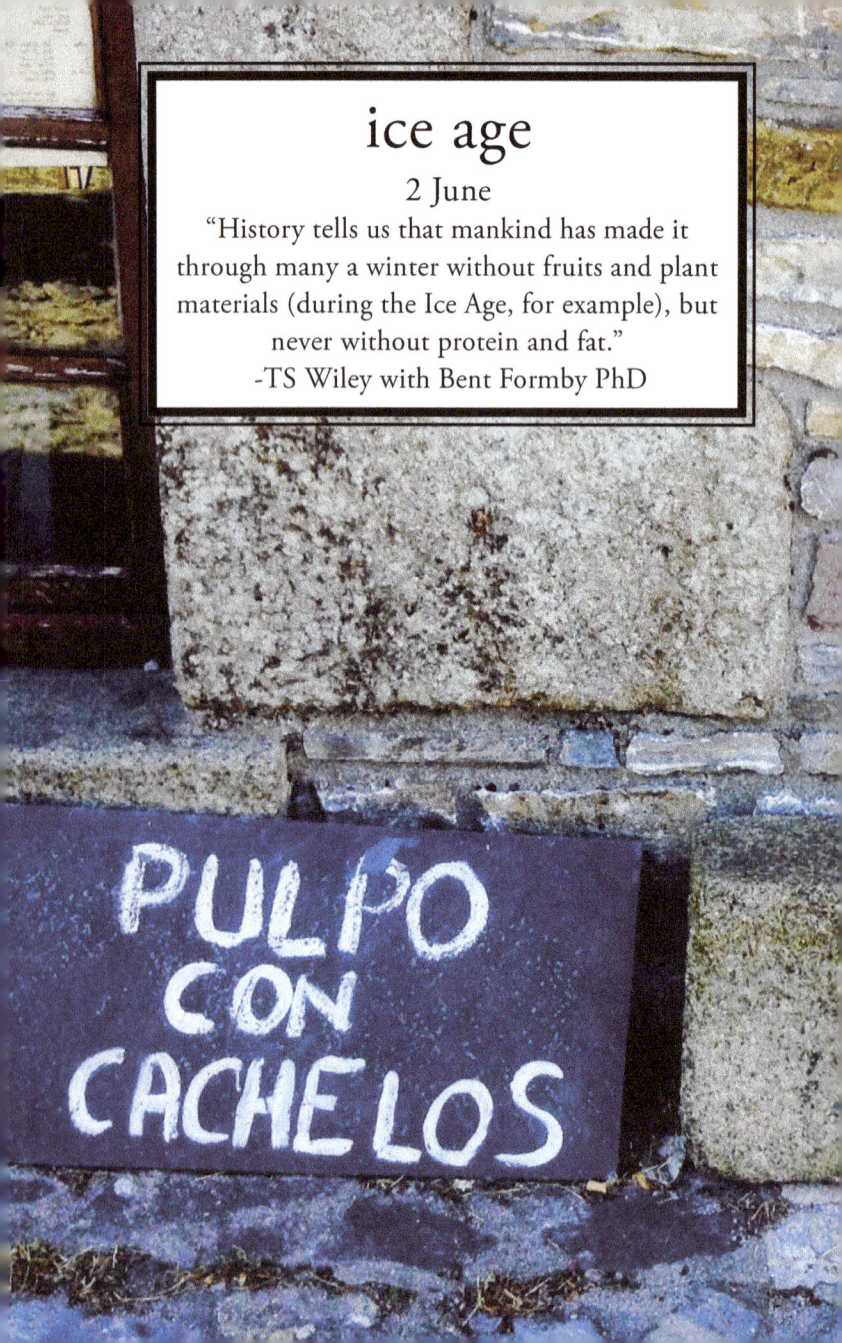

ice age

2 June

"History tells us that mankind has made it through many a winter without fruits and plant materials (during the Ice Age, for example), but never without protein and fat."
-TS Wiley with Bent Formby PhD

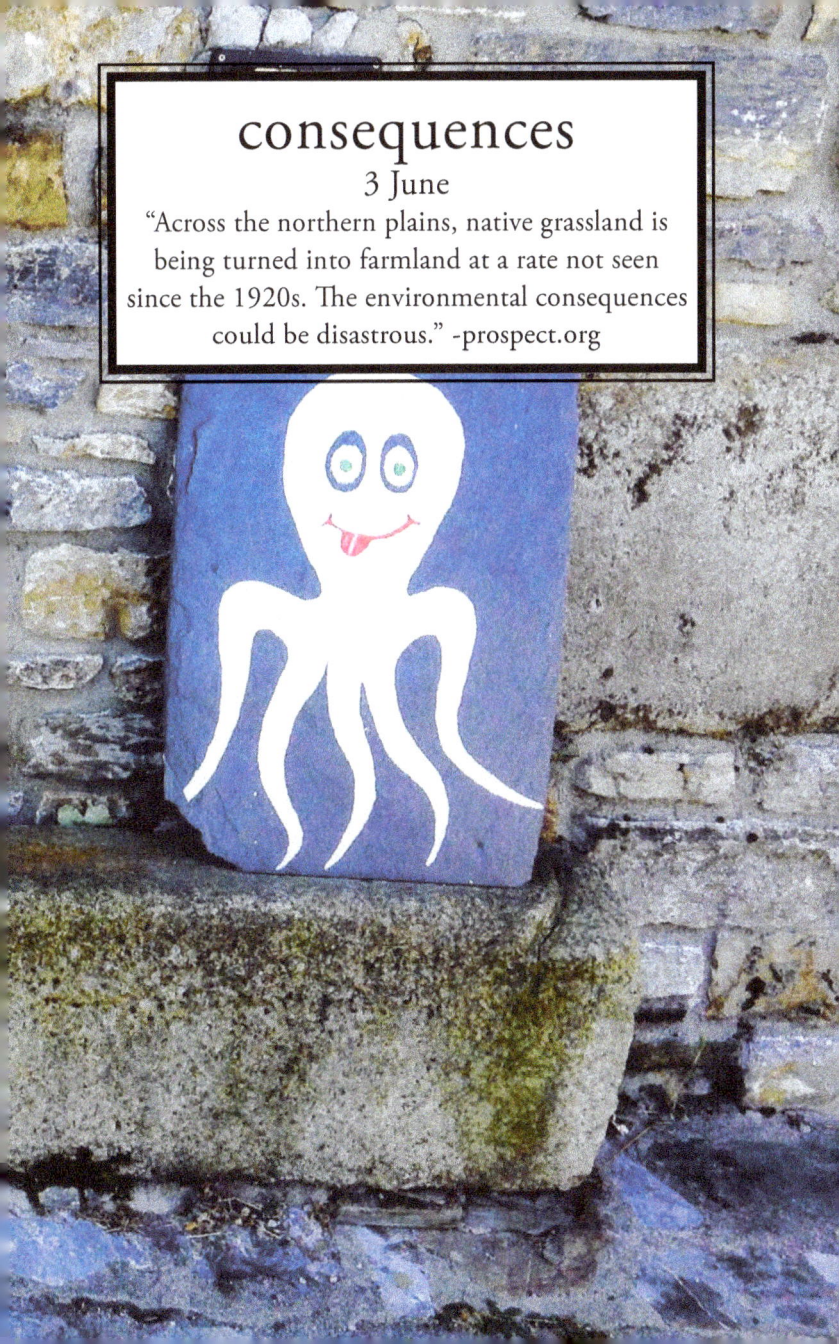

consequences
3 June
"Across the northern plains, native grassland is being turned into farmland at a rate not seen since the 1920s. The environmental consequences could be disastrous." -prospect.org

shine

4 June

"I have questioned my thinking, and I've discovered that it doesn't mean a thing. I shine internally with the joy of understanding...when there's no story, no past or future, nothing to worry about, nothing to do, nowhere to go, no one to be, it's all good." -Byron Katie

say it again

5 June

"There's no actual stress or anxiety in the world; it's your thoughts that create these false beliefs. You can't package stress, touch it, or see it. There are only people engaged in stressful thinking."
-Wayne Dyer

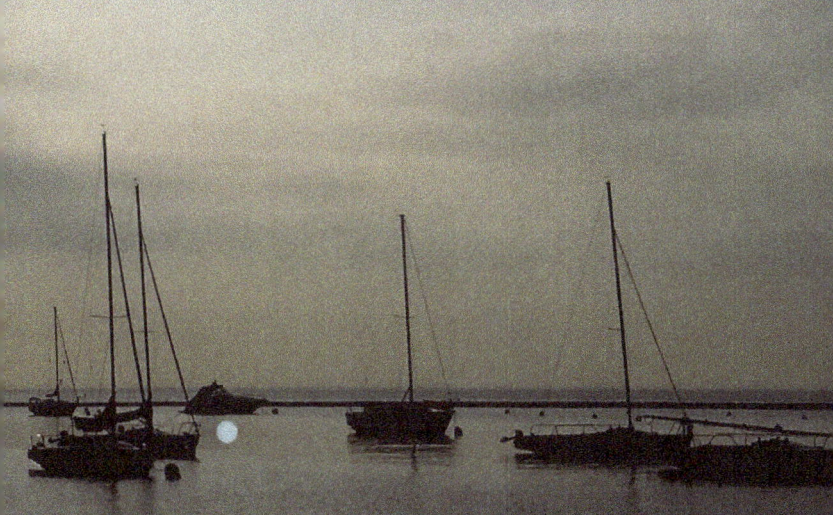

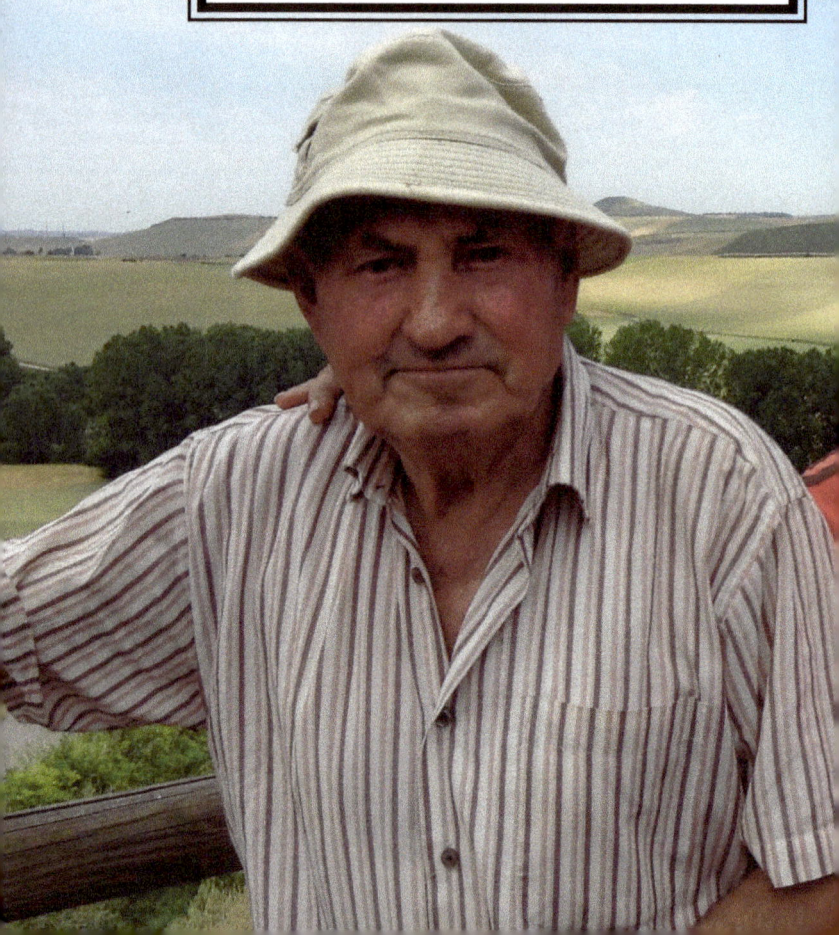

calling all angels!

6 June
Calling all angels! Please help!
For the good of all concerned!
Thank you so much!
Love, Laura (Jean Slatter)

to the Y chromosome, with love

7 June

To the Y chromosome, How do I love thee? Let me count the ways. Strong, decisive, courageous, powerful, funny, fun! With love, Laura (Deepak Chopra)

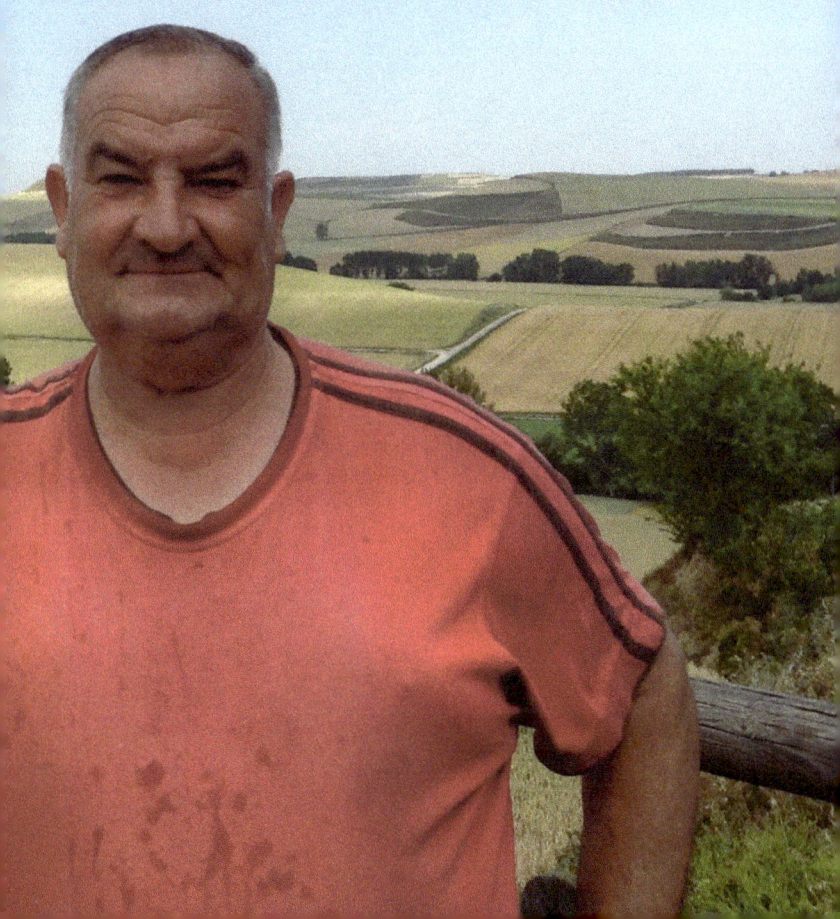

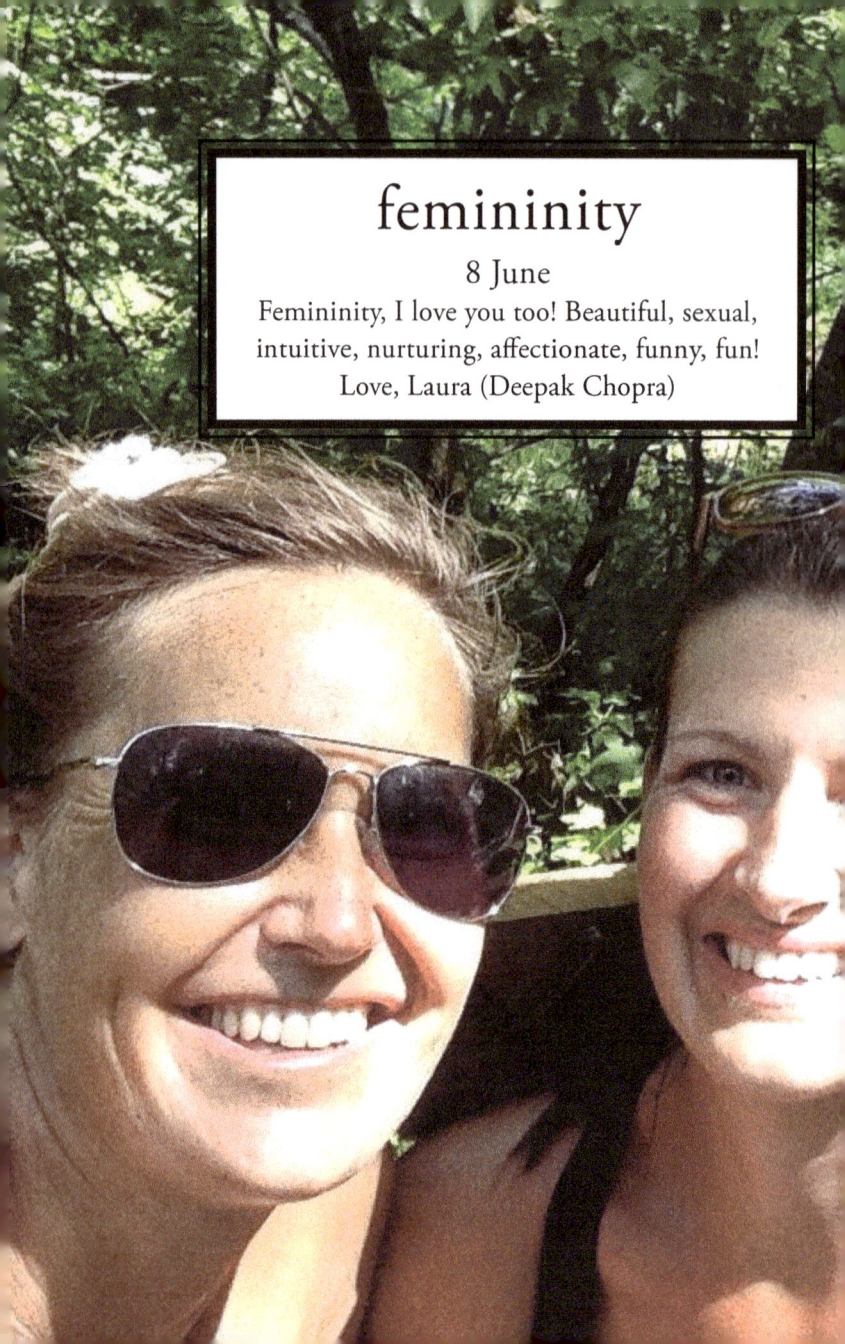

femininity

8 June

Femininity, I love you too! Beautiful, sexual, intuitive, nurturing, affectionate, funny, fun! Love, Laura (Deepak Chopra)

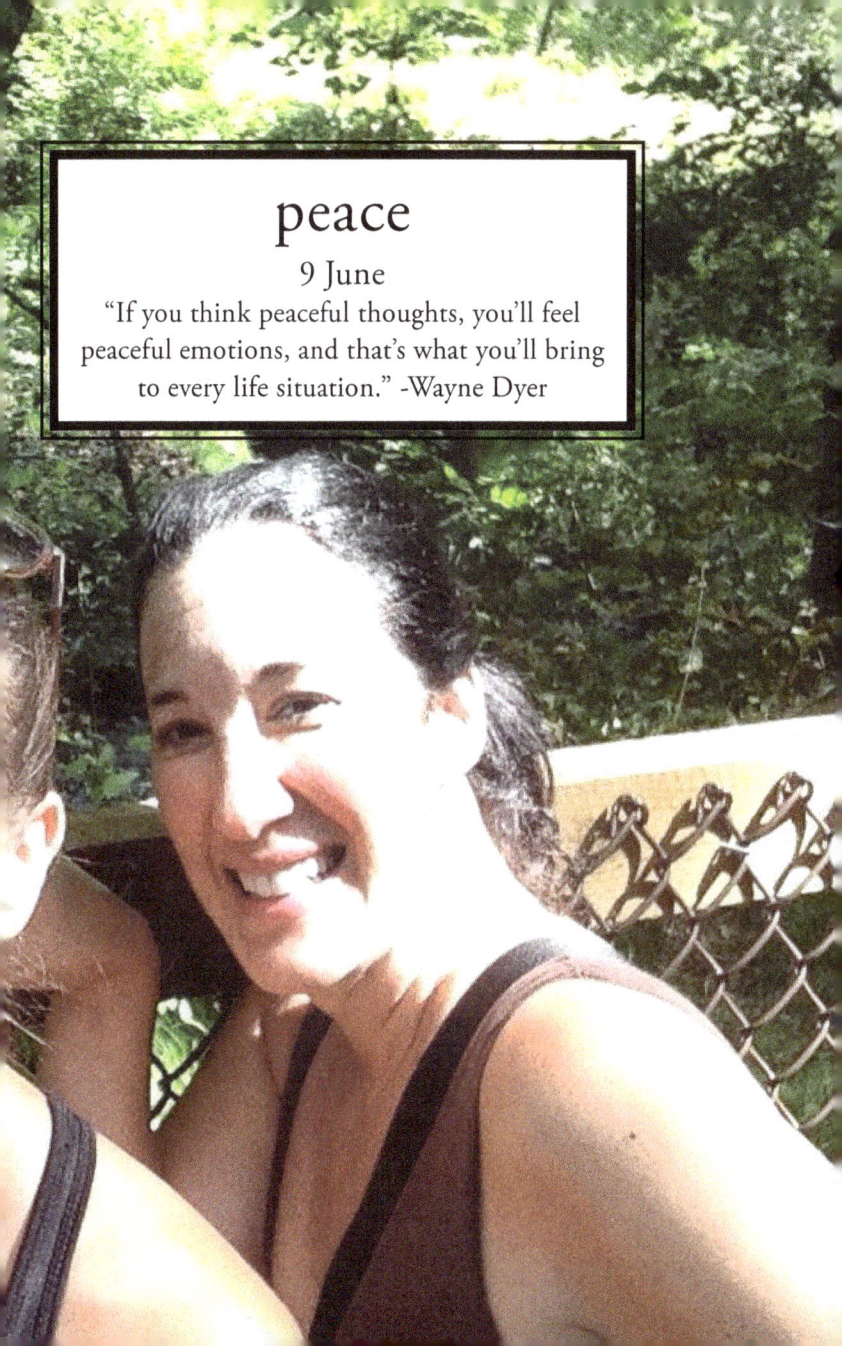

peace

9 June

"If you think peaceful thoughts, you'll feel peaceful emotions, and that's what you'll bring to every life situation." -Wayne Dyer

fermented foods

10 June

"It makes sense that fermented foods might improve digestive health...filled with 'friendly' bacteria...because the gut is the largest component of your immune system, introducing friendly bacteria into your digestive system may also help keep illness away. Evidence suggests that gut health could affect inflammation, allergies and autoimmune disorders." -Tufts University

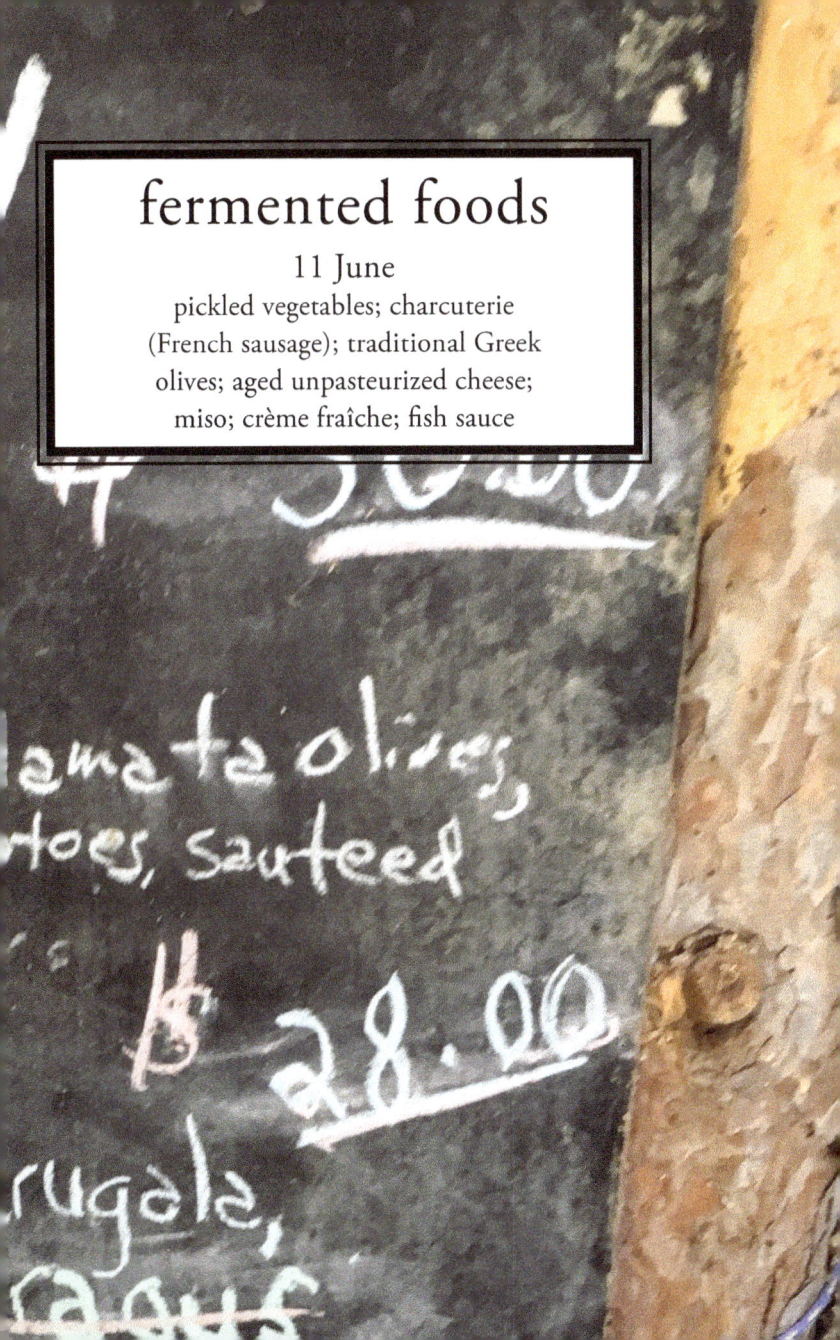

fermented foods

11 June
pickled vegetables; charcuterie (French sausage); traditional Greek olives; aged unpasteurized cheese; miso; crème fraîche; fish sauce

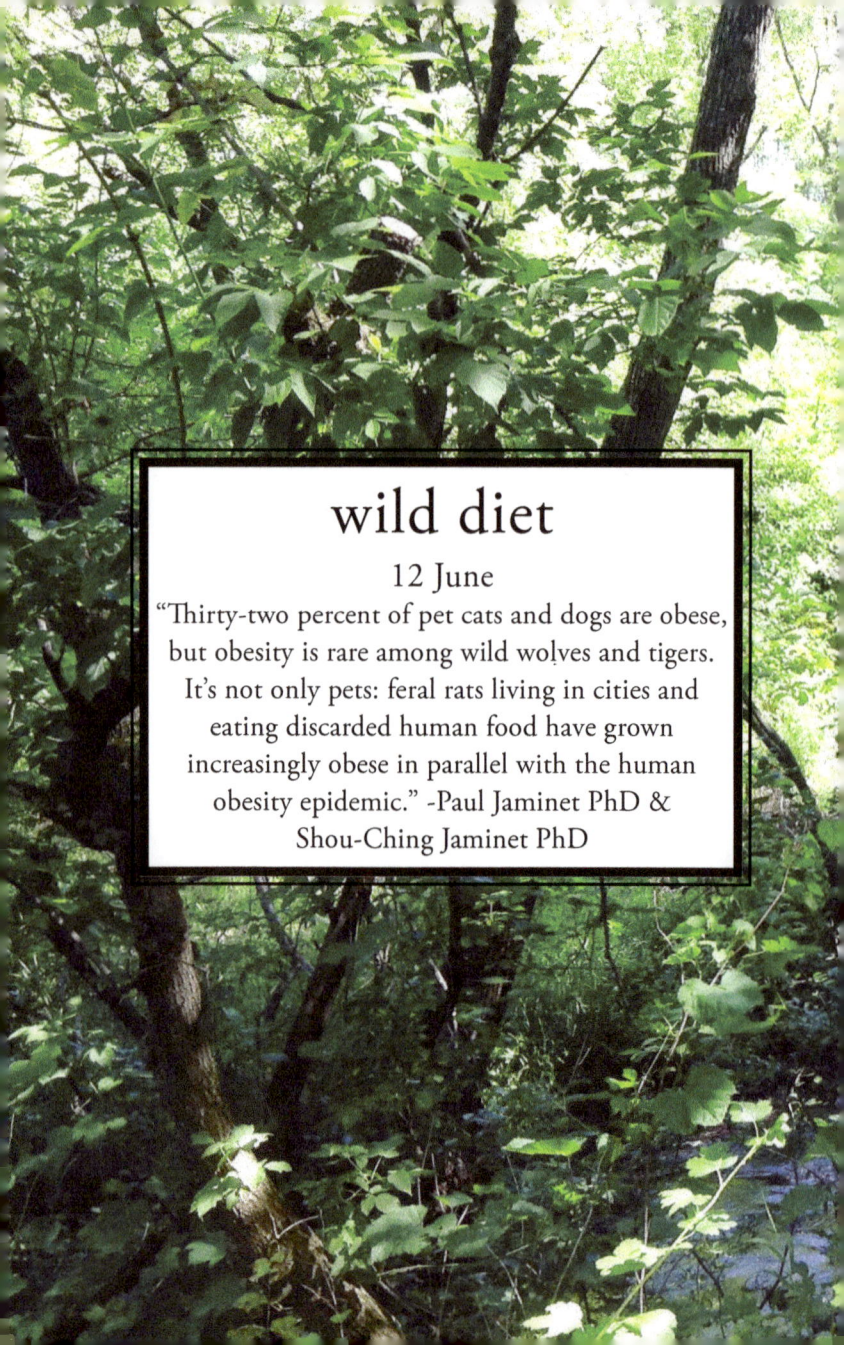

wild diet

12 June

"Thirty-two percent of pet cats and dogs are obese, but obesity is rare among wild wolves and tigers. It's not only pets: feral rats living in cities and eating discarded human food have grown increasingly obese in parallel with the human obesity epidemic." -Paul Jaminet PhD & Shou-Ching Jaminet PhD

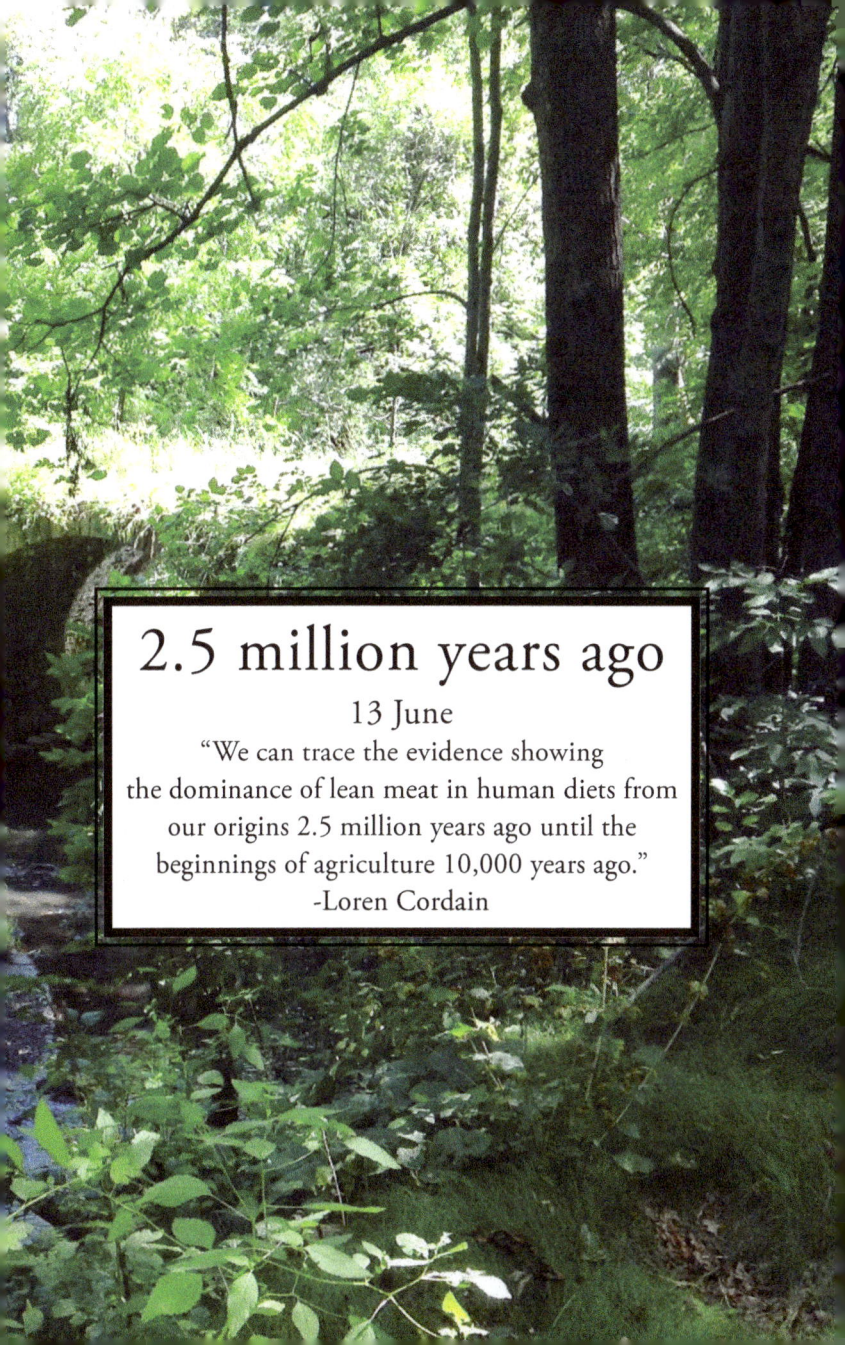

2.5 million years ago

13 June

"We can trace the evidence showing the dominance of lean meat in human diets from our origins 2.5 million years ago until the beginnings of agriculture 10,000 years ago."
-Loren Cordain

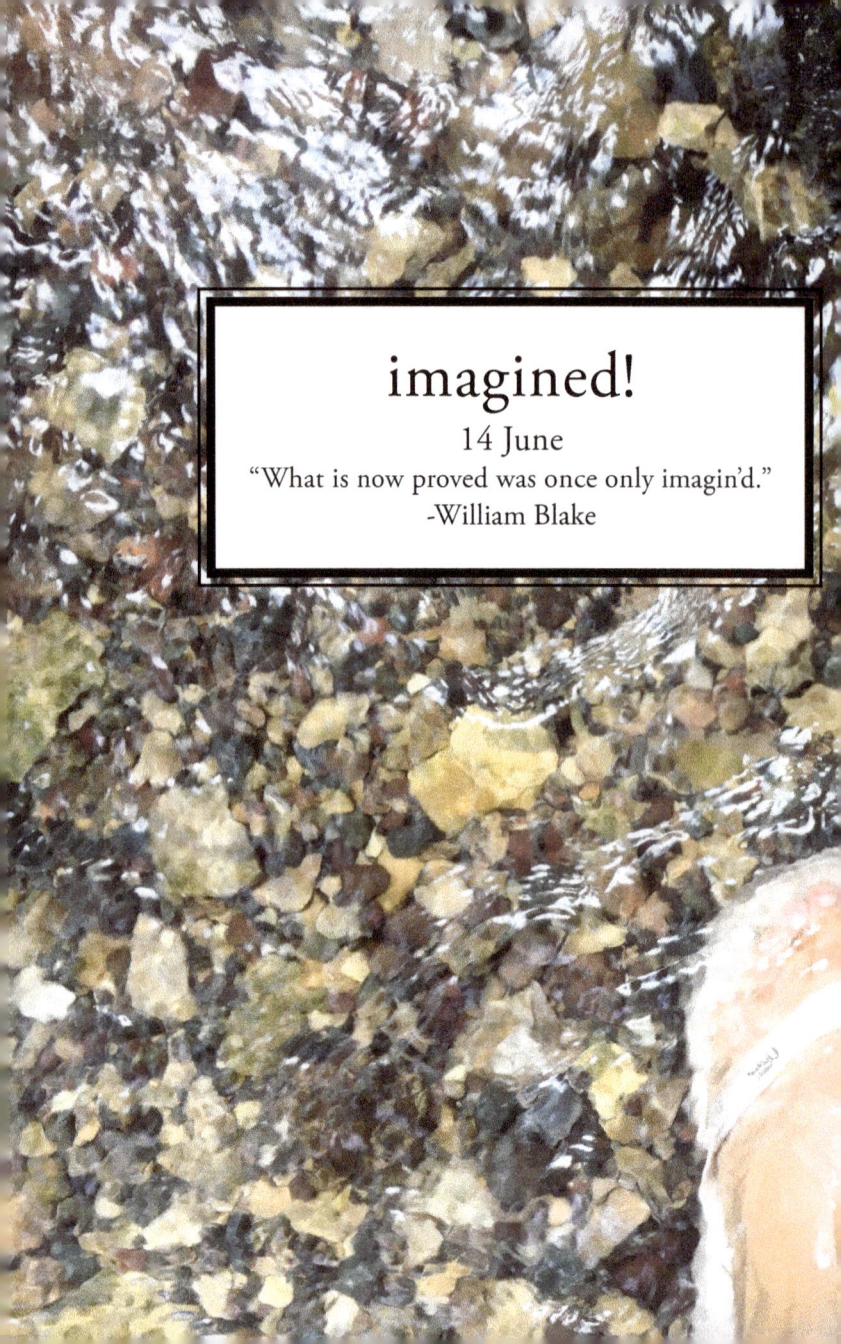

imagined!
14 June
"What is now proved was once only imagin'd."
-William Blake

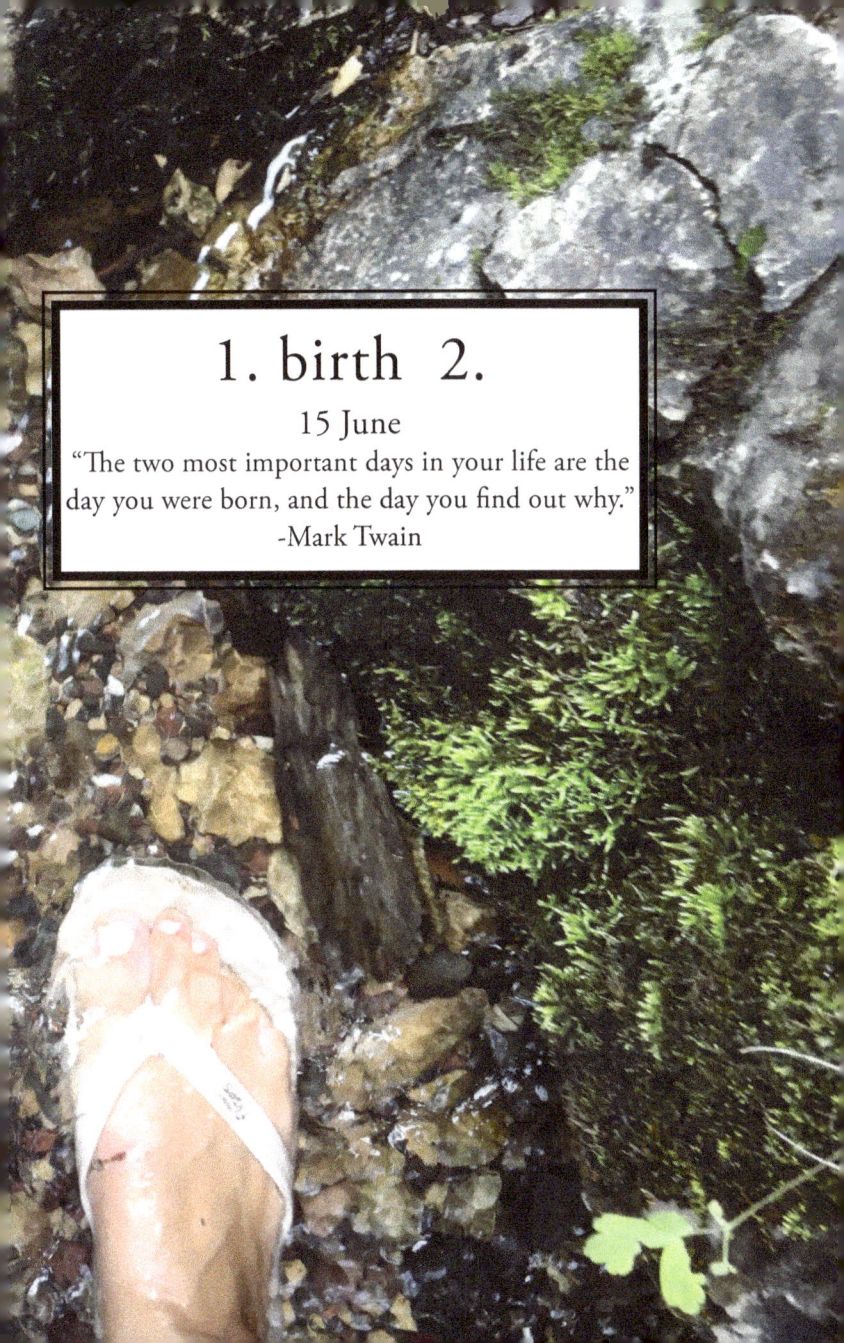

1. birth 2.
15 June
"The two most important days in your life are the day you were born, and the day you find out why."
-Mark Twain

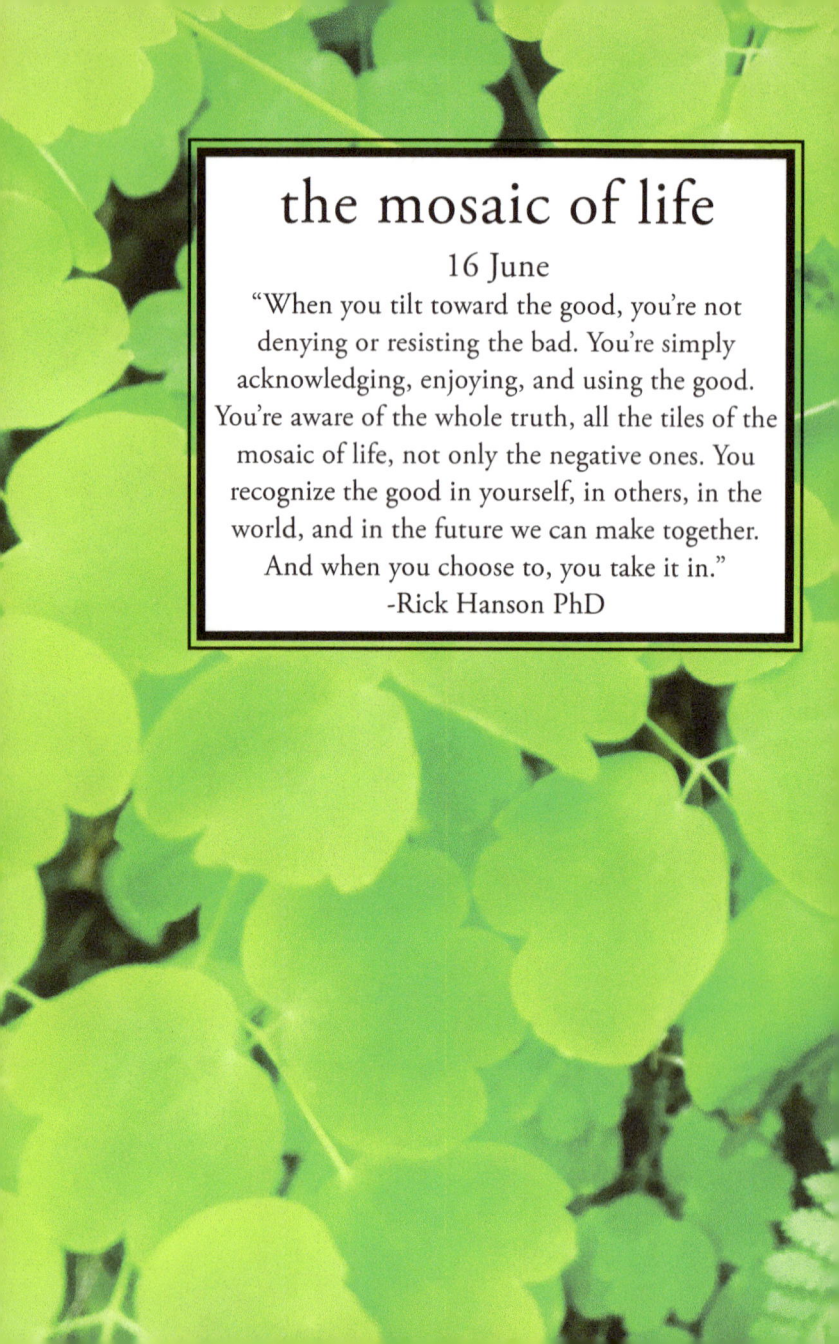

the mosaic of life

16 June

"When you tilt toward the good, you're not denying or resisting the bad. You're simply acknowledging, enjoying, and using the good. You're aware of the whole truth, all the tiles of the mosaic of life, not only the negative ones. You recognize the good in yourself, in others, in the world, and in the future we can make together. And when you choose to, you take it in."
-Rick Hanson PhD

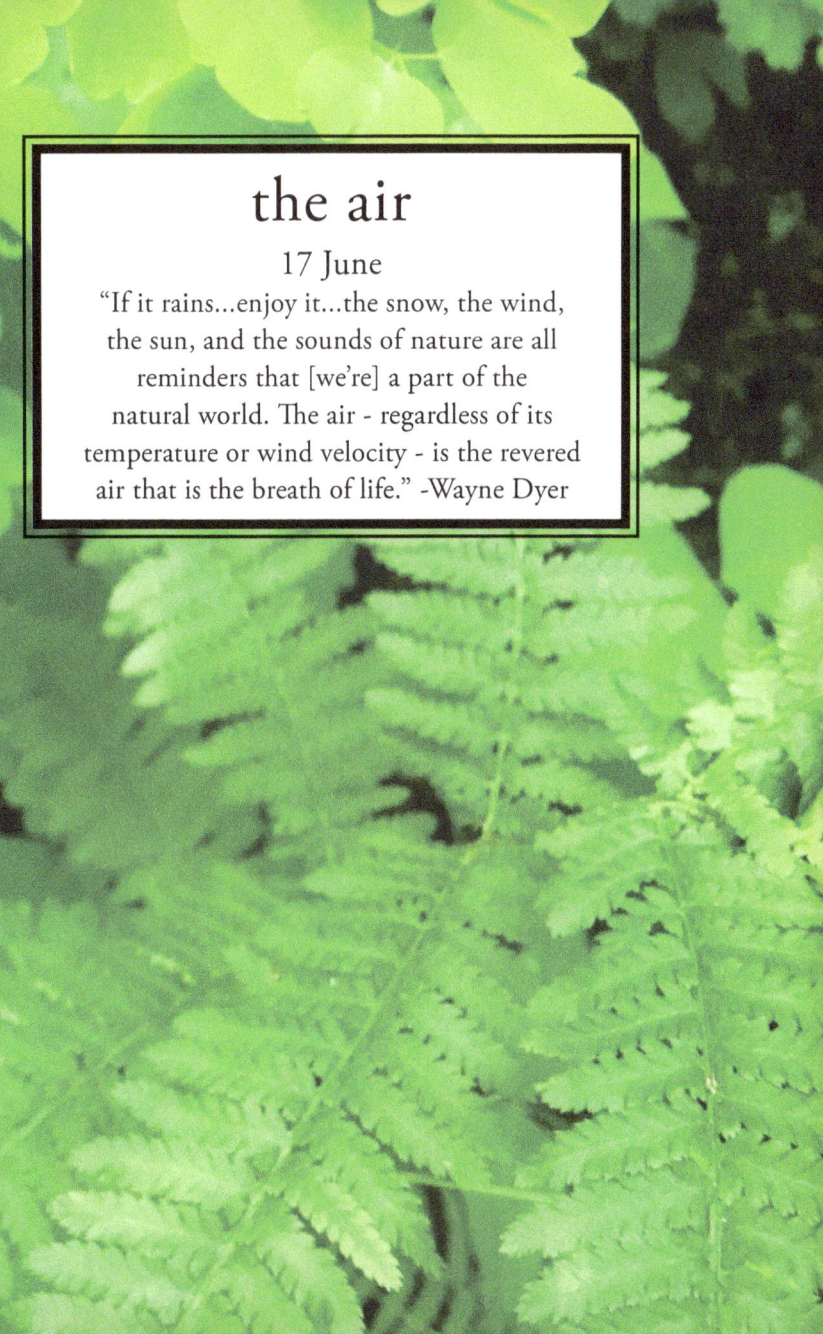

the air

17 June

"If it rains...enjoy it...the snow, the wind, the sun, and the sounds of nature are all reminders that [we're] a part of the natural world. The air - regardless of its temperature or wind velocity - is the revered air that is the breath of life." -Wayne Dyer

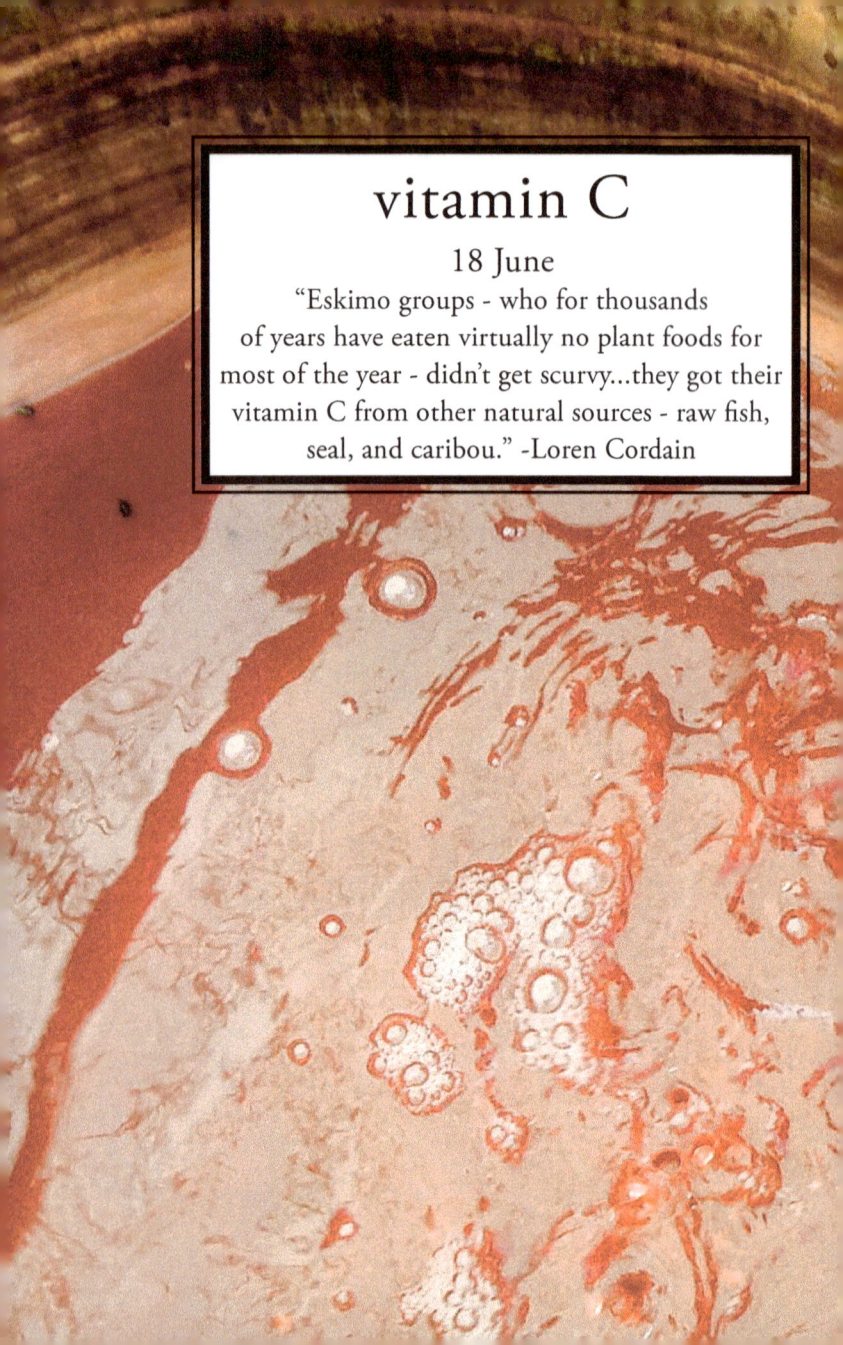

vitamin C

18 June

"Eskimo groups - who for thousands of years have eaten virtually no plant foods for most of the year - didn't get scurvy...they got their vitamin C from other natural sources - raw fish, seal, and caribou." -Loren Cordain

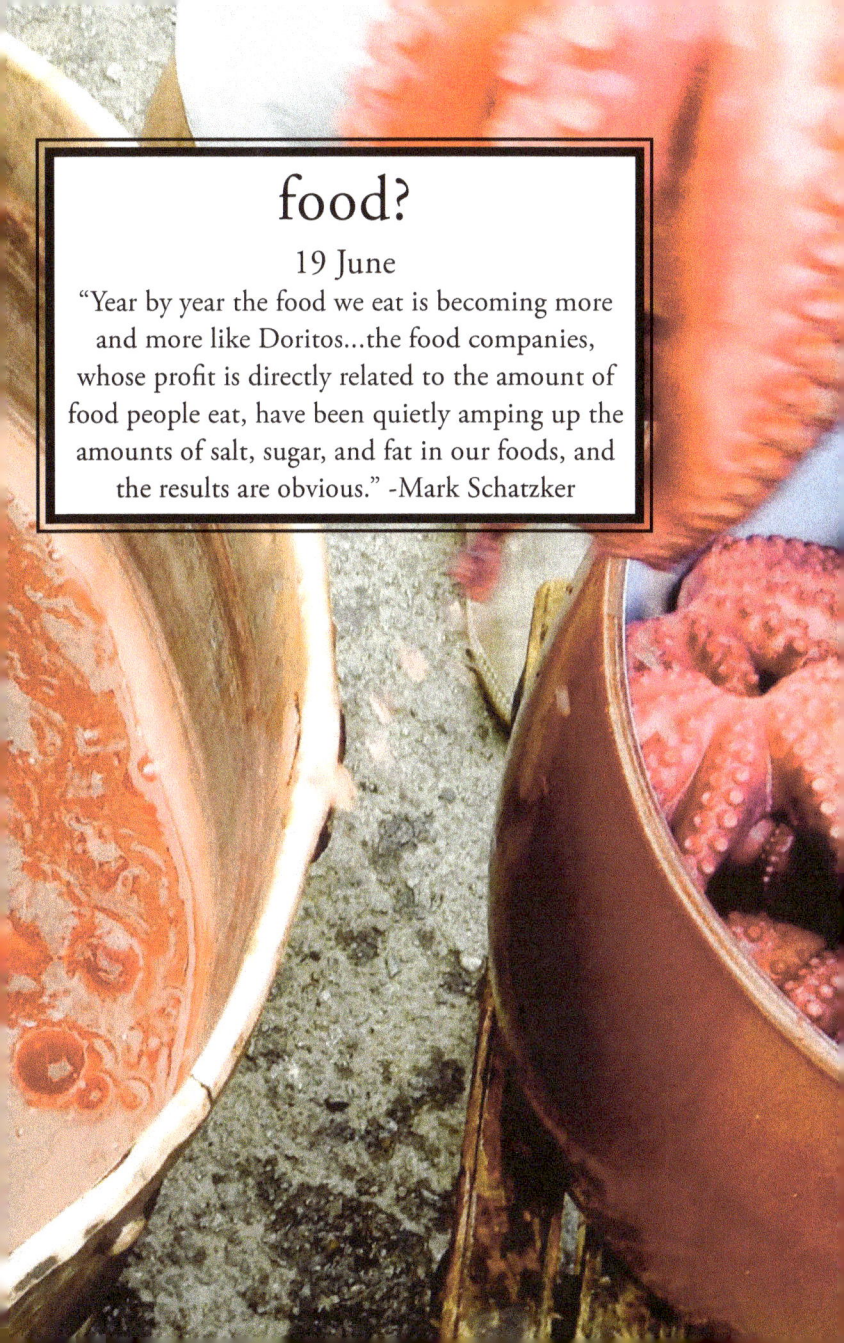

food?
19 June

"Year by year the food we eat is becoming more and more like Doritos...the food companies, whose profit is directly related to the amount of food people eat, have been quietly amping up the amounts of salt, sugar, and fat in our foods, and the results are obvious." -Mark Schatzker

closer

20 June
"Virtuous thoughts bring us happiness. Instead of separating us and making us feel more cut off and afraid, they bring us closer to others."
-Pema Chödrön

creatures!

21 June
"Loving the creator in the creature." -Eckhart Tolle

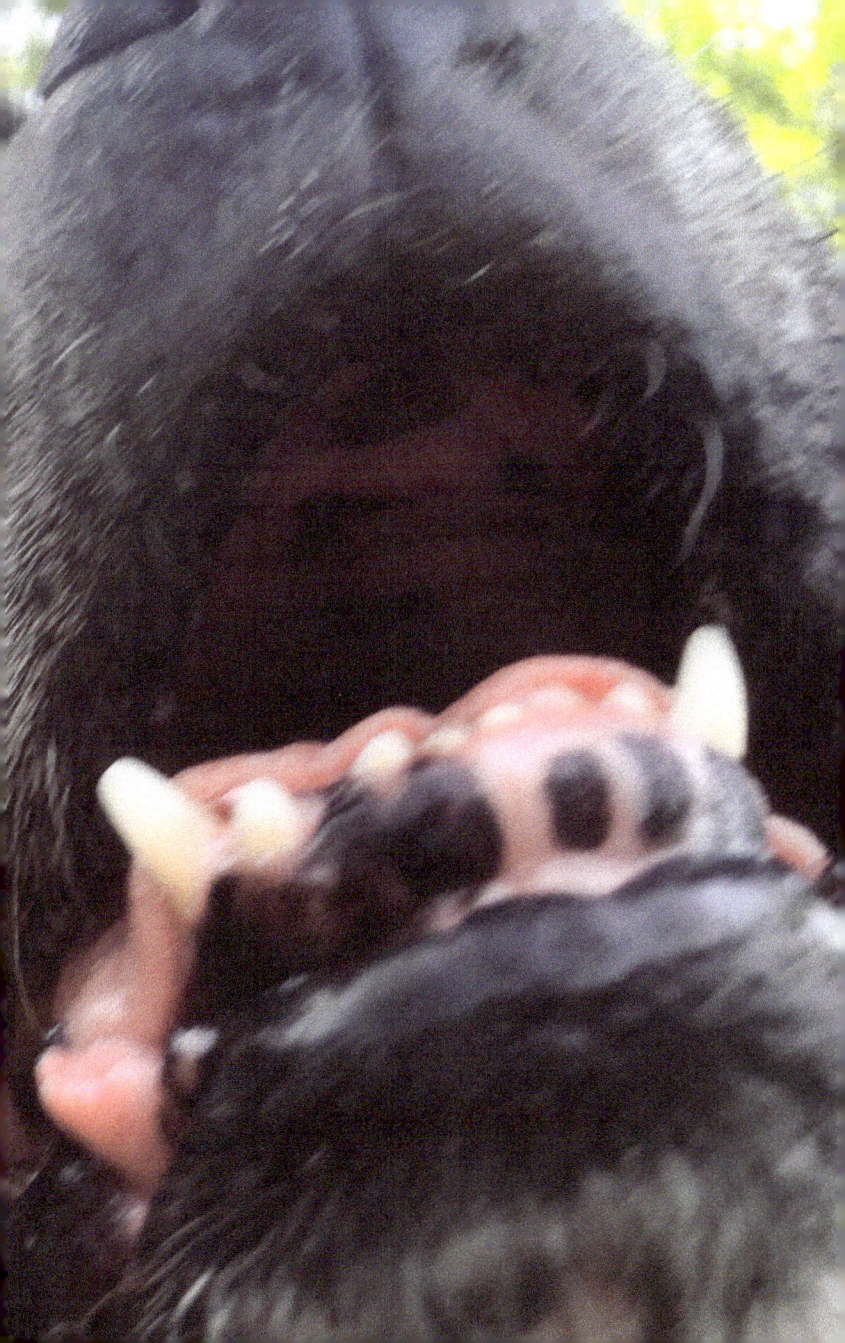

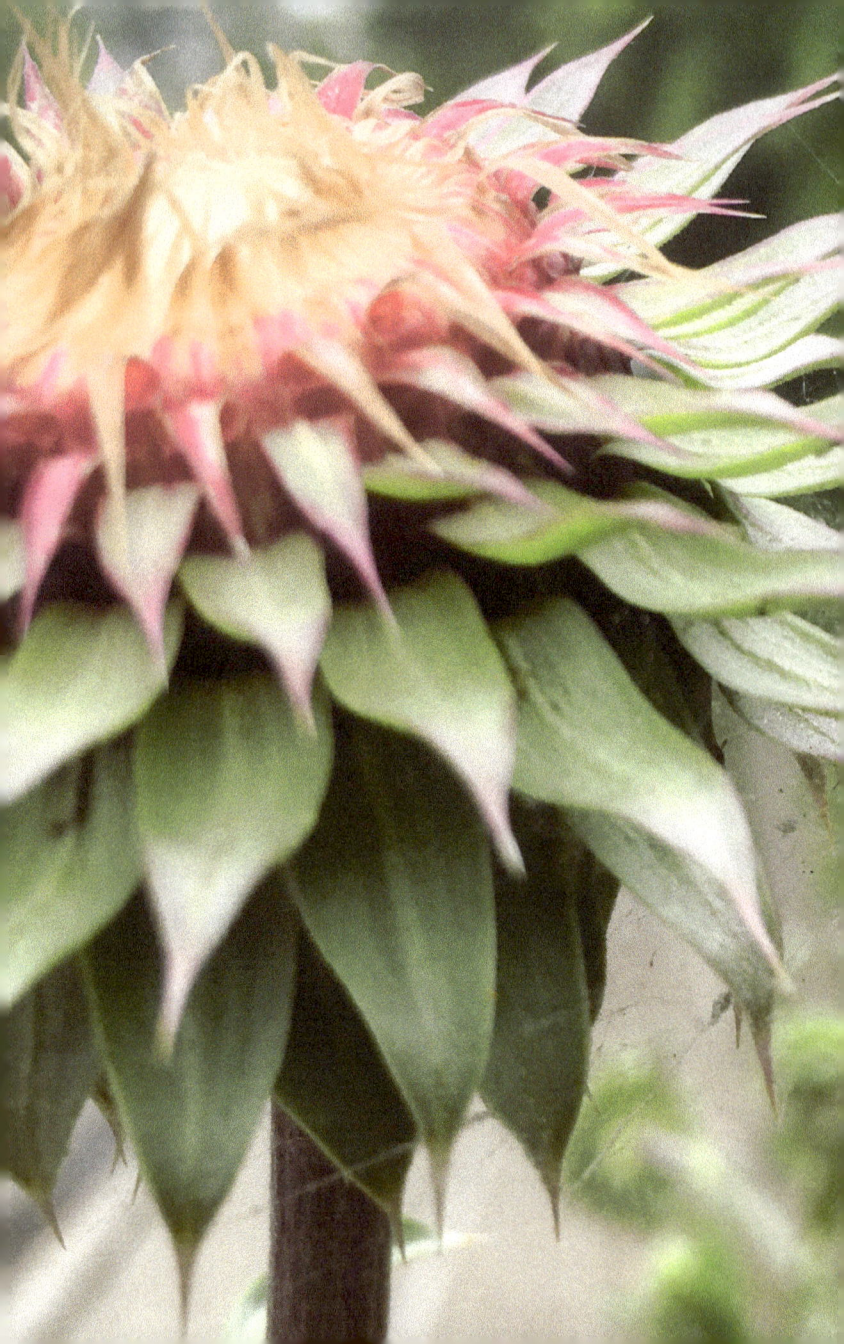

good news!
22 June
"I noticed that things happen with or without me, people approve of me or they don't. It has nothing to do with me. This is really good news, since it leaves me responsible for my own happiness. It leaves me to do nothing but live my life as kindly and intelligently as I can." -Byron Katie

anything you want!
23 June
"The real point of doing anything is to be happy, so do only what makes you happy." -Derek Sivers

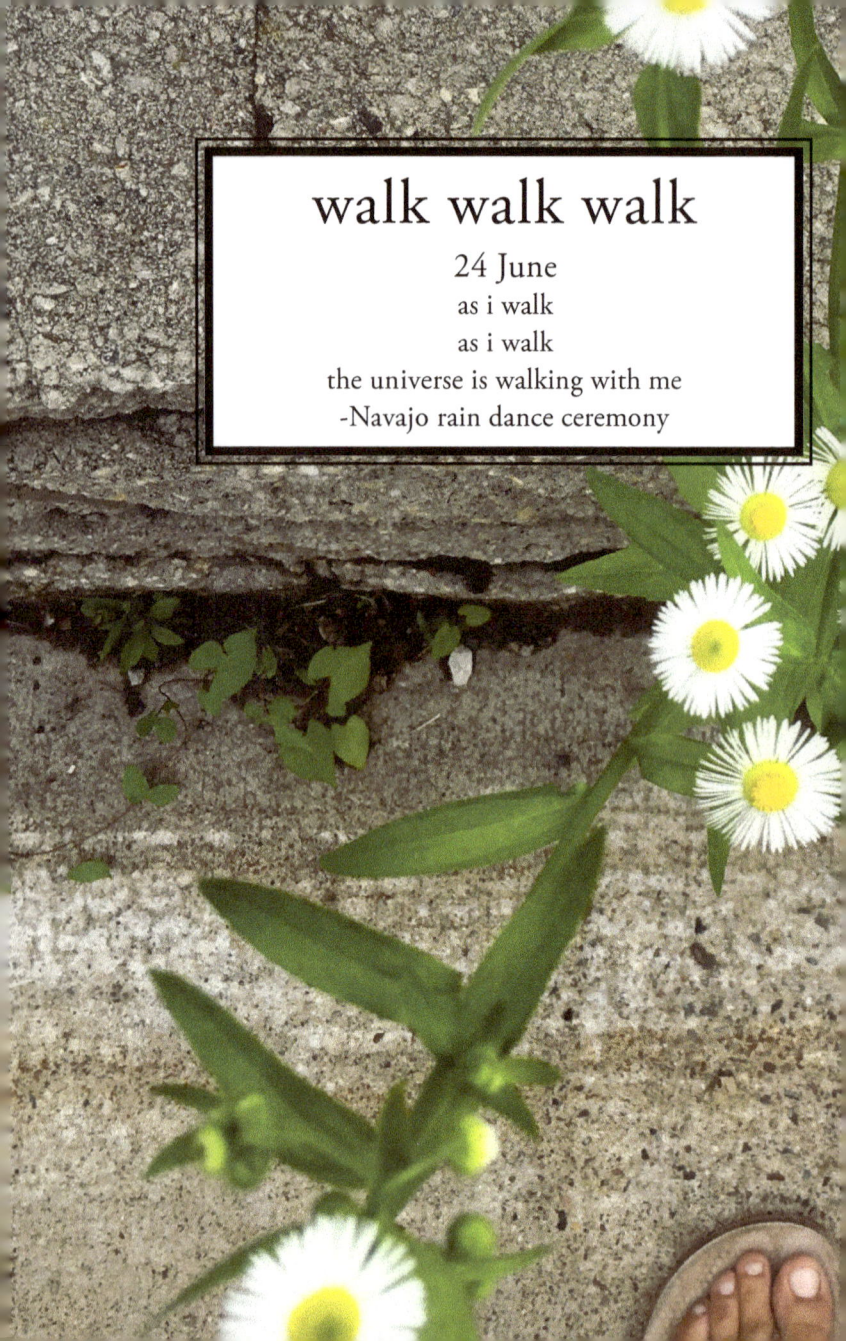

walk walk walk

24 June
as i walk
as i walk
the universe is walking with me
-Navajo rain dance ceremony

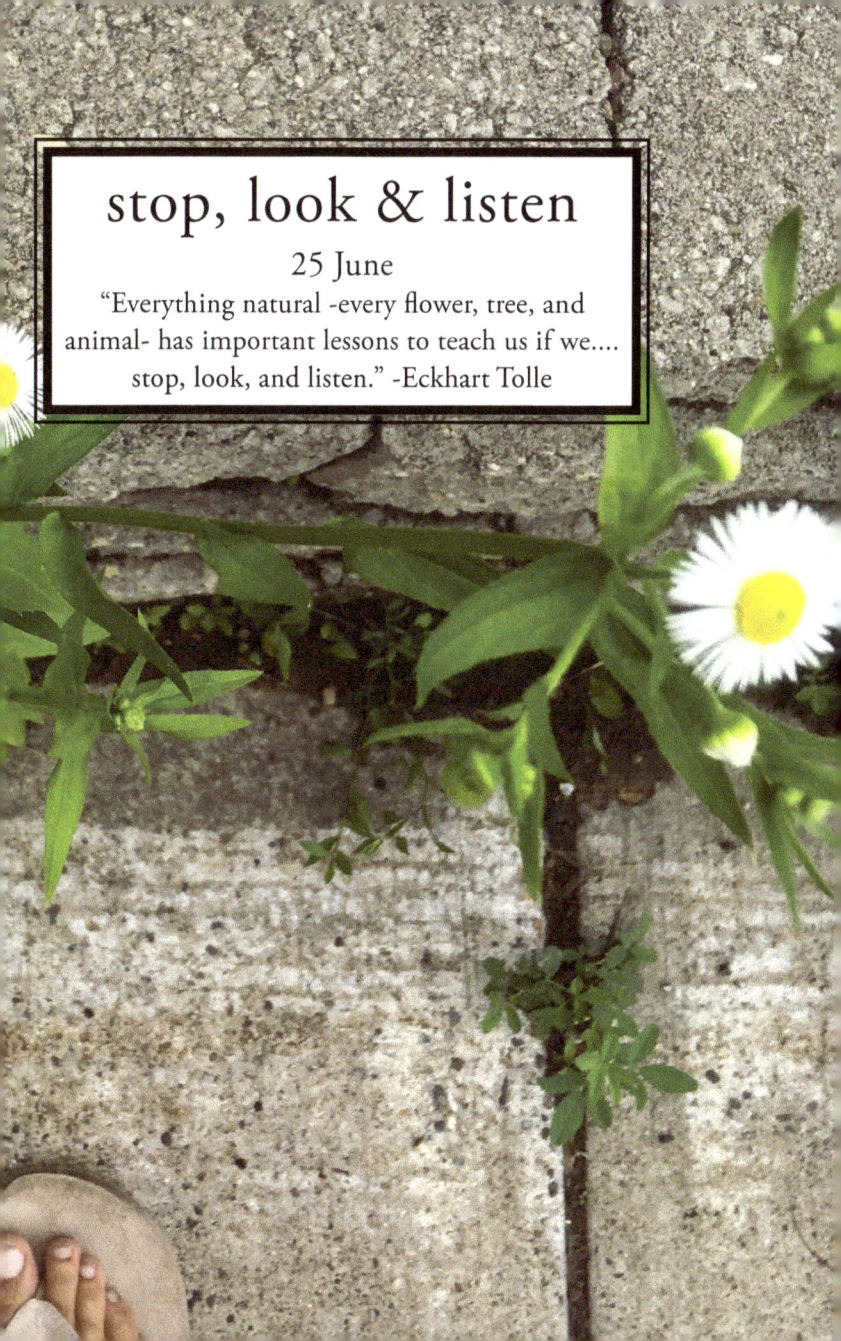

stop, look & listen

25 June

"Everything natural -every flower, tree, and animal- has important lessons to teach us if we.... stop, look, and listen." -Eckhart Tolle

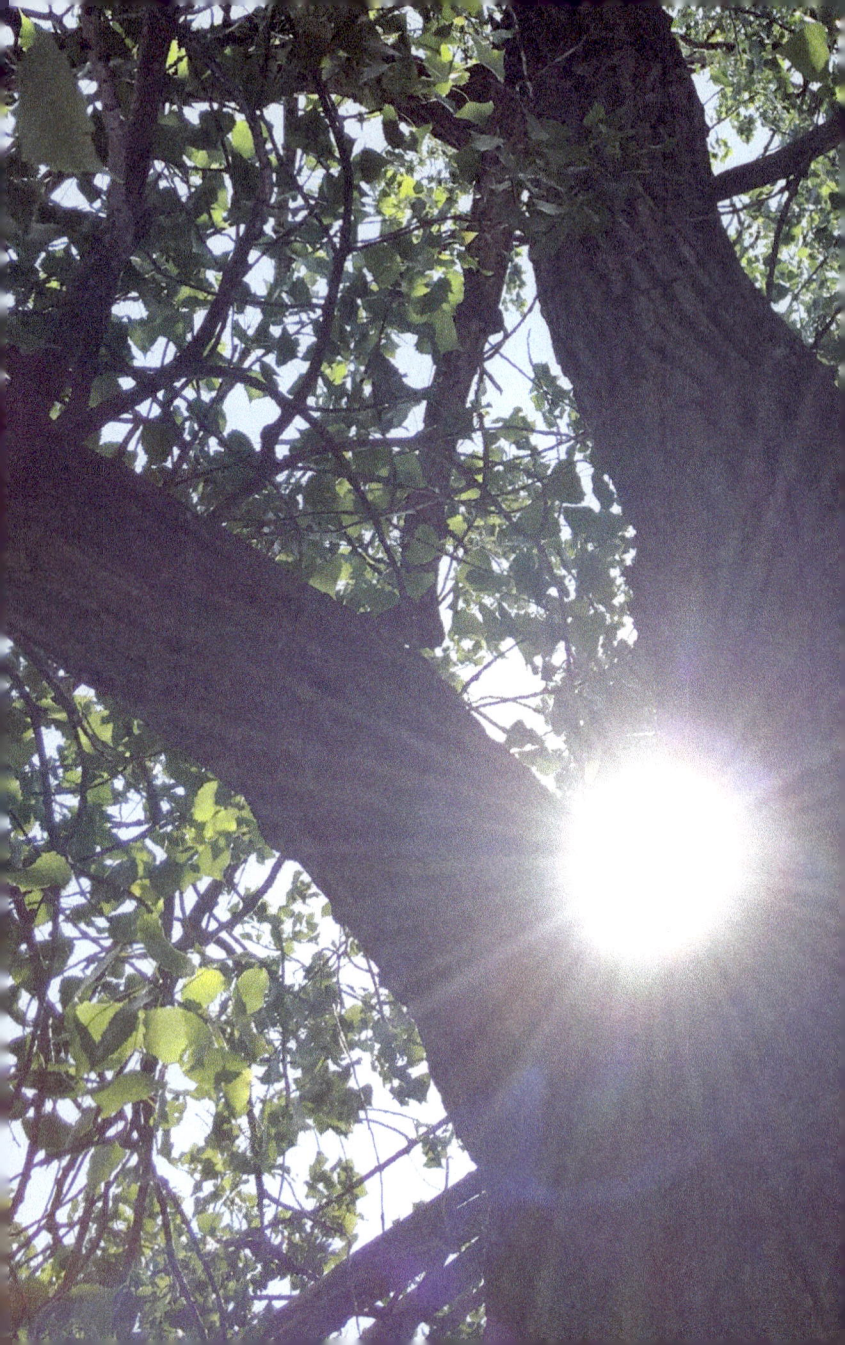

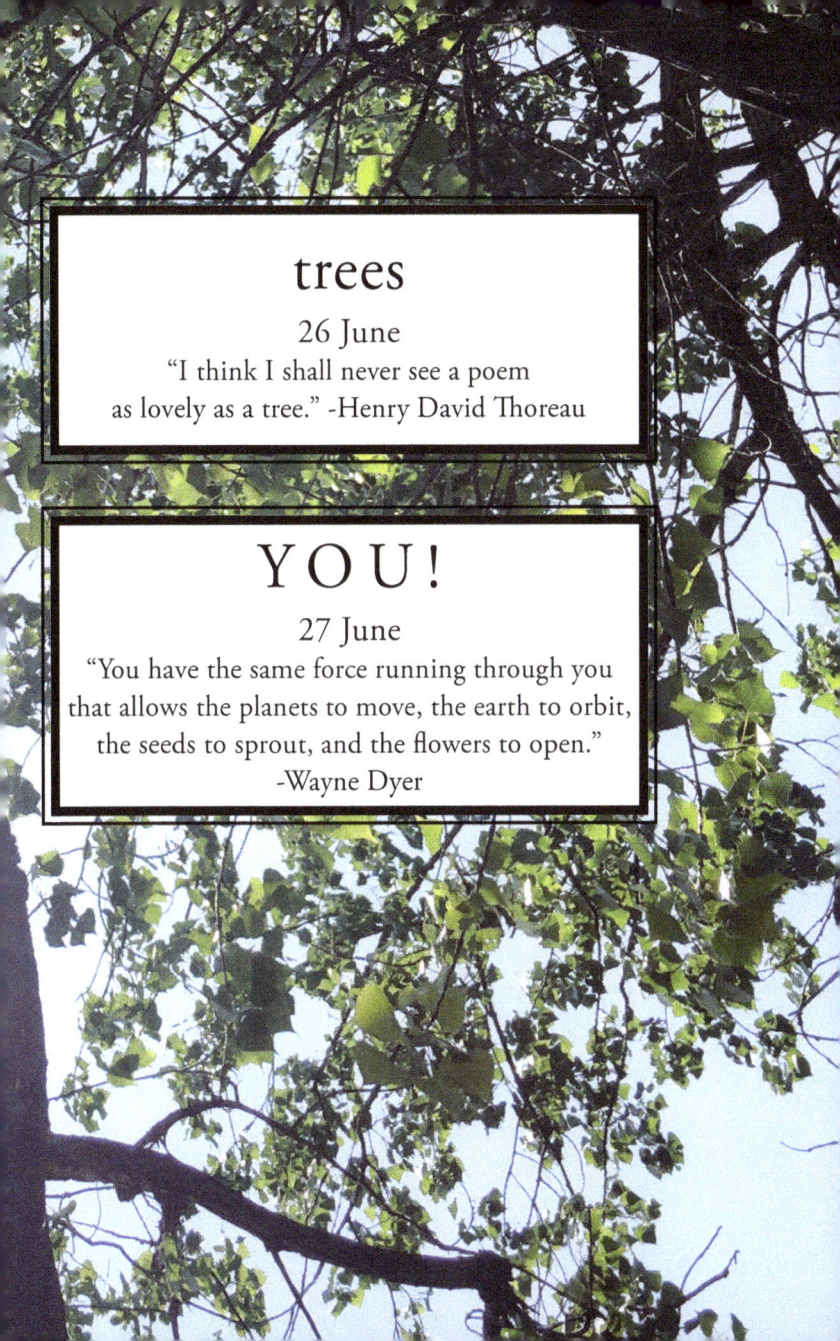

trees

26 June
"I think I shall never see a poem
as lovely as a tree." -Henry David Thoreau

YOU!

27 June
"You have the same force running through you
that allows the planets to move, the earth to orbit,
the seeds to sprout, and the flowers to open."
-Wayne Dyer

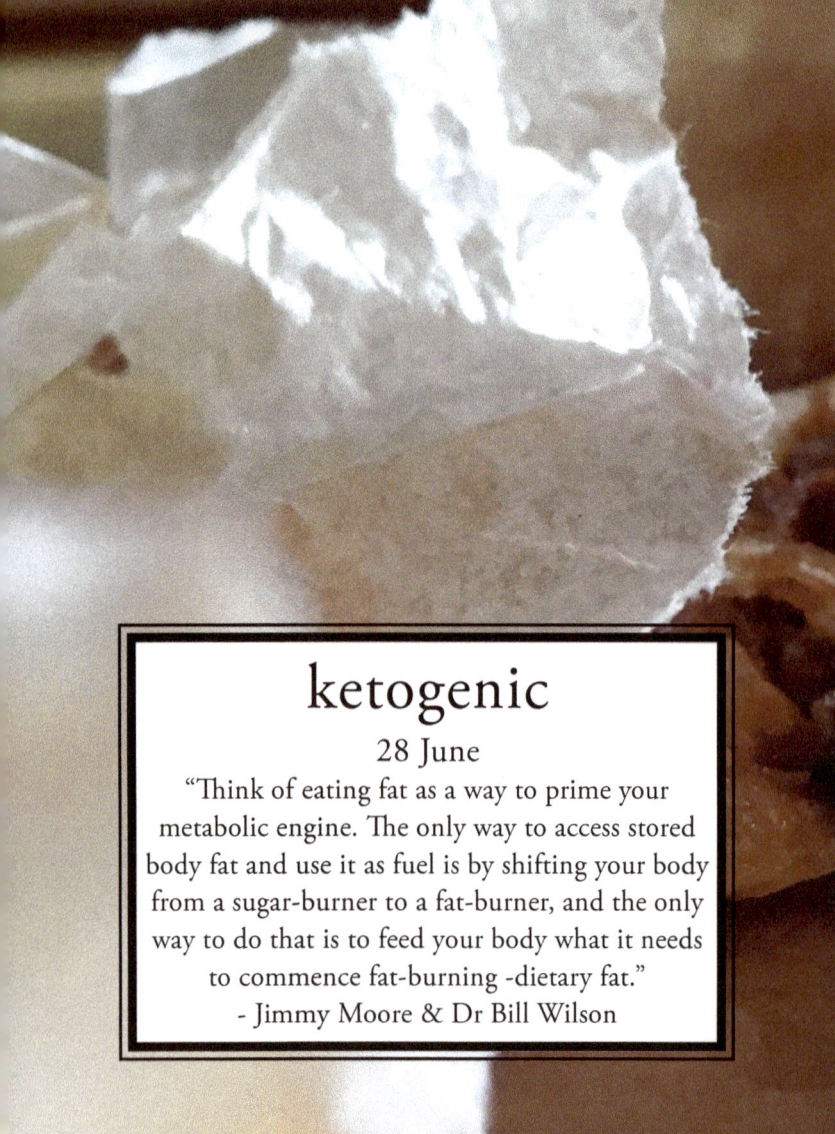

ketogenic
28 June

"Think of eating fat as a way to prime your metabolic engine. The only way to access stored body fat and use it as fuel is by shifting your body from a sugar-burner to a fat-burner, and the only way to do that is to feed your body what it needs to commence fat-burning -dietary fat."

- Jimmy Moore & Dr Bill Wilson

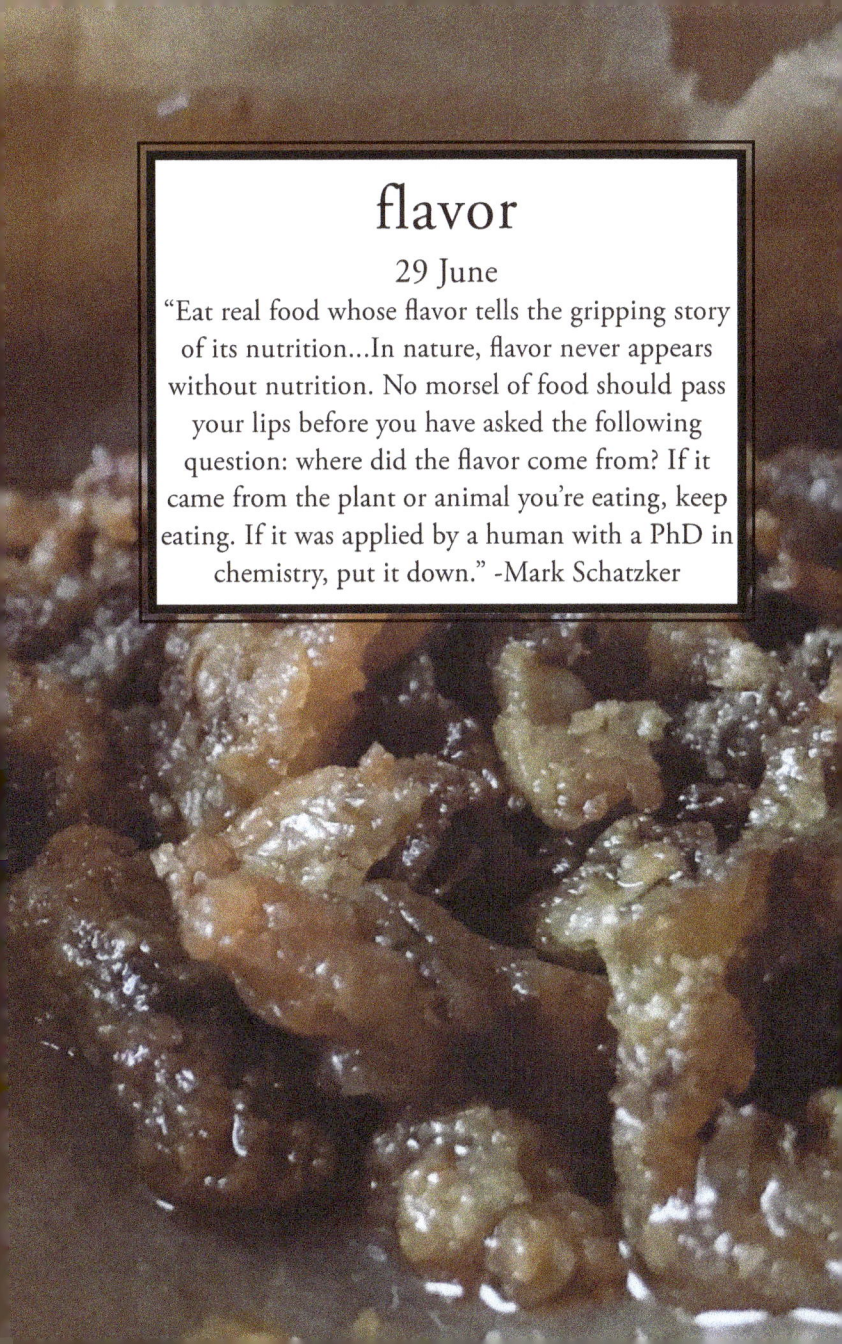

flavor

29 June

"Eat real food whose flavor tells the gripping story of its nutrition...In nature, flavor never appears without nutrition. No morsel of food should pass your lips before you have asked the following question: where did the flavor come from? If it came from the plant or animal you're eating, keep eating. If it was applied by a human with a PhD in chemistry, put it down." -Mark Schatzker

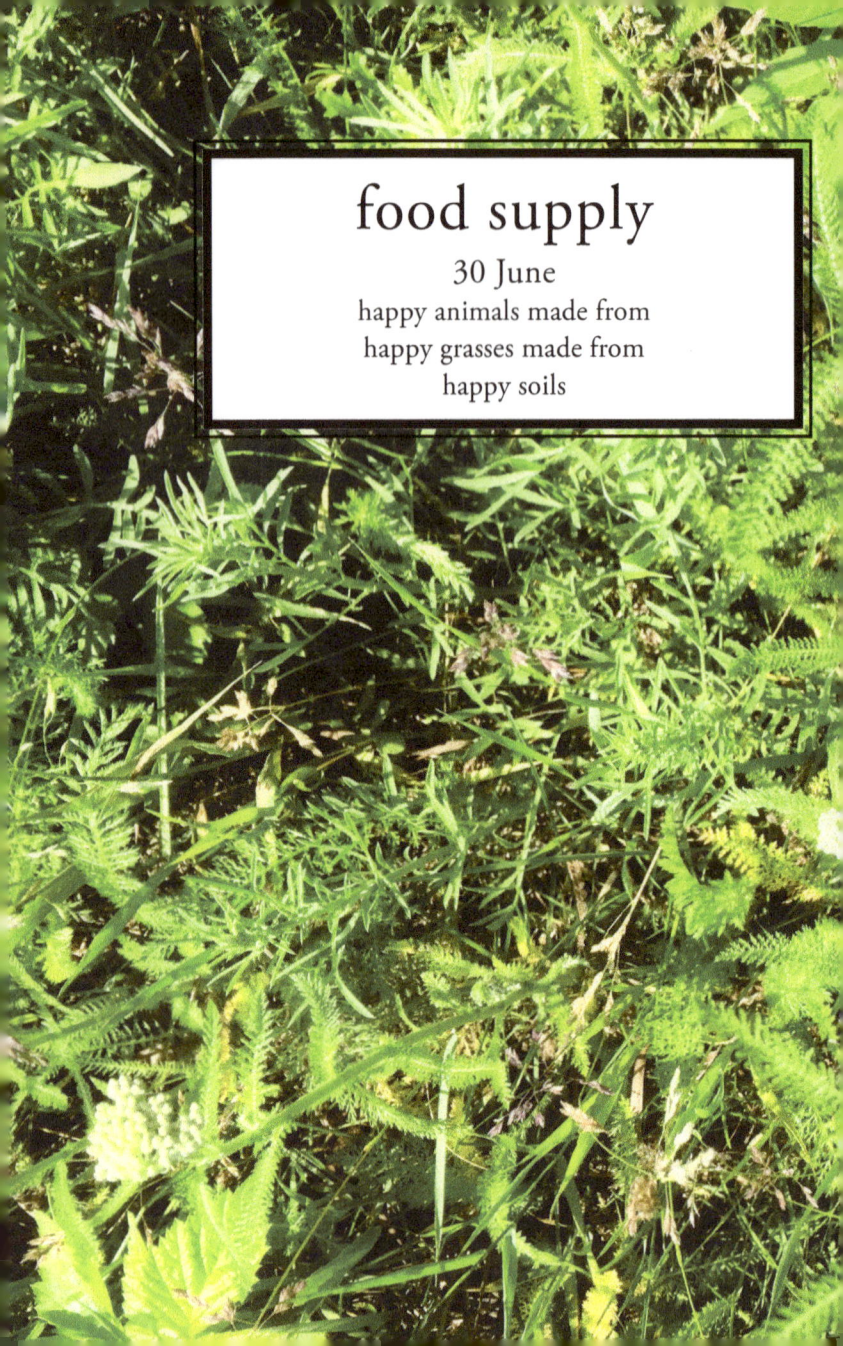

food supply

30 June
happy animals made from
happy grasses made from
happy soils

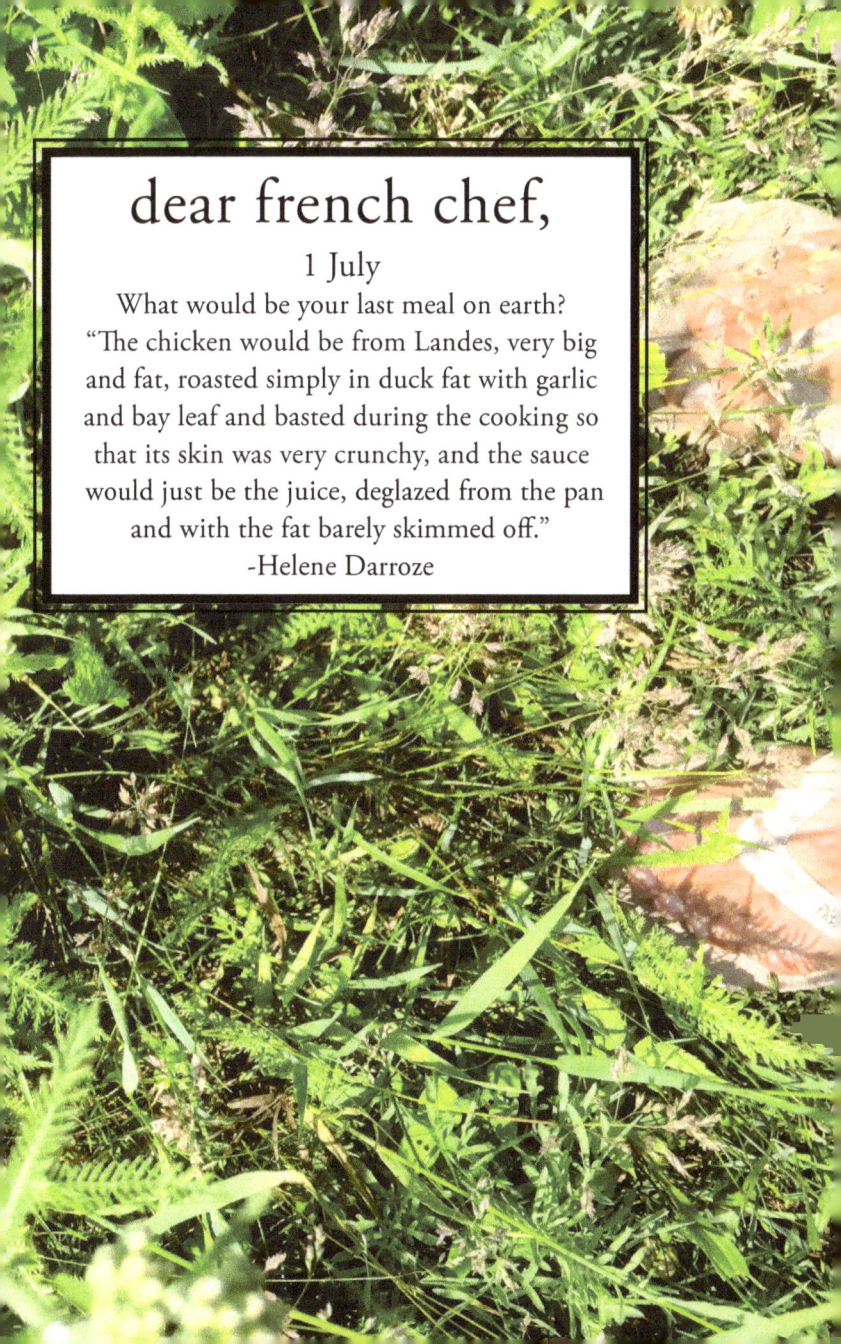

dear french chef,

1 July

What would be your last meal on earth?
"The chicken would be from Landes, very big and fat, roasted simply in duck fat with garlic and bay leaf and basted during the cooking so that its skin was very crunchy, and the sauce would just be the juice, deglazed from the pan and with the fat barely skimmed off."
-Helene Darroze

forces

2 July
gravity-electromagnetic
strong nuclear-weak nuclear

intention-desire/destiny
synchronicity-love

wealth

3 July
"The material wealth of the world can never fill the void we feel within us." -James Twyman

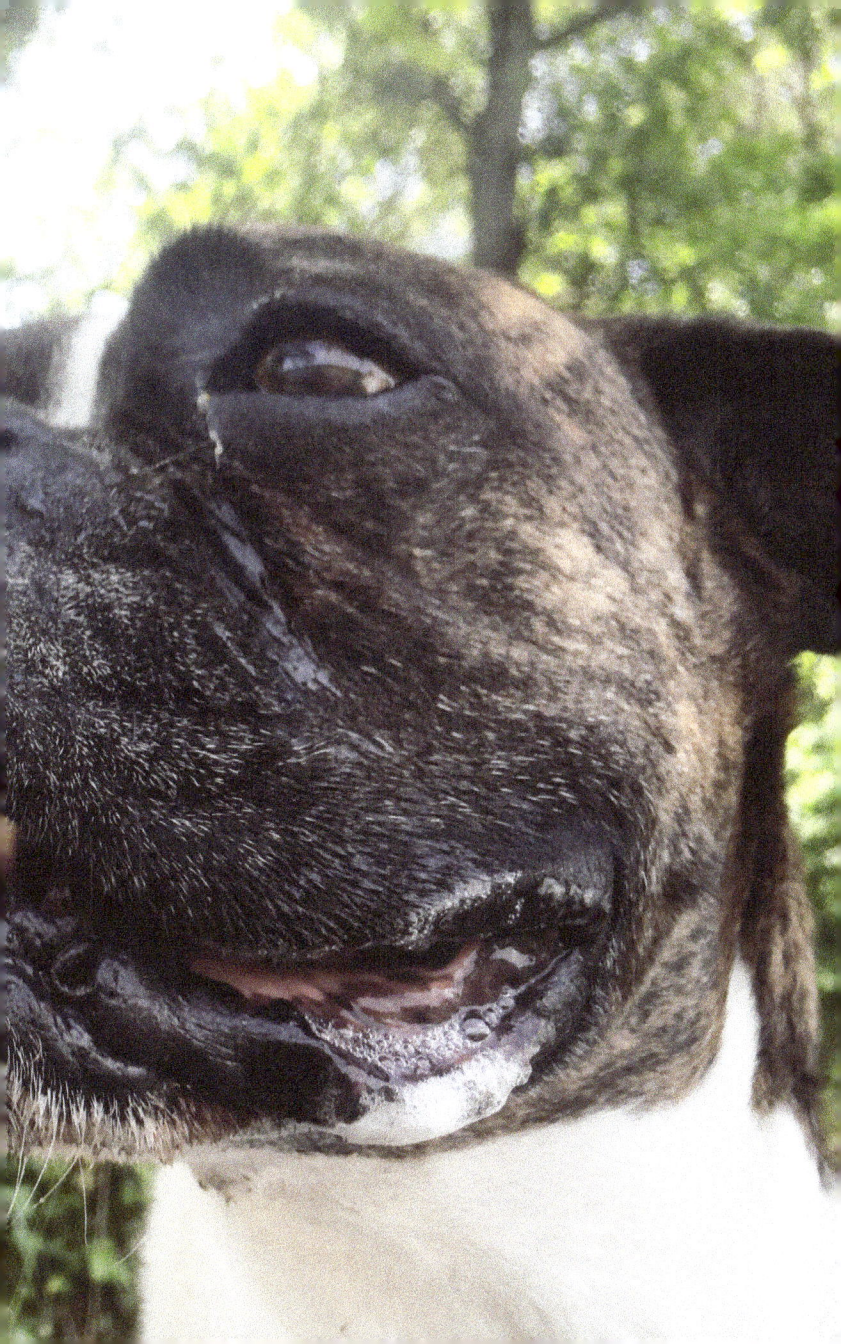

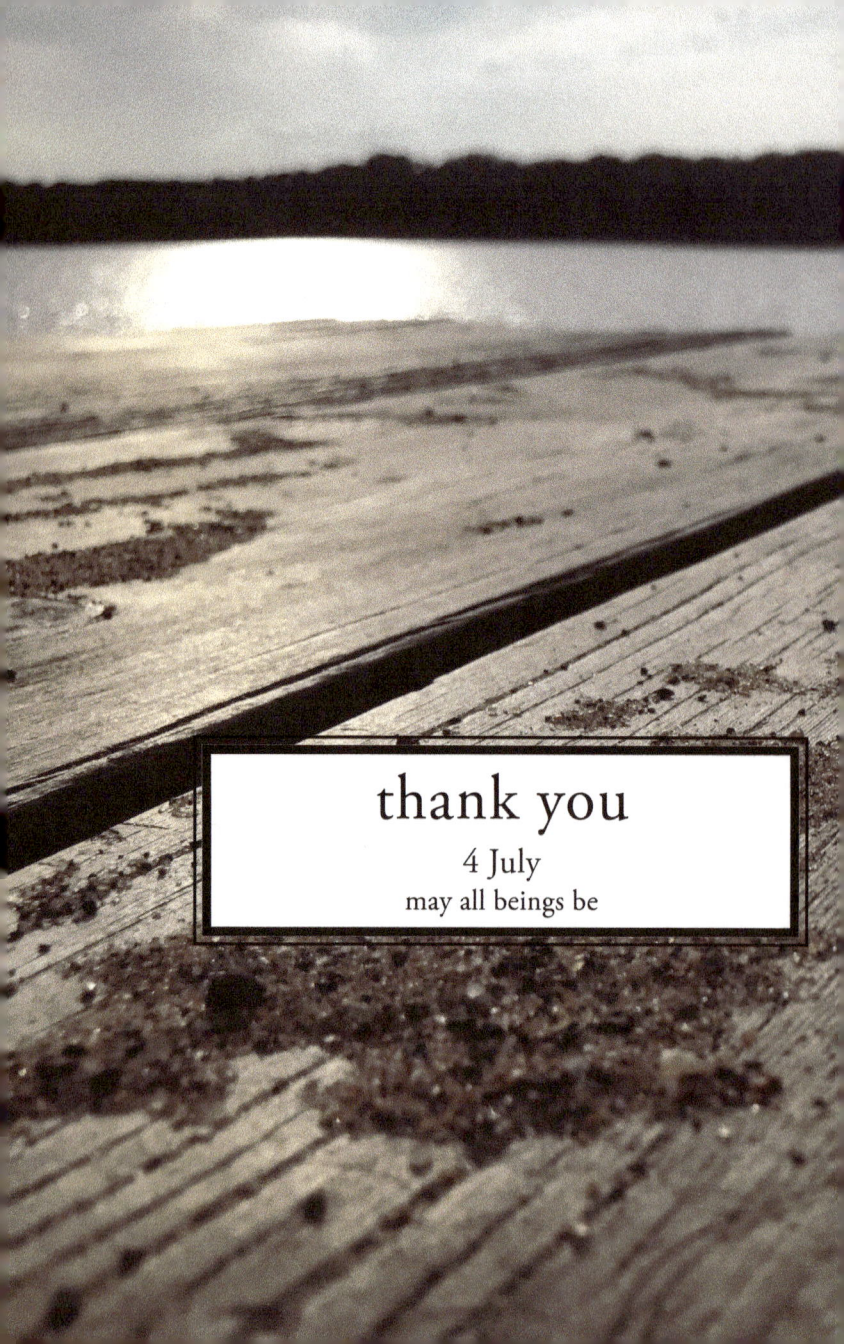

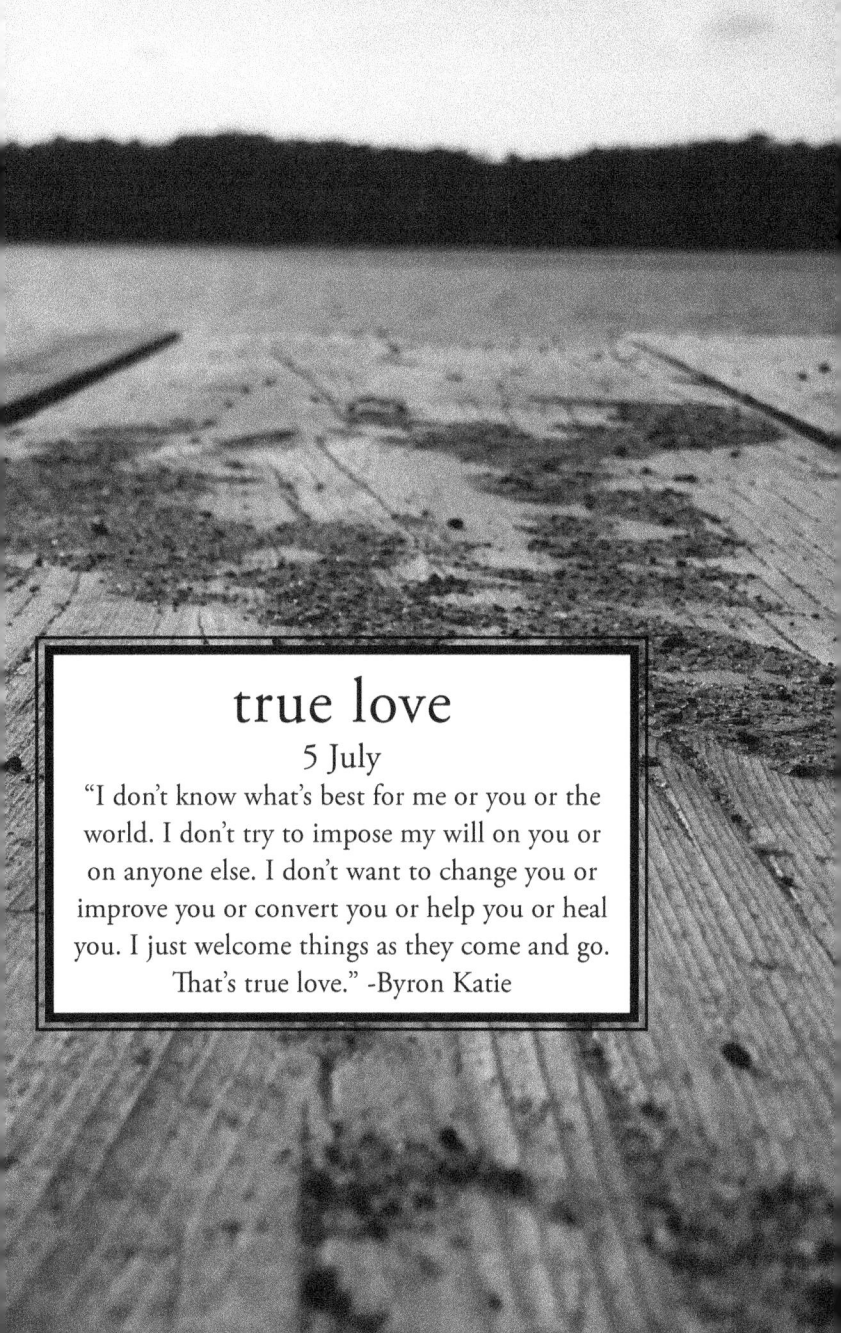

true love

5 July

"I don't know what's best for me or you or the world. I don't try to impose my will on you or on anyone else. I don't want to change you or improve you or convert you or help you or heal you. I just welcome things as they come and go. That's true love." -Byron Katie

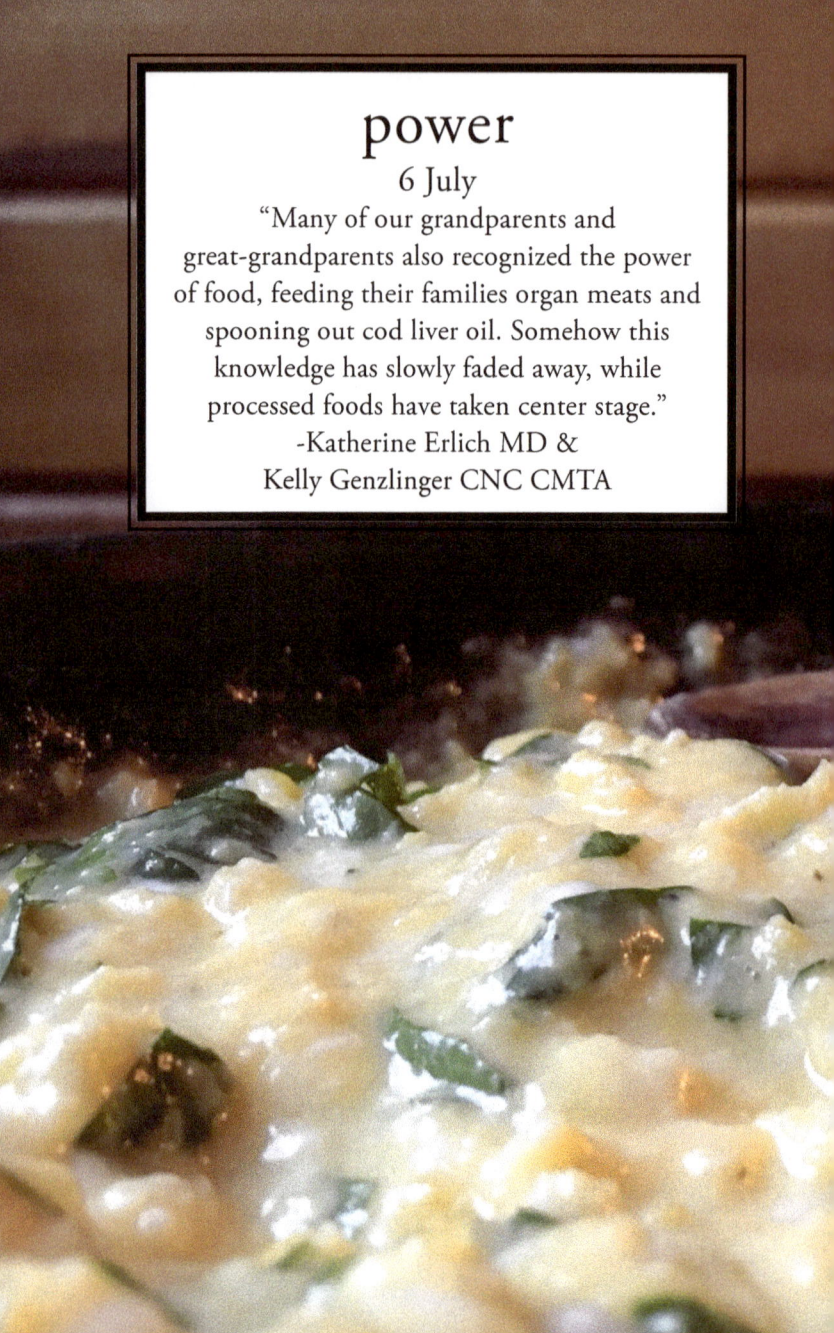

power
6 July

"Many of our grandparents and great-grandparents also recognized the power of food, feeding their families organ meats and spooning out cod liver oil. Somehow this knowledge has slowly faded away, while processed foods have taken center stage."
-Katherine Erlich MD &
Kelly Genzlinger CNC CMTA

privilege
7 July
"I had the great privilege of learning that food comes from the earth not from a factory."
-Sarah Fragoso

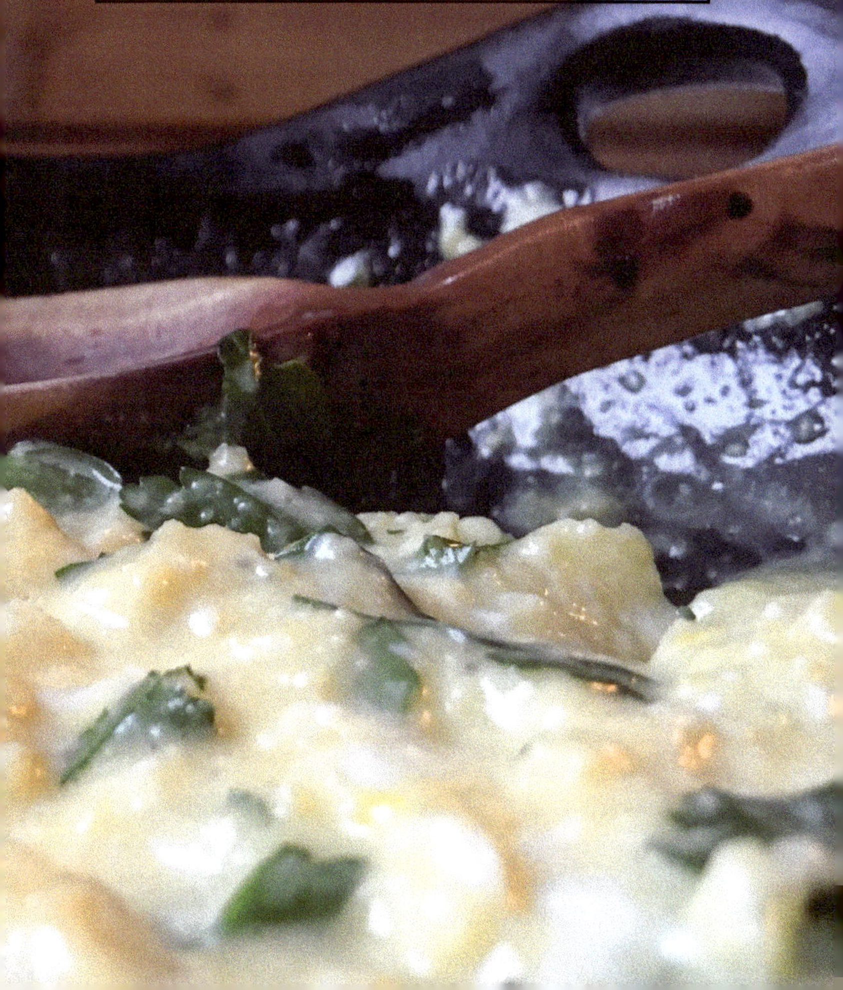

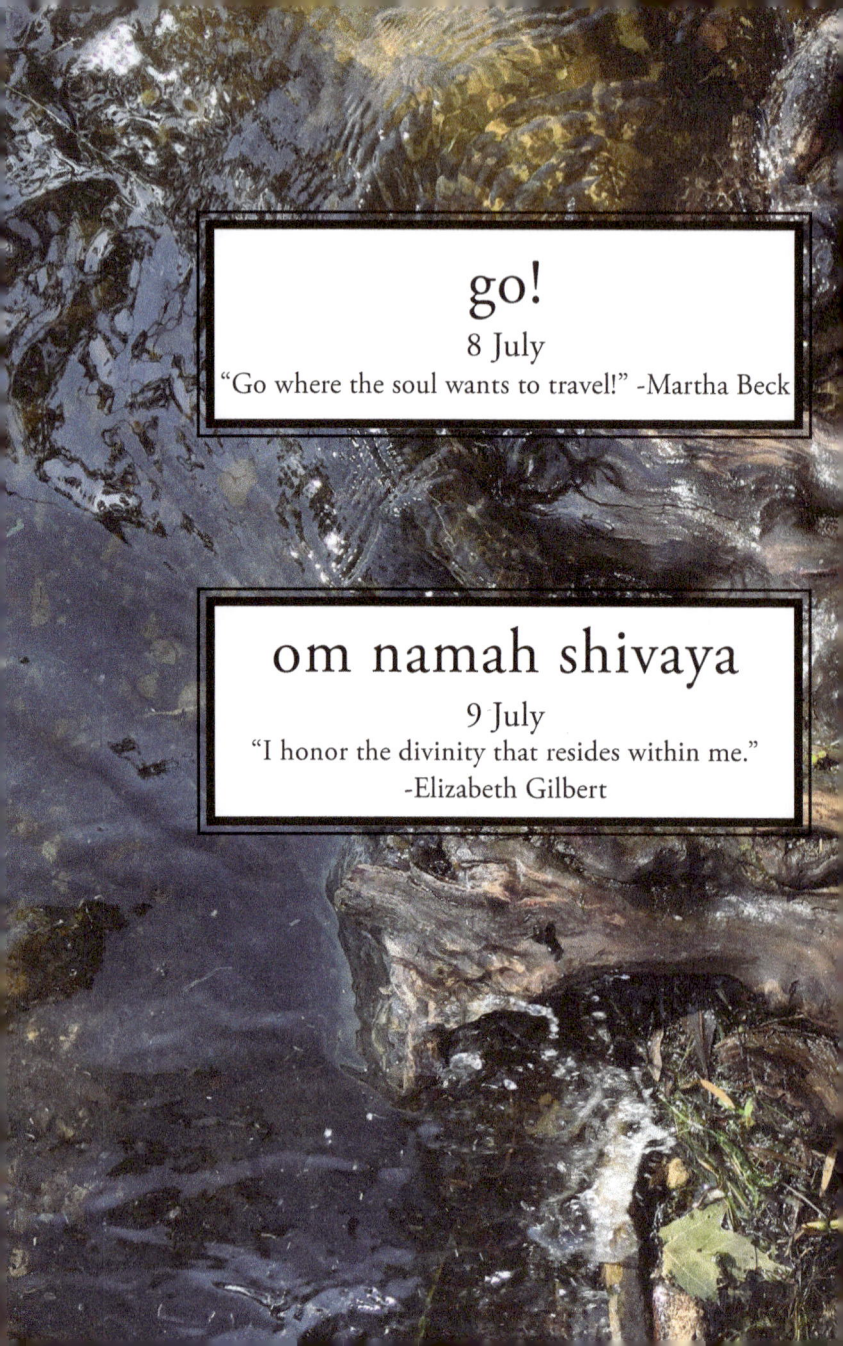

go!
8 July
"Go where the soul wants to travel!" -Martha Beck

om namah shivaya
9 July
"I honor the divinity that resides within me."
-Elizabeth Gilbert

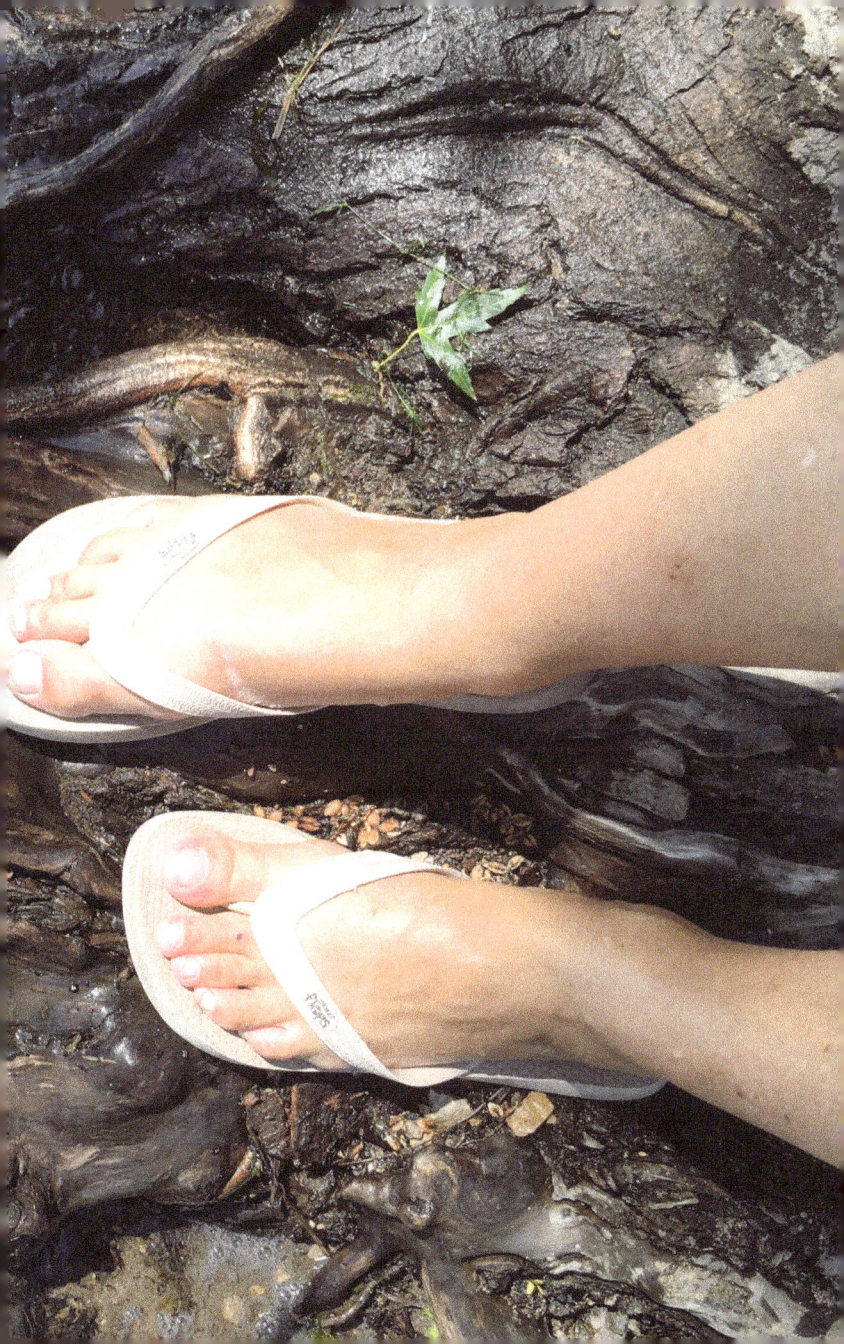

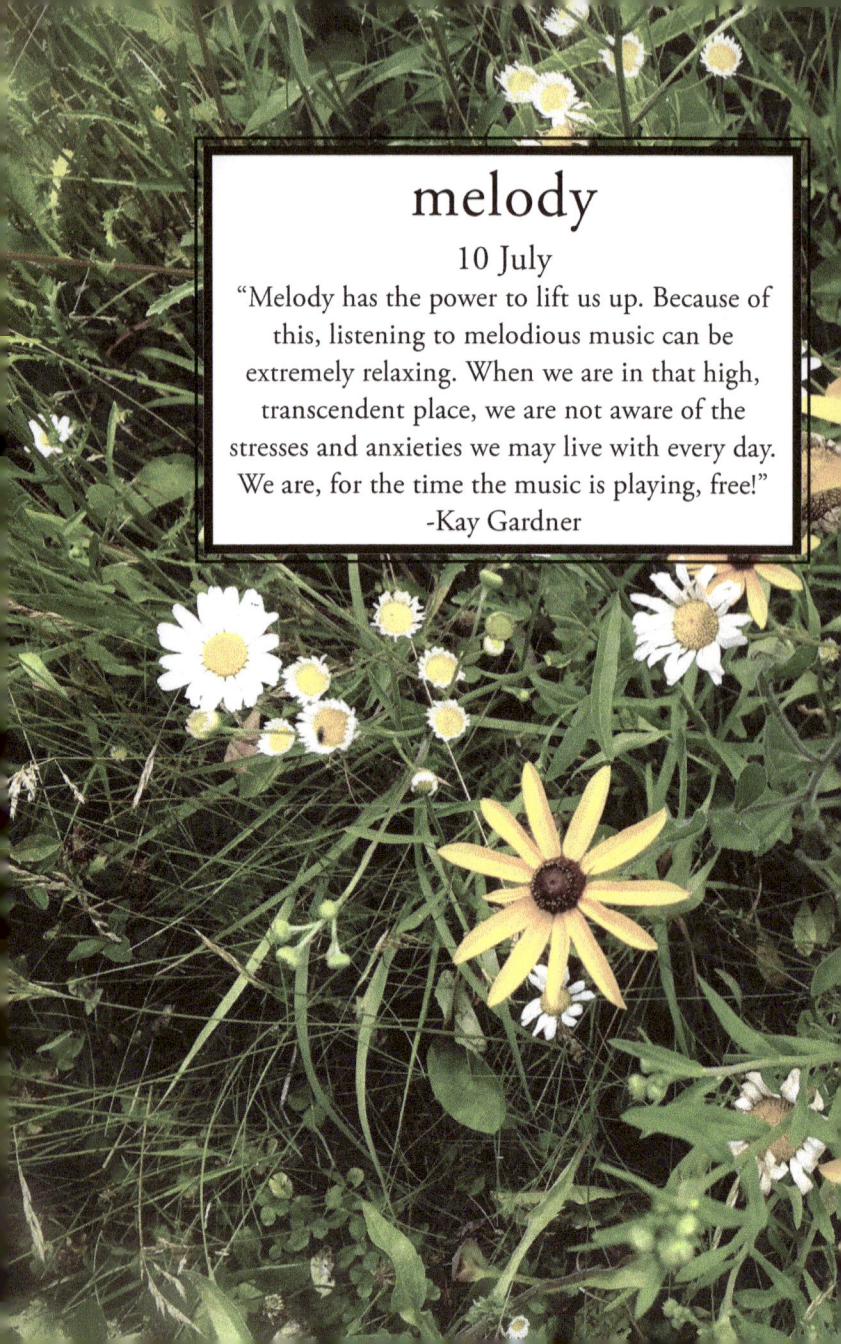

melody

10 July

"Melody has the power to lift us up. Because of this, listening to melodious music can be extremely relaxing. When we are in that high, transcendent place, we are not aware of the stresses and anxieties we may live with every day. We are, for the time the music is playing, free!"
-Kay Gardner

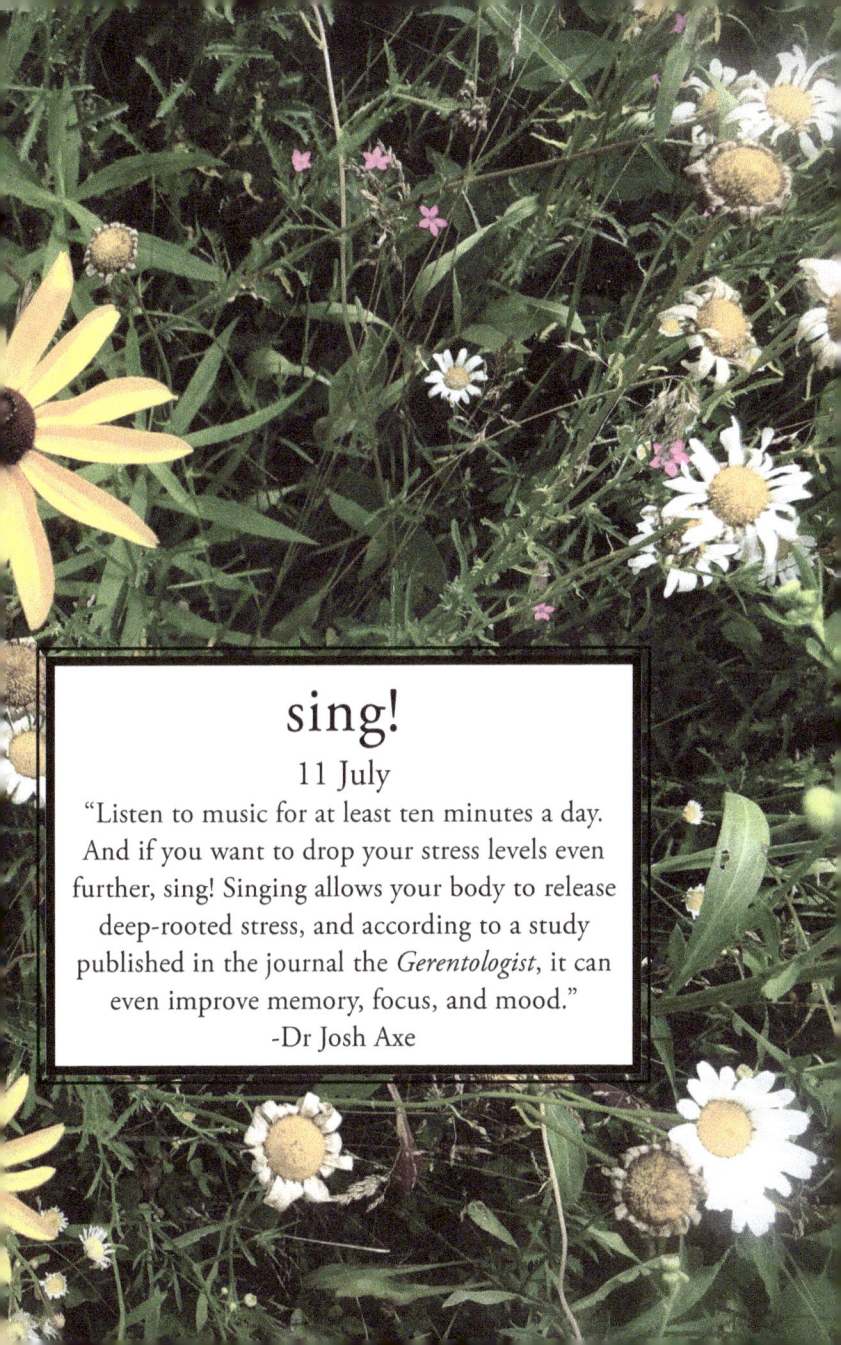

sing!
11 July

"Listen to music for at least ten minutes a day. And if you want to drop your stress levels even further, sing! Singing allows your body to release deep-rooted stress, and according to a study published in the journal the *Gerentologist*, it can even improve memory, focus, and mood."
-Dr Josh Axe

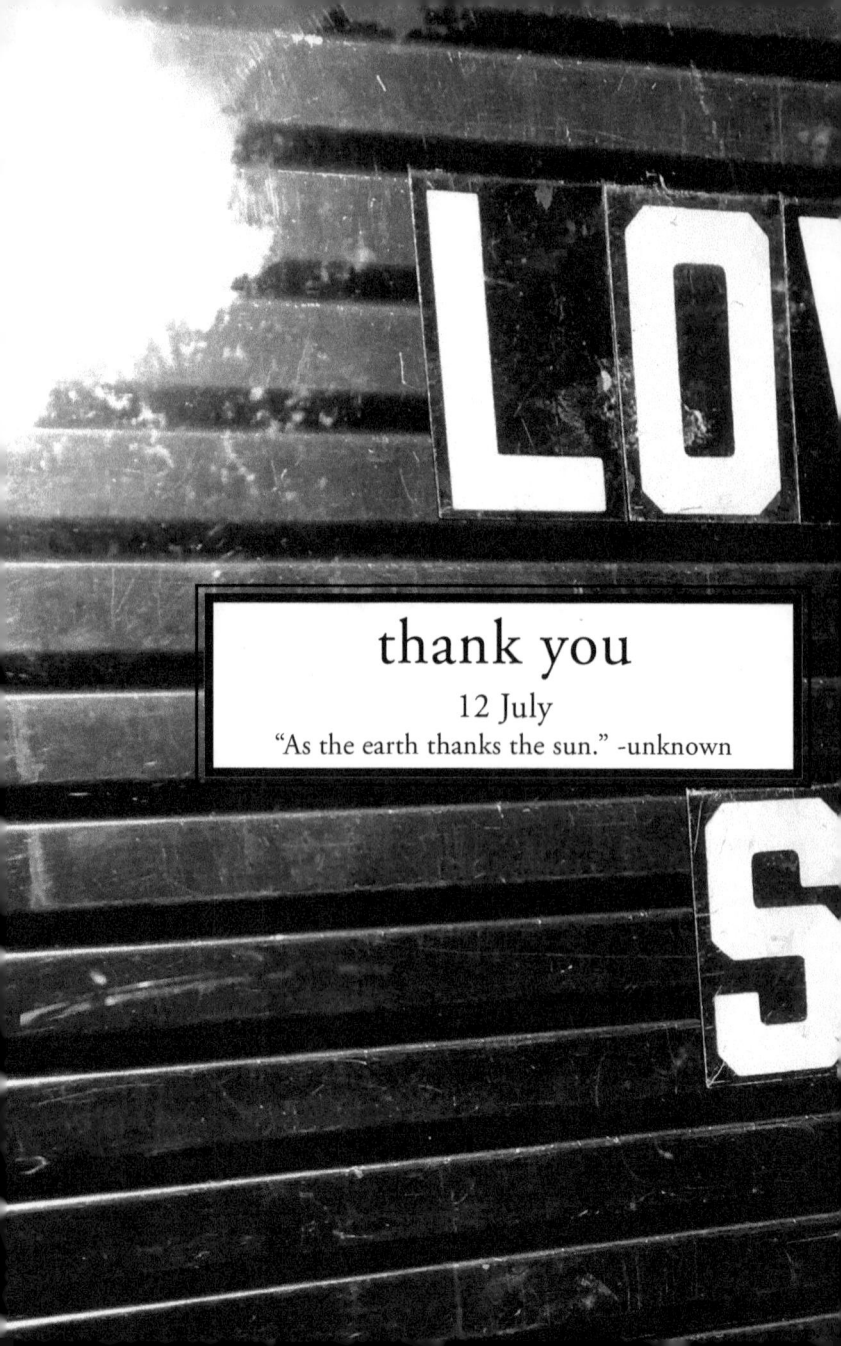

thank you

12 July
"As the earth thanks the sun." -unknown

gratitude

13 July
grateful for gratitude

happiness class

14 July
follow heart
it knows the WAY

lauraness

15 July
being laura

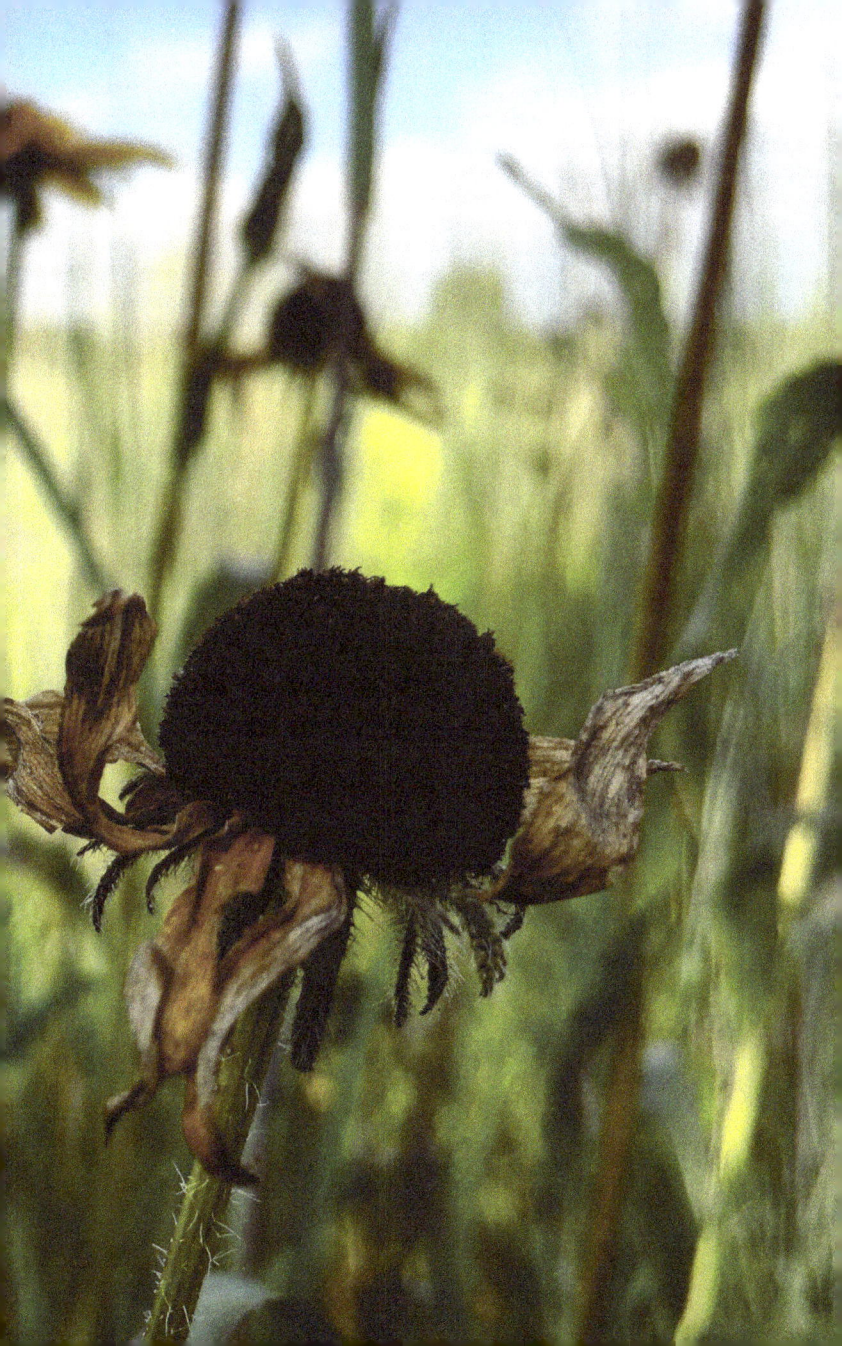

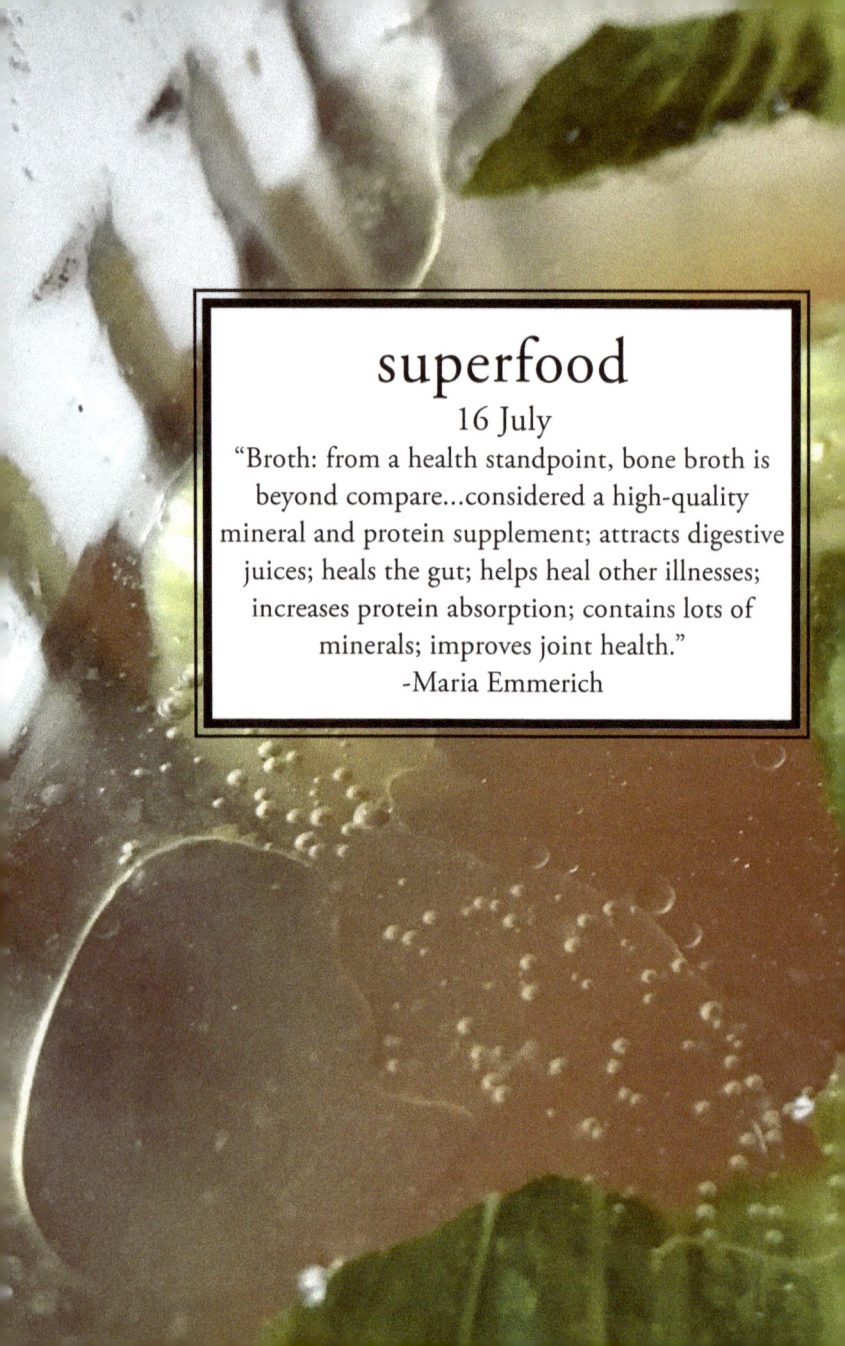

superfood
16 July
"Broth: from a health standpoint, bone broth is beyond compare...considered a high-quality mineral and protein supplement; attracts digestive juices; heals the gut; helps heal other illnesses; increases protein absorption; contains lots of minerals; improves joint health."
-Maria Emmerich

gelatin bouillon

17 July

"Sally Fallon: when broth is cooled, it congeals due to the presence of gelatin. The use of gelatin as a therapeutic agent goes back to the ancient Chinese...although gelatin is not a complete protein, containing only the amino acids agrinine and glycine in large amounts, it acts as a protein sparer, helping the poor stretch a few morsels of meat into a complete meal. During the siege of Paris, when vegetables and meat were scarce, a doctor named Guerard put his patients on gelatin bouillon with some added fat and they survived in good health." -Kristen Michaelis

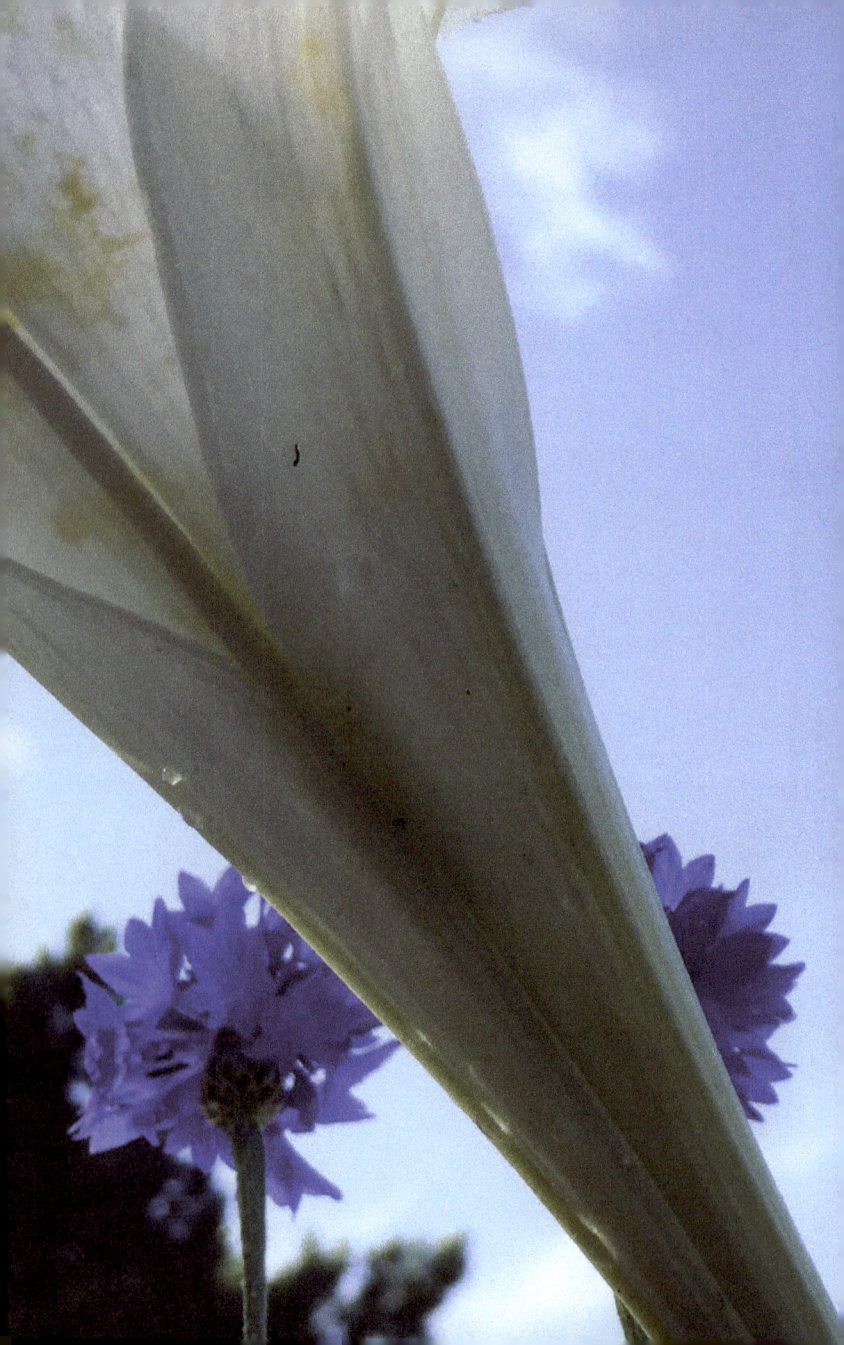

imagination
18 July
"Passionately believe in that which is in your imagination and which does not yet exist on the physical plane." -Wayne Dyer

dear thoughts,
19 July
Dear thoughts, Please let me listen while I'm listening, drive while I'm driving, drink water while I'm drinking water, play while I'm playing, eat while I'm eating, sleep while I'm sleeping, shower while I'm showering, love while I'm loving, read while I'm reading, cook while I'm cooking, brush my teeth while I'm brushing my teeth, see nature while I'm seeing nature.
Thank you. Love, Laura

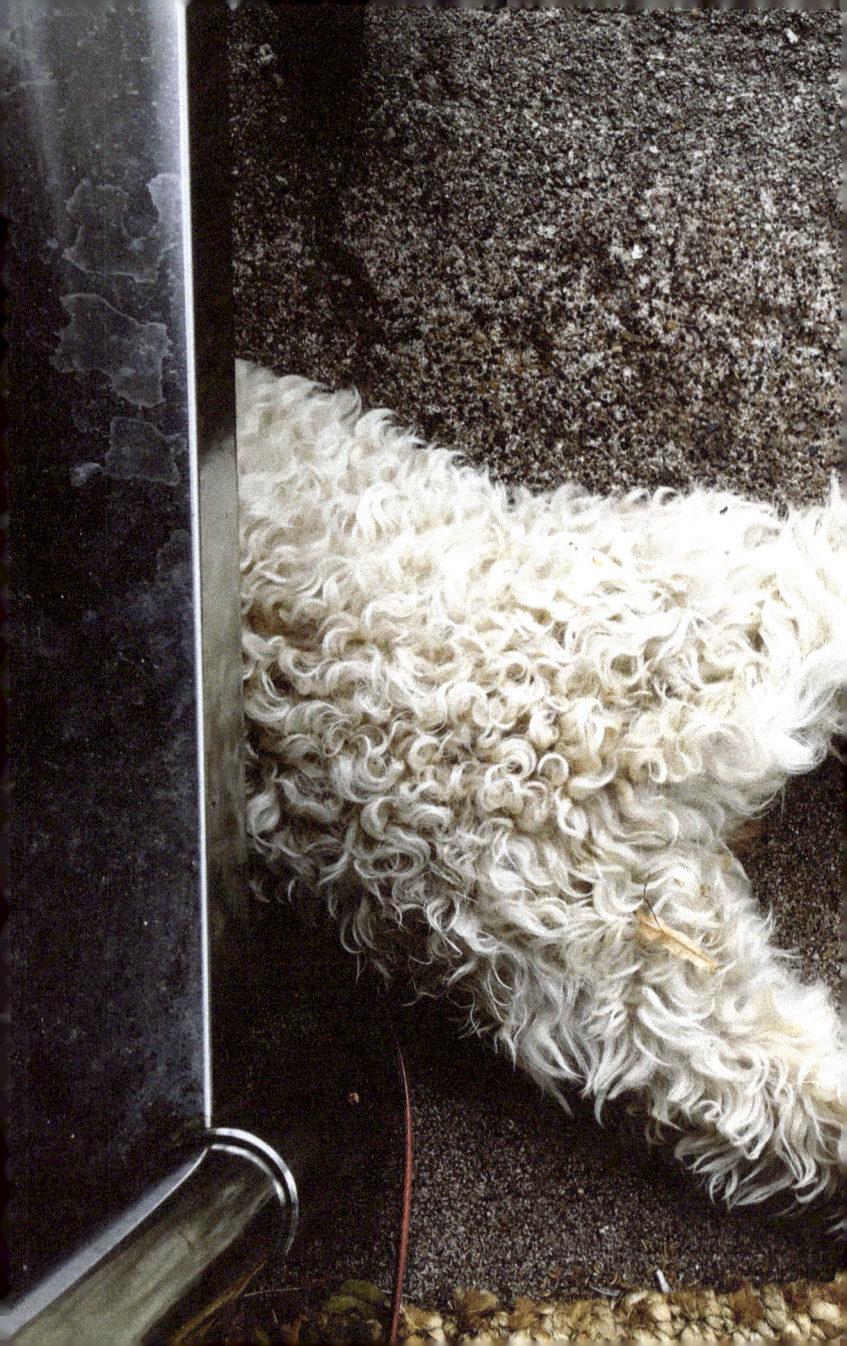

nothing!
20 July
"In my world, nothing ever goes wrong."
-Sri Nisargadatta Maharaj

hehe
21 July
"Mark Twain: 'I am an old man and have known a great many troubles, but most of them never happened.'" -Timothy Ferriss

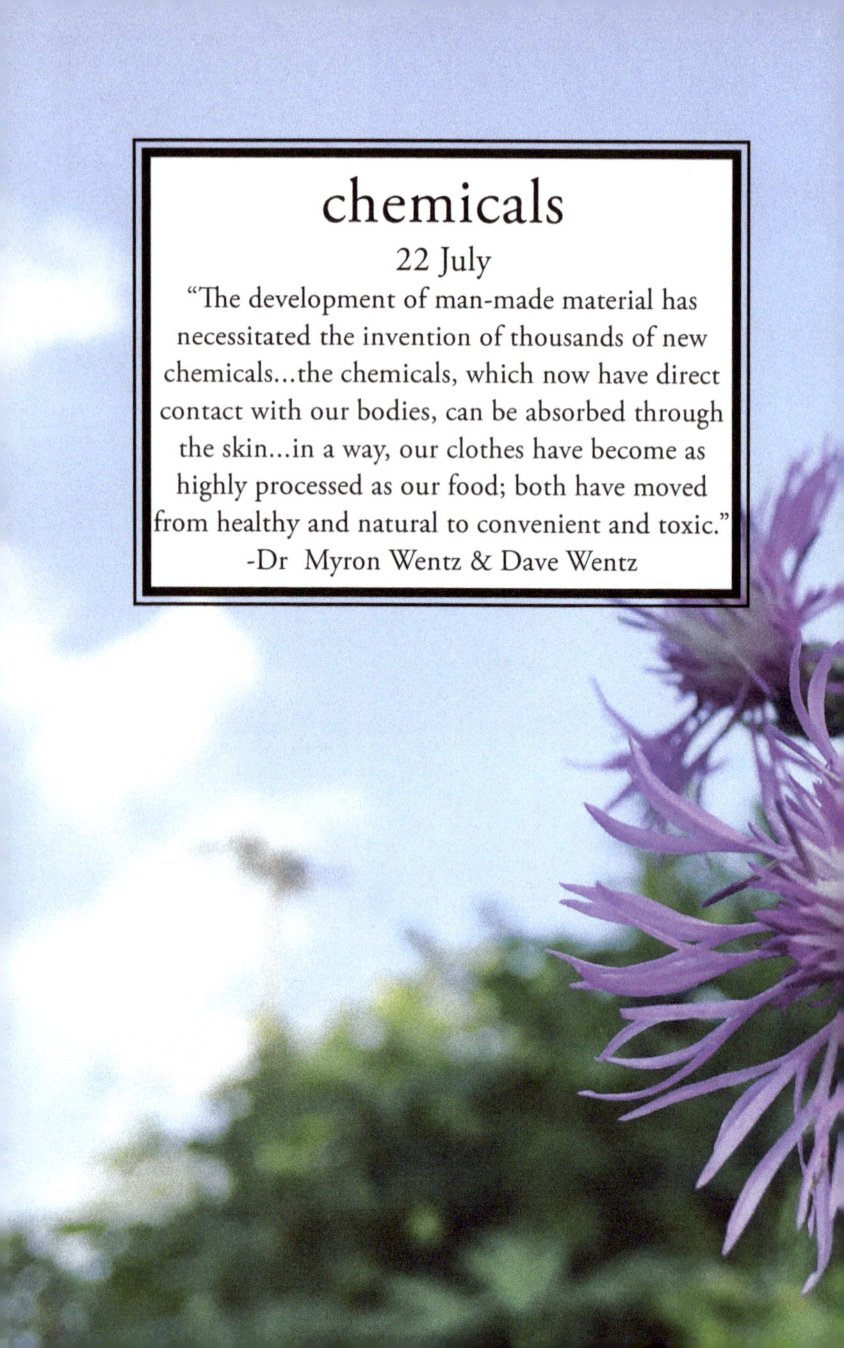

chemicals

22 July

"The development of man-made material has necessitated the invention of thousands of new chemicals...the chemicals, which now have direct contact with our bodies, can be absorbed through the skin...in a way, our clothes have become as highly processed as our food; both have moved from healthy and natural to convenient and toxic."

-Dr Myron Wentz & Dave Wentz

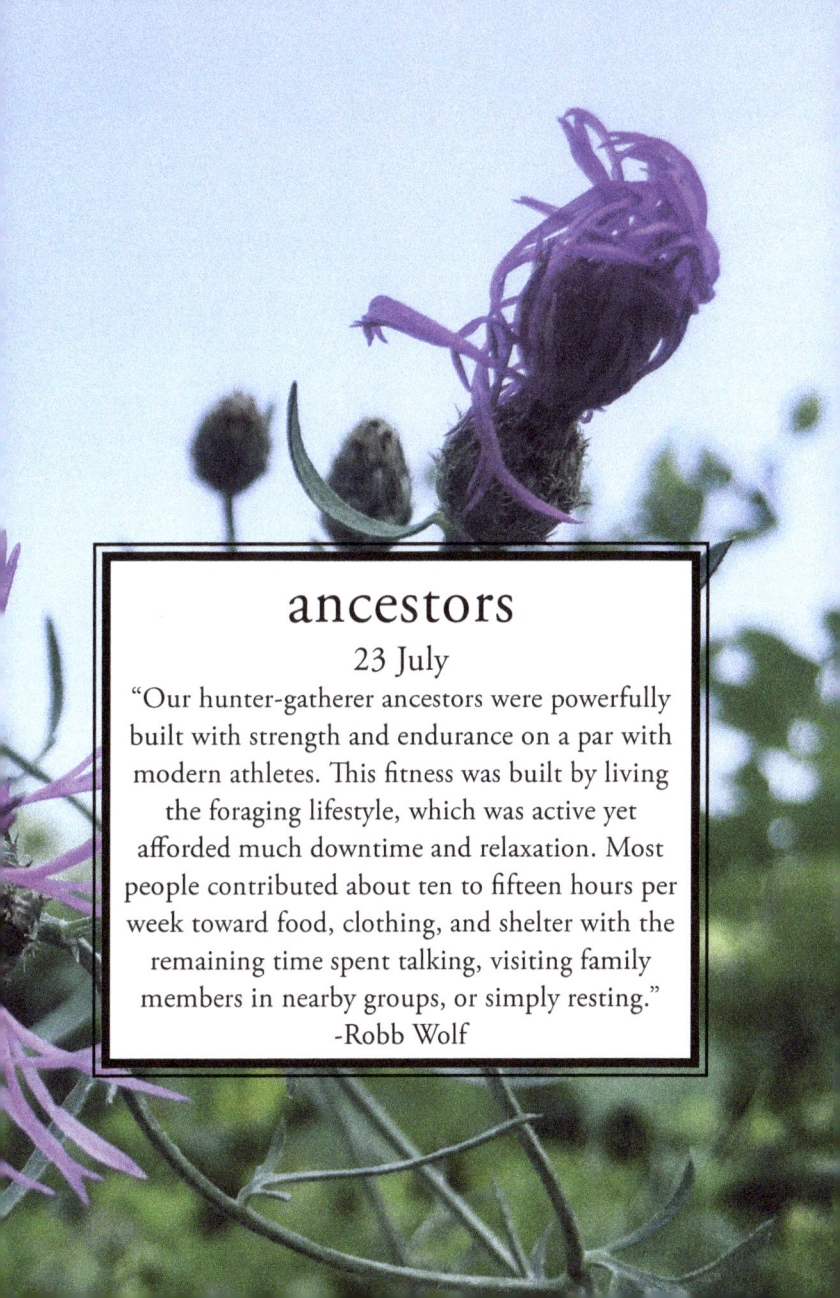

ancestors
23 July
"Our hunter-gatherer ancestors were powerfully built with strength and endurance on a par with modern athletes. This fitness was built by living the foraging lifestyle, which was active yet afforded much downtime and relaxation. Most people contributed about ten to fifteen hours per week toward food, clothing, and shelter with the remaining time spent talking, visiting family members in nearby groups, or simply resting."
-Robb Wolf

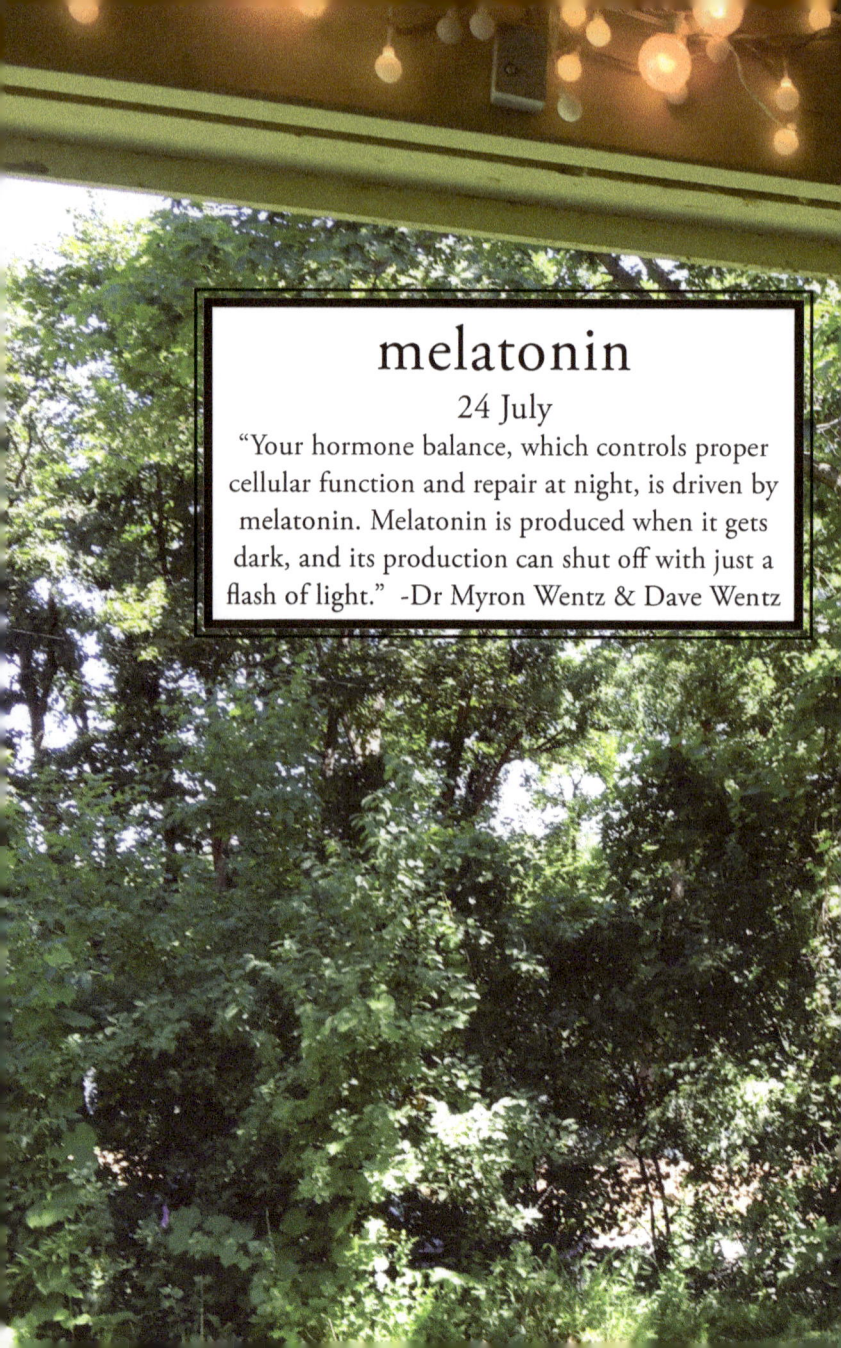

melatonin

24 July

"Your hormone balance, which controls proper cellular function and repair at night, is driven by melatonin. Melatonin is produced when it gets dark, and its production can shut off with just a flash of light." -Dr Myron Wentz & Dave Wentz

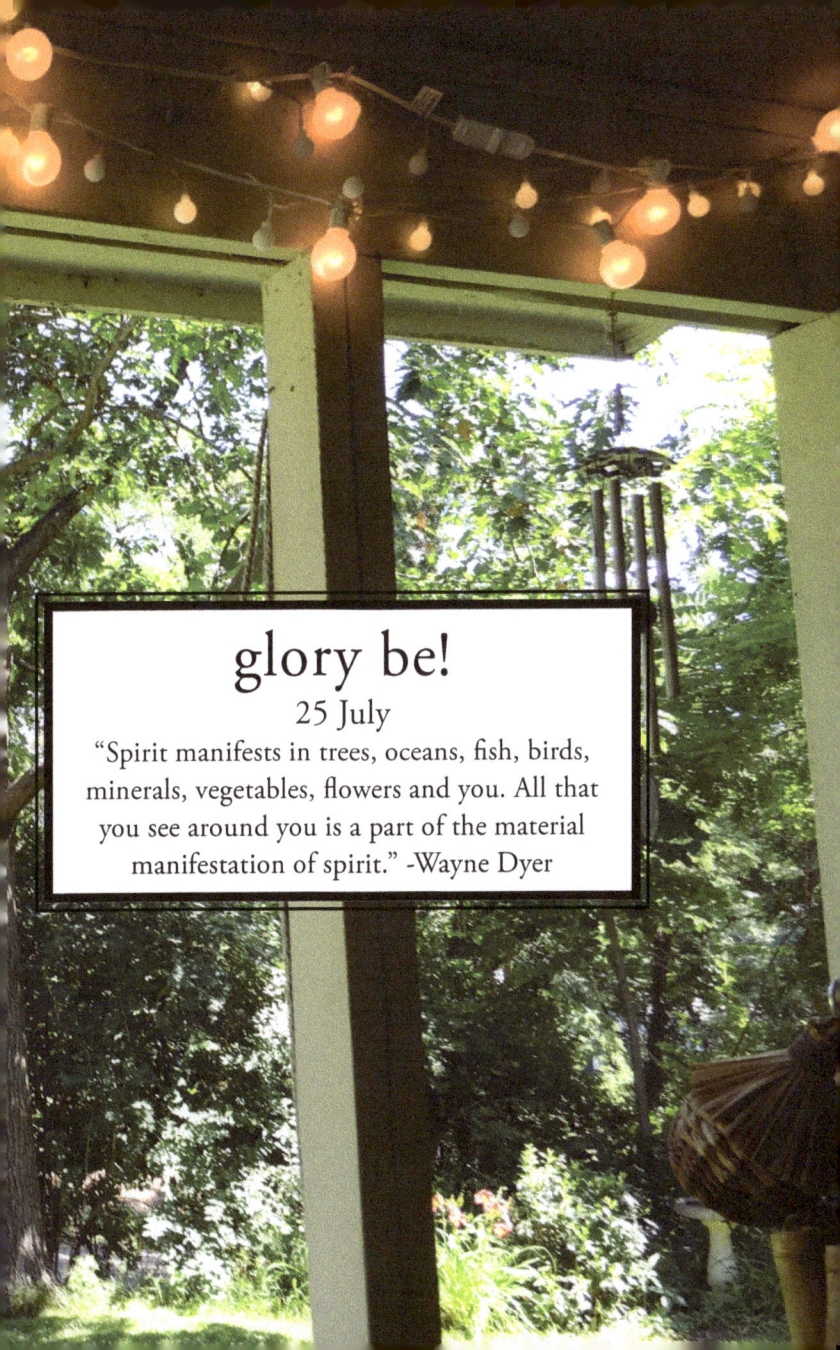

glory be!
25 July
"Spirit manifests in trees, oceans, fish, birds, minerals, vegetables, flowers and you. All that you see around you is a part of the material manifestation of spirit." -Wayne Dyer

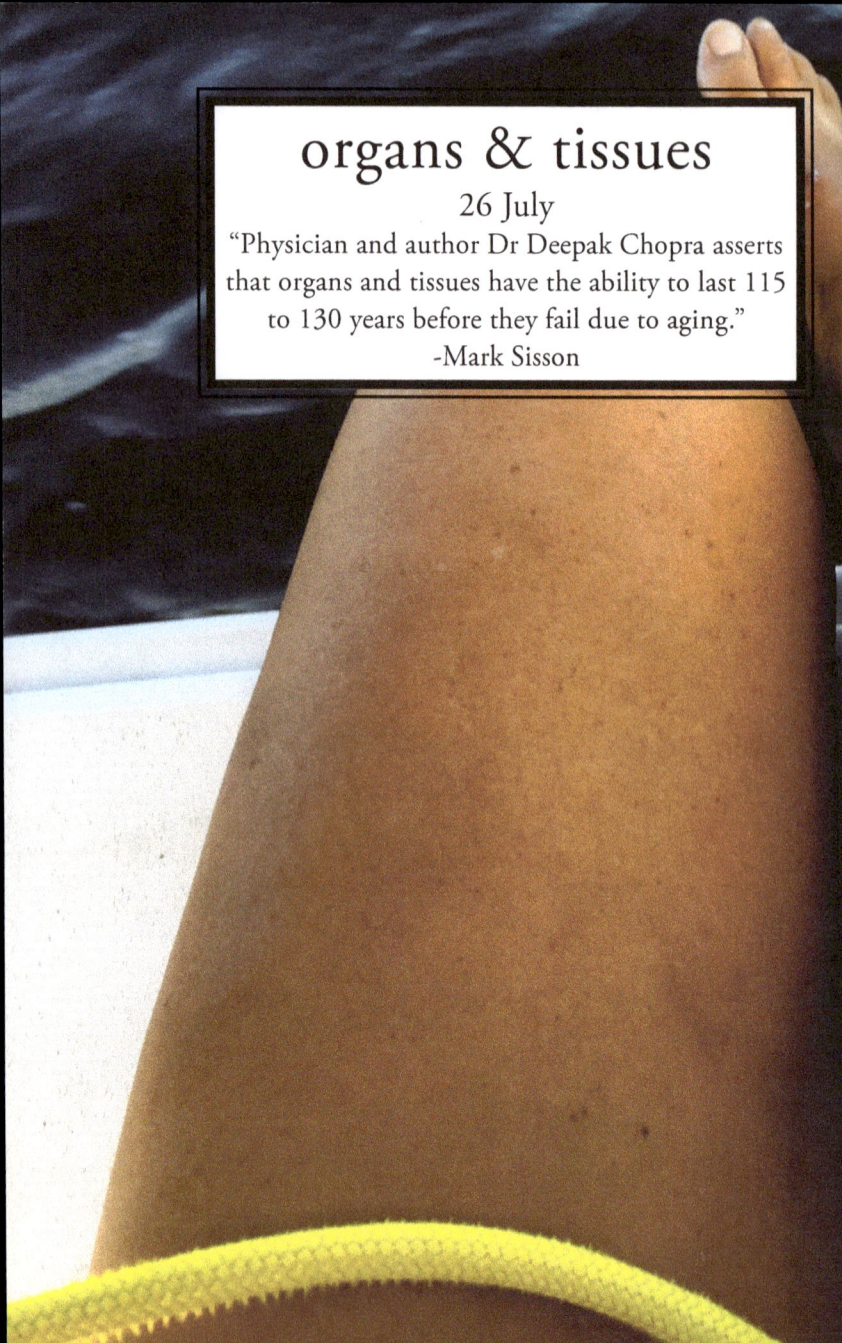

organs & tissues

26 July

"Physician and author Dr Deepak Chopra asserts that organs and tissues have the ability to last 115 to 130 years before they fail due to aging."

-Mark Sisson

lowest cholesterol
27 July
"Populations, who live almost entirely on animal food have the lowest cholesterol ever measured."
-Uffe Ravnskov MD, PhD

the head & the heart

28 July

The head always trying to prove its Divine worthiness that it knows is its heart.

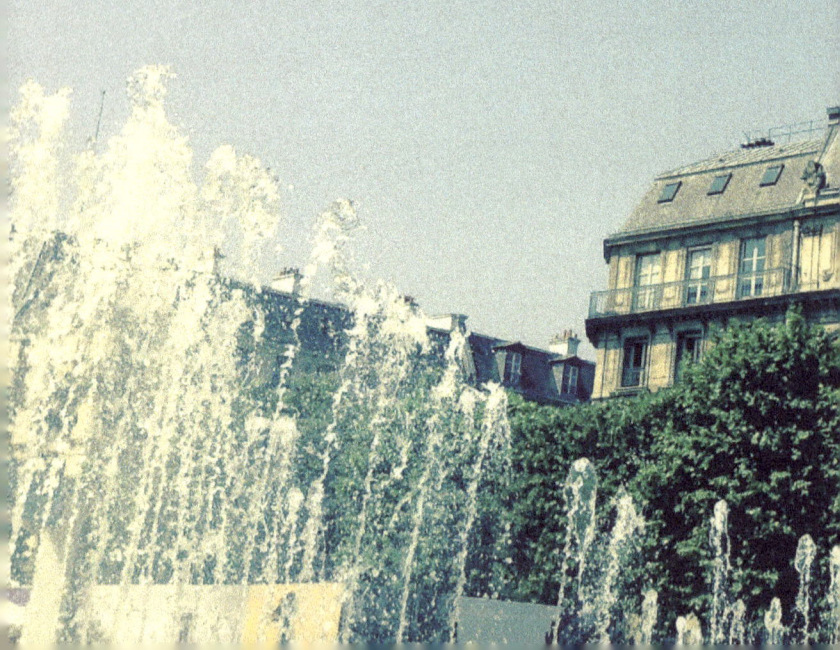

oui
29 July
you
me
oui

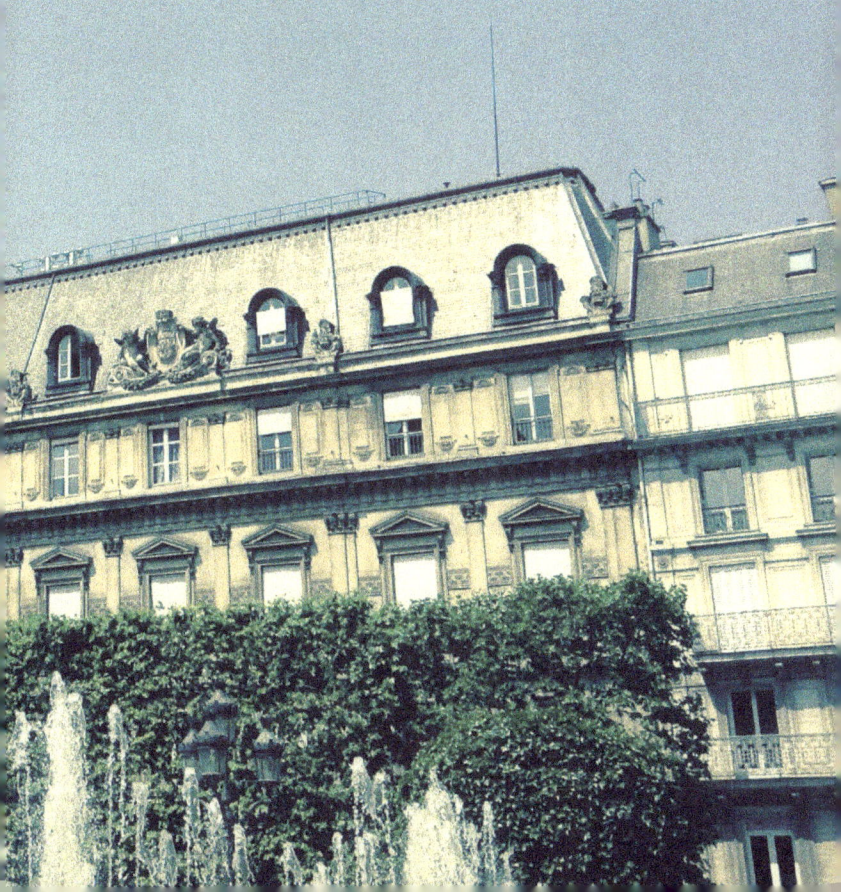

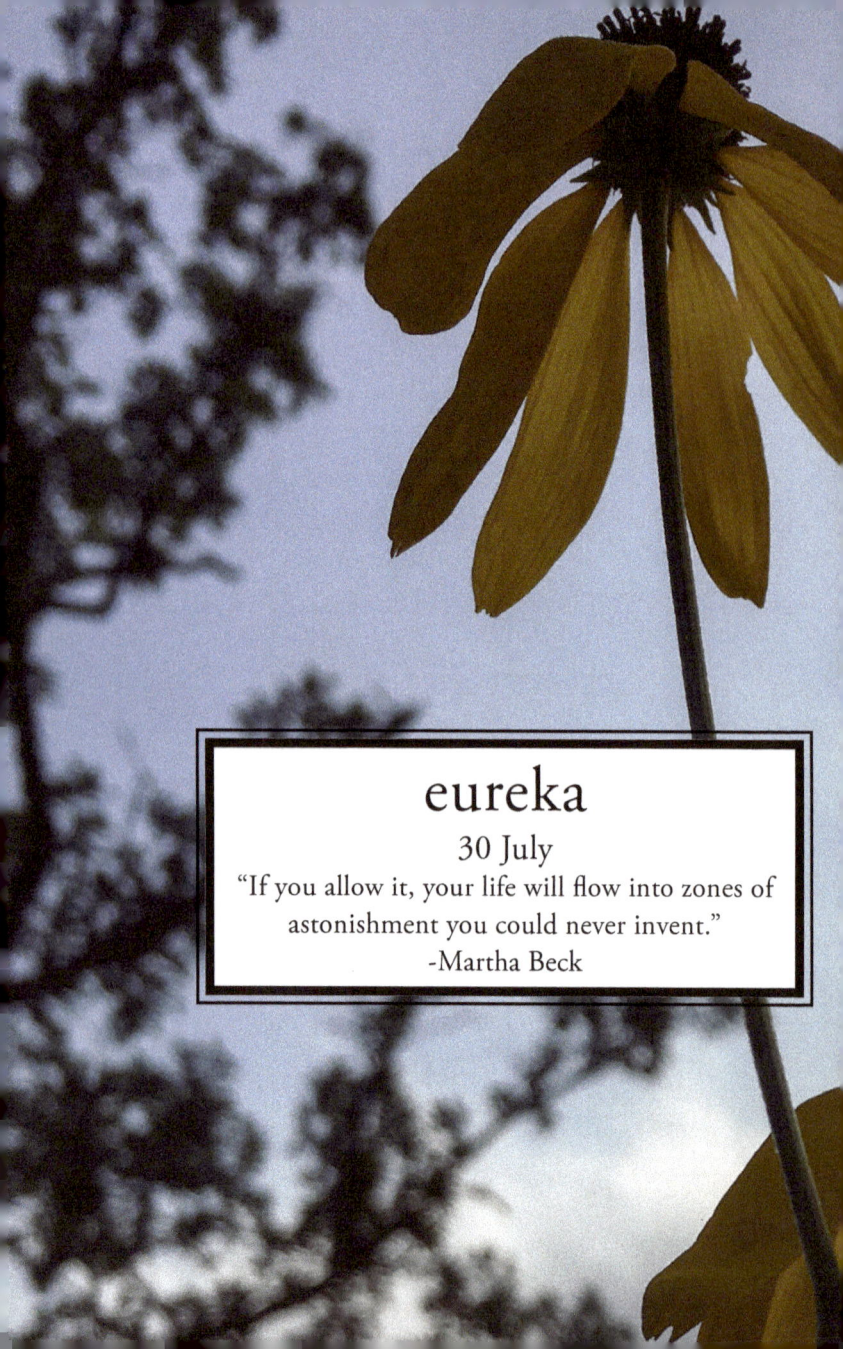

eureka
30 July
"If you allow it, your life will flow into zones of astonishment you could never invent."
-Martha Beck

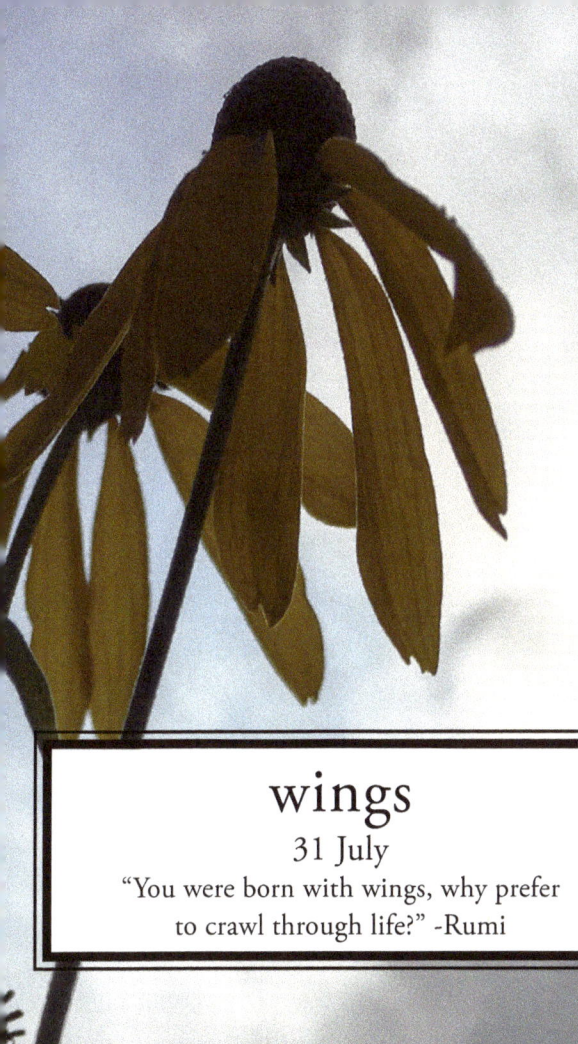

wings
31 July
"You were born with wings, why prefer to crawl through life?" -Rumi

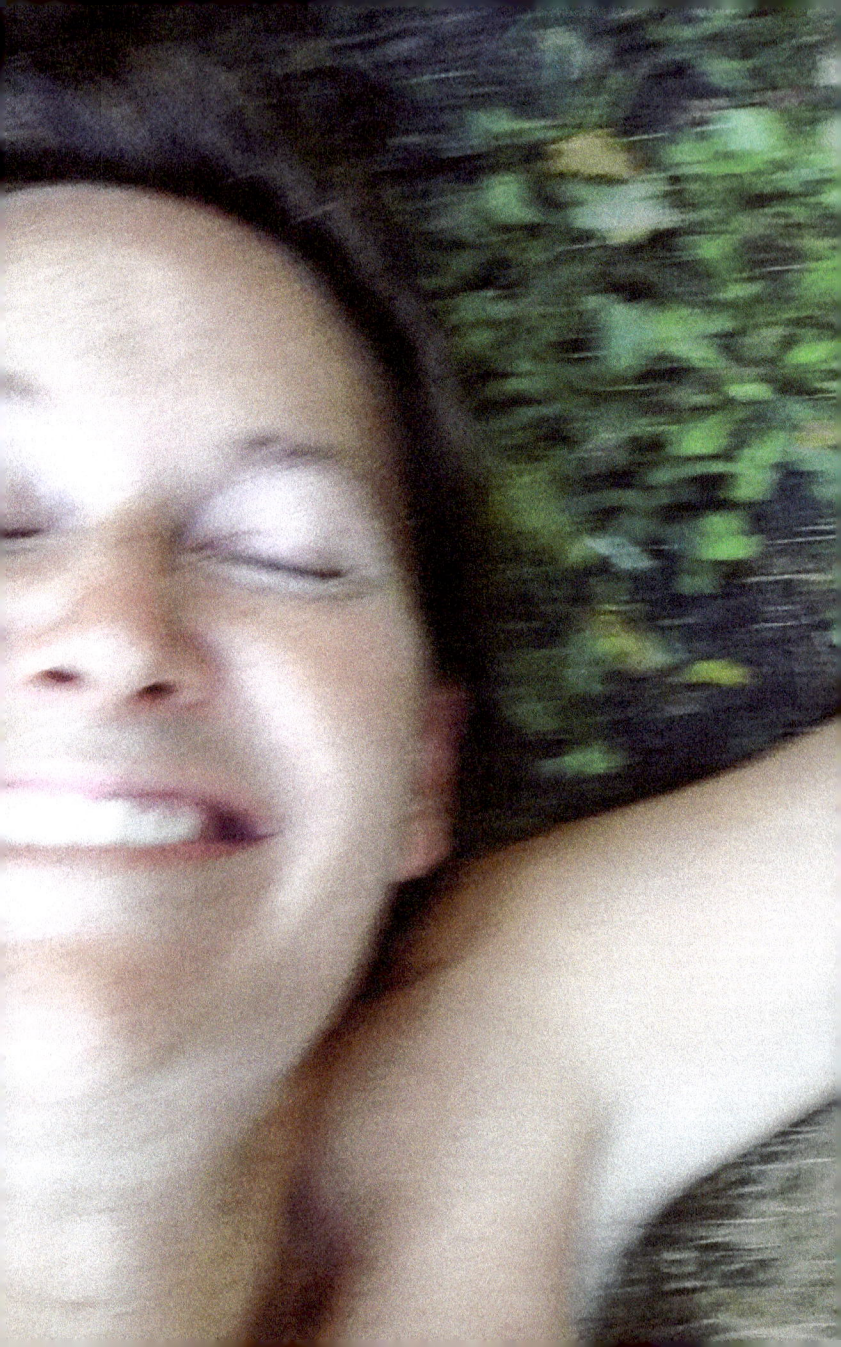

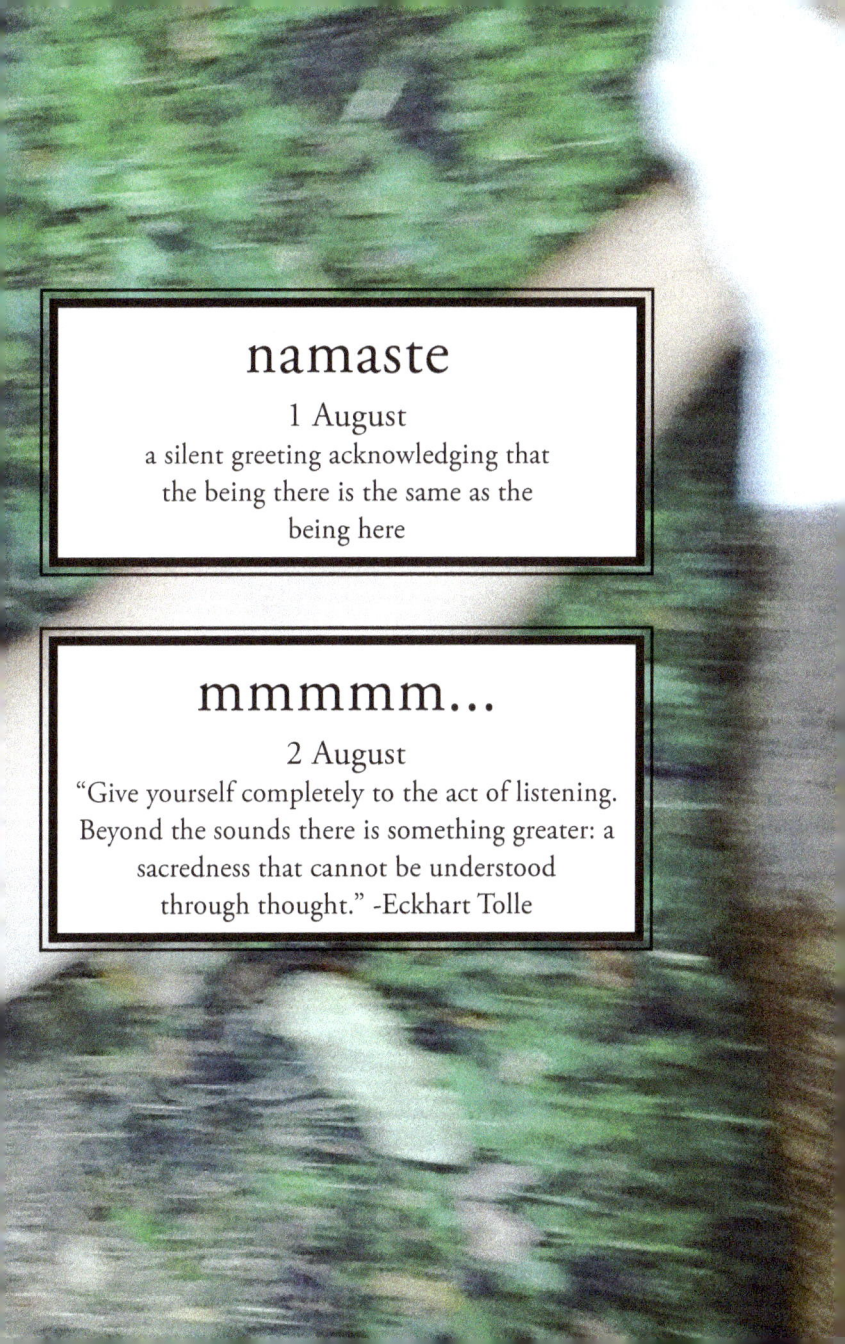

namaste

1 August
a silent greeting acknowledging that
the being there is the same as the
being here

mmmmm...

2 August
"Give yourself completely to the act of listening.
Beyond the sounds there is something greater: a
sacredness that cannot be understood
through thought." -Eckhart Tolle

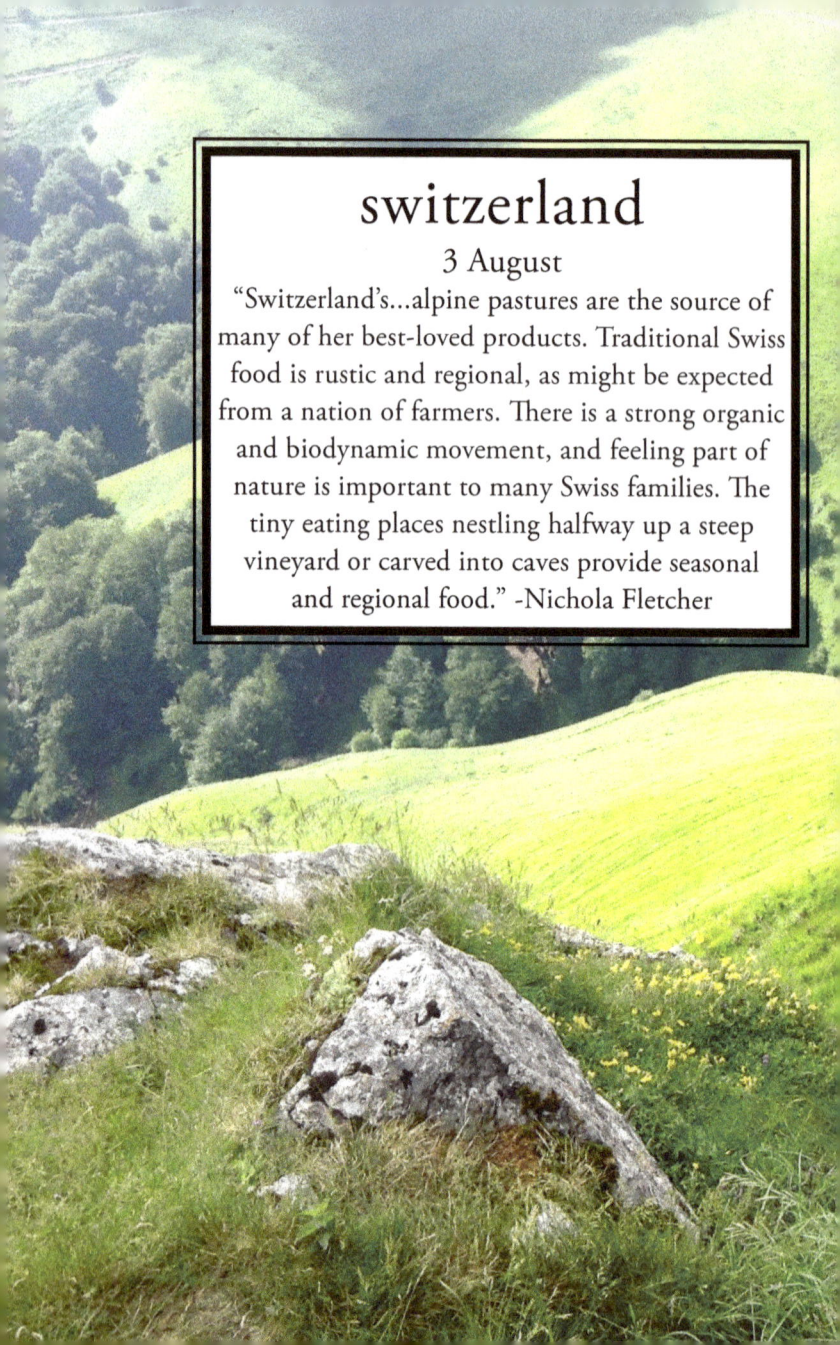

switzerland

3 August

"Switzerland's...alpine pastures are the source of many of her best-loved products. Traditional Swiss food is rustic and regional, as might be expected from a nation of farmers. There is a strong organic and biodynamic movement, and feeling part of nature is important to many Swiss families. The tiny eating places nestling halfway up a steep vineyard or carved into caves provide seasonal and regional food." -Nichola Fletcher

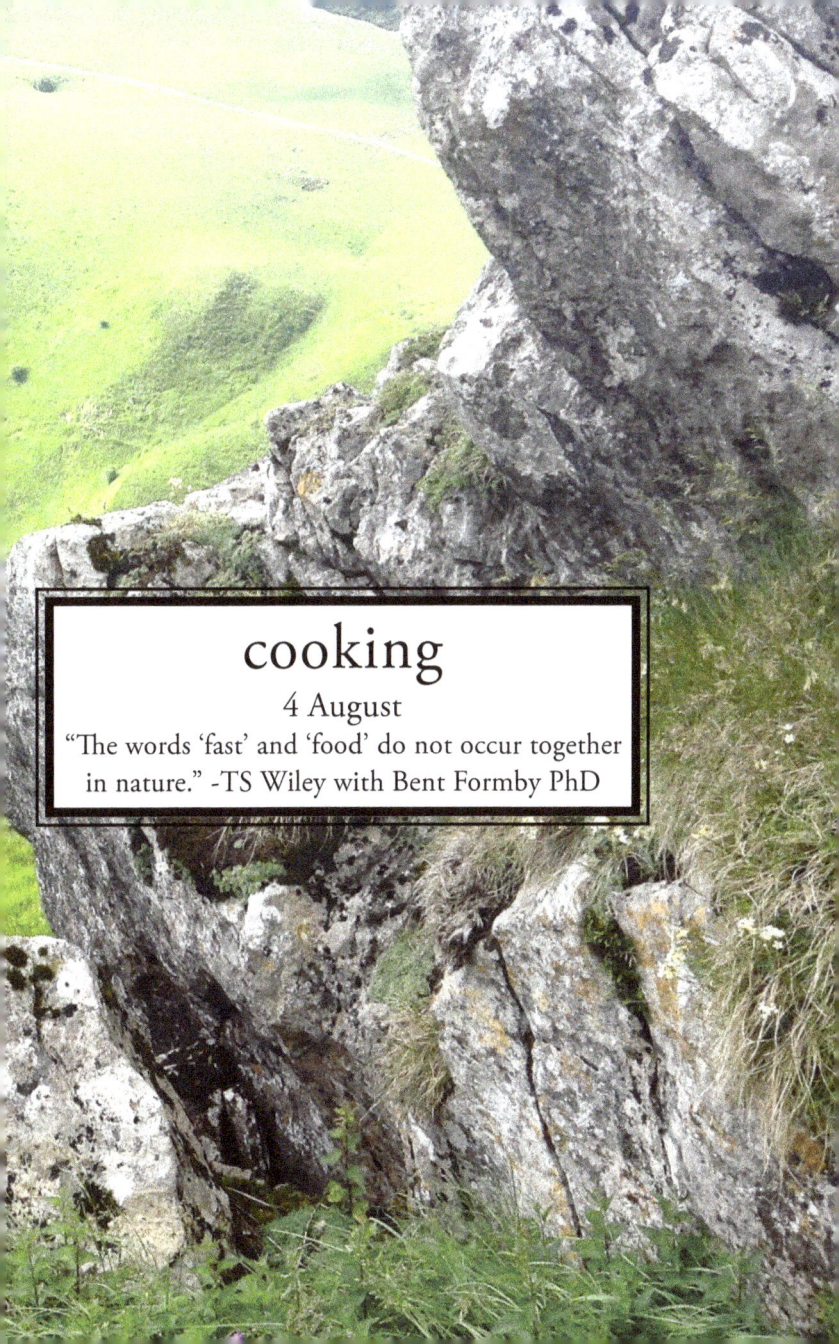

cooking
4 August
"The words 'fast' and 'food' do not occur together in nature." -TS Wiley with Bent Formby PhD

lovelution
5 August
revolution of love

god
6 August
"God is the word we use for infinite love."
-Jim Finley

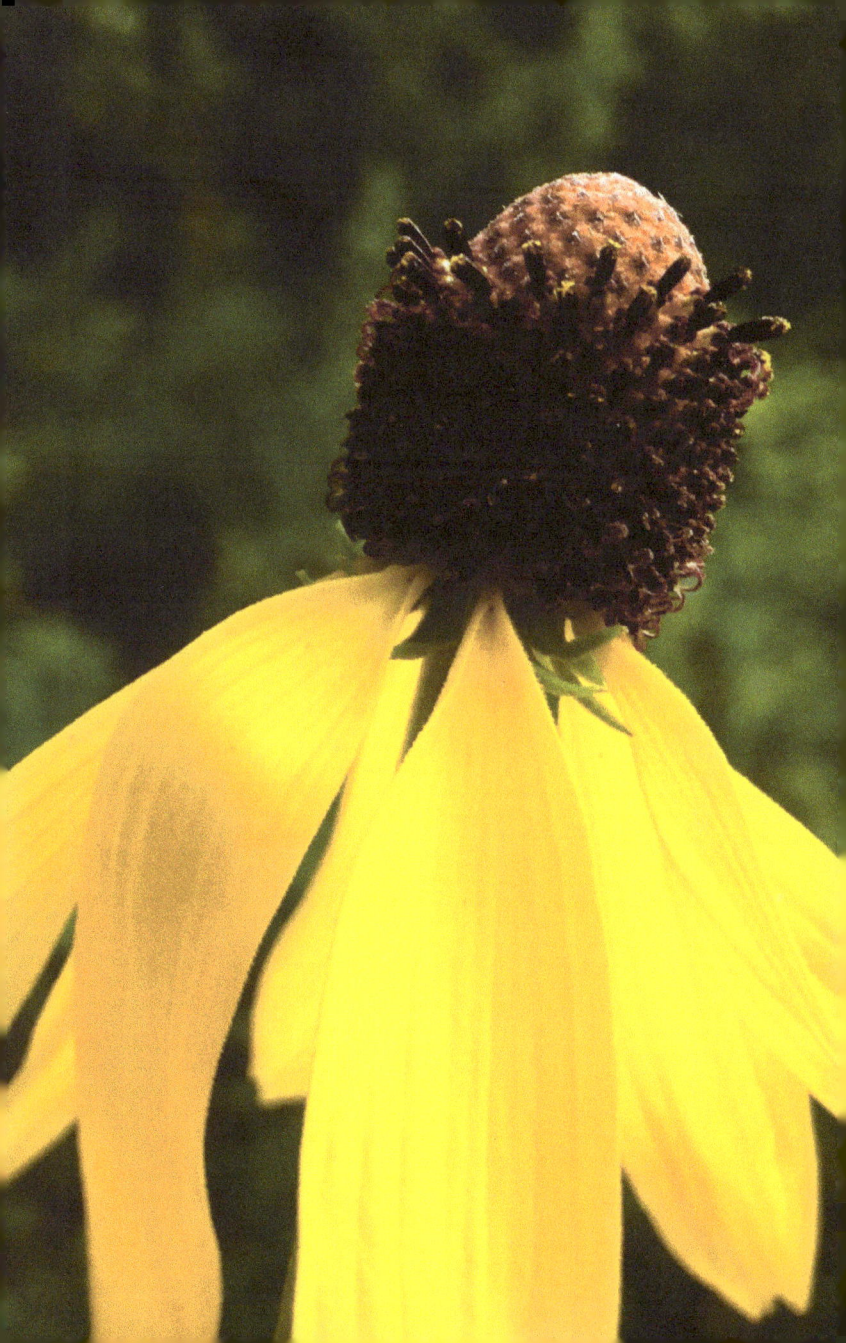

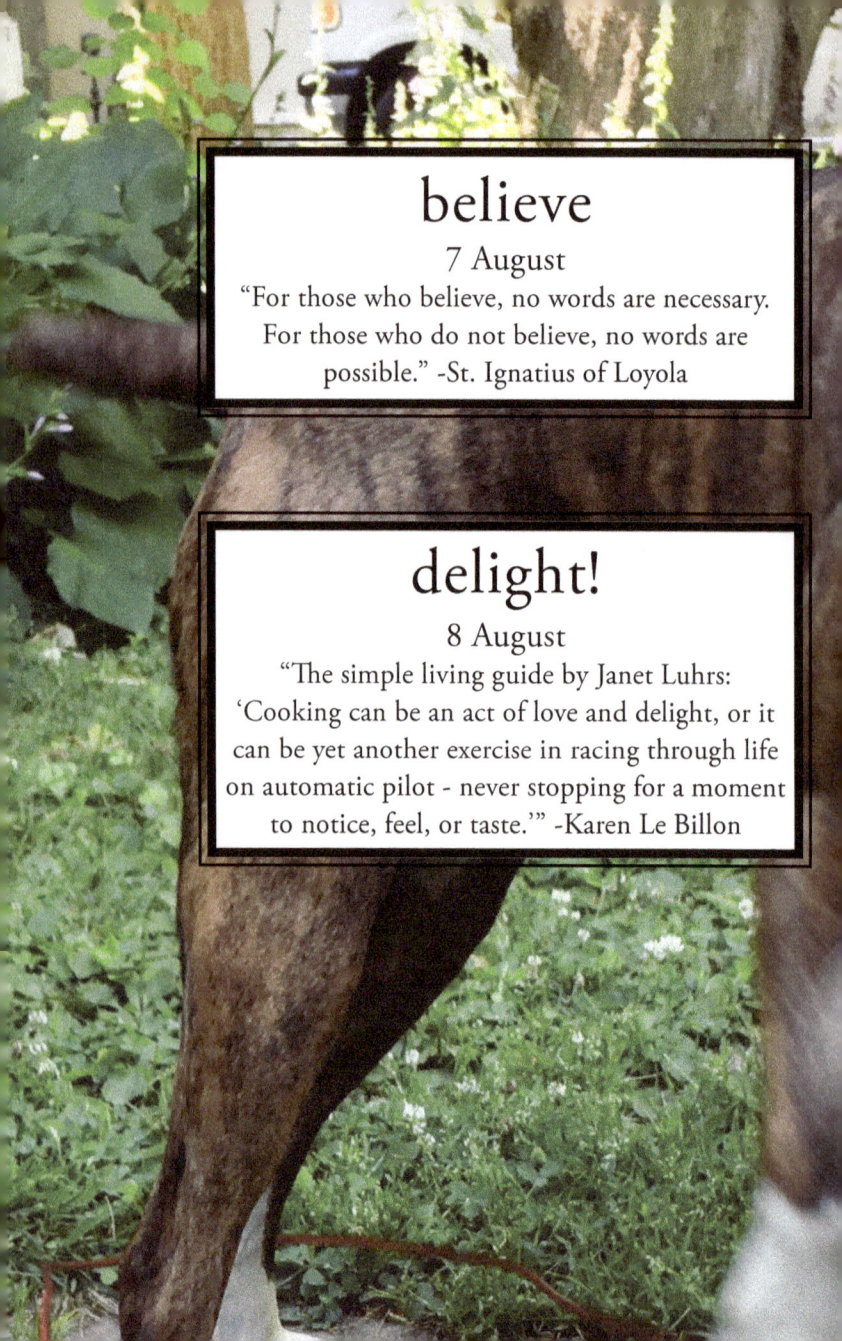

believe
7 August
"For those who believe, no words are necessary. For those who do not believe, no words are possible." -St. Ignatius of Loyola

delight!
8 August
"The simple living guide by Janet Luhrs: 'Cooking can be an act of love and delight, or it can be yet another exercise in racing through life on automatic pilot - never stopping for a moment to notice, feel, or taste.'" -Karen Le Billon

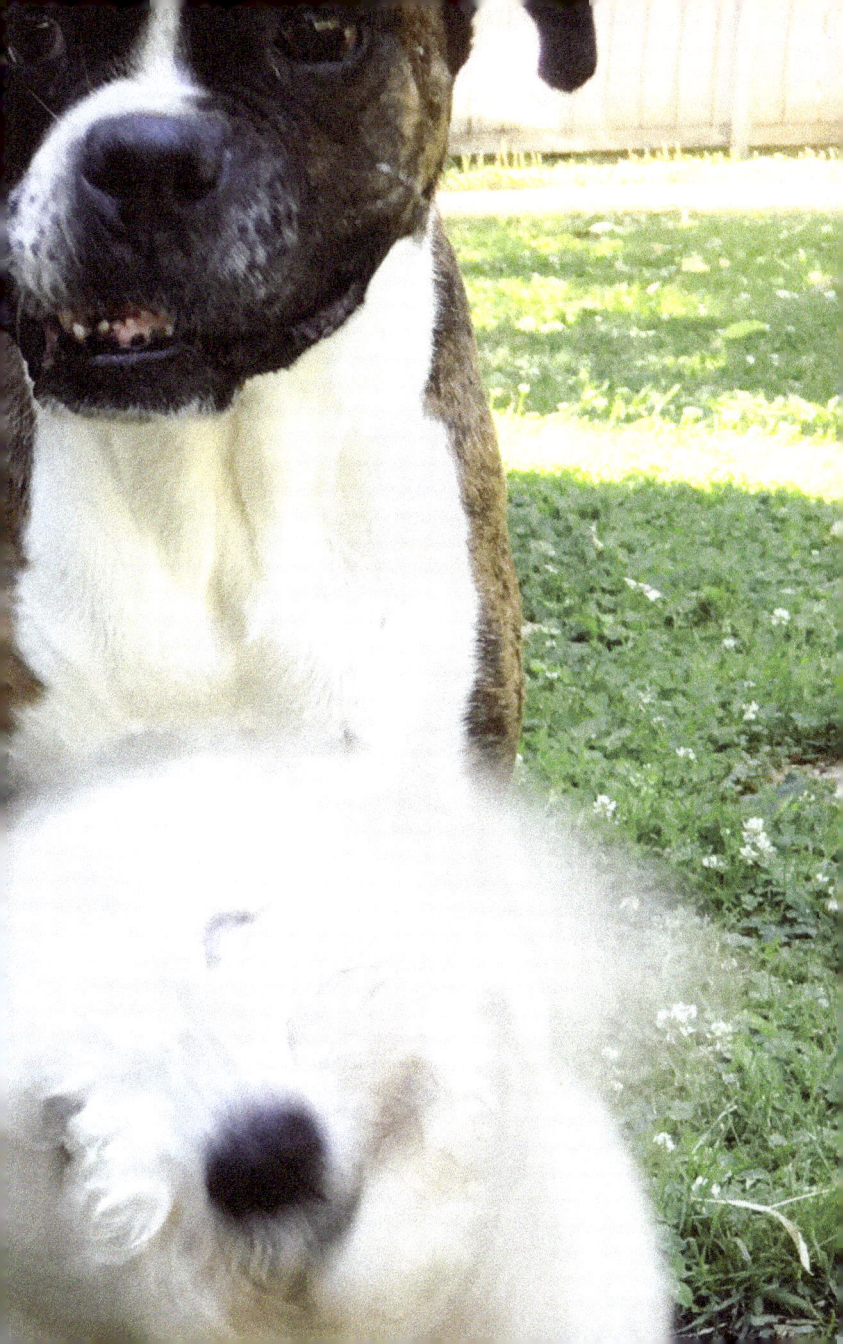

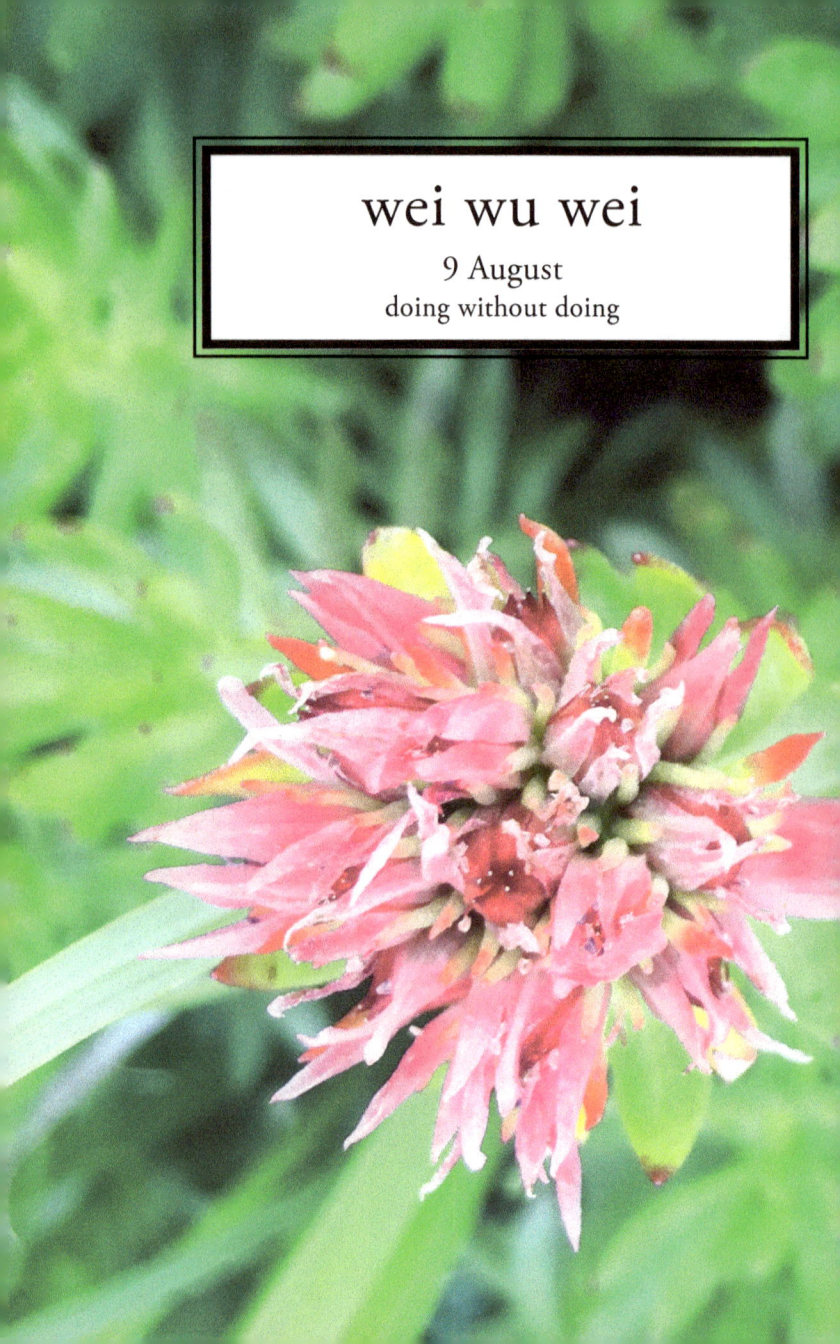

wei wu wei

9 August
doing without doing

munificence

10 August
very liberal in giving or bestowing

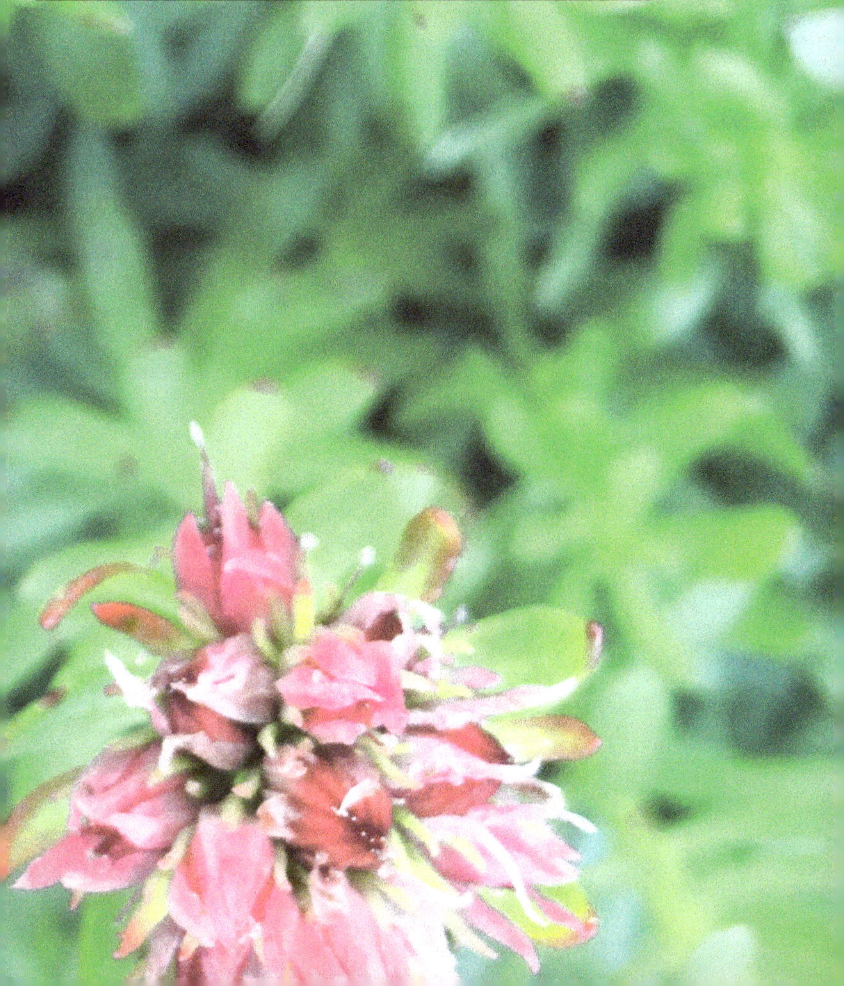

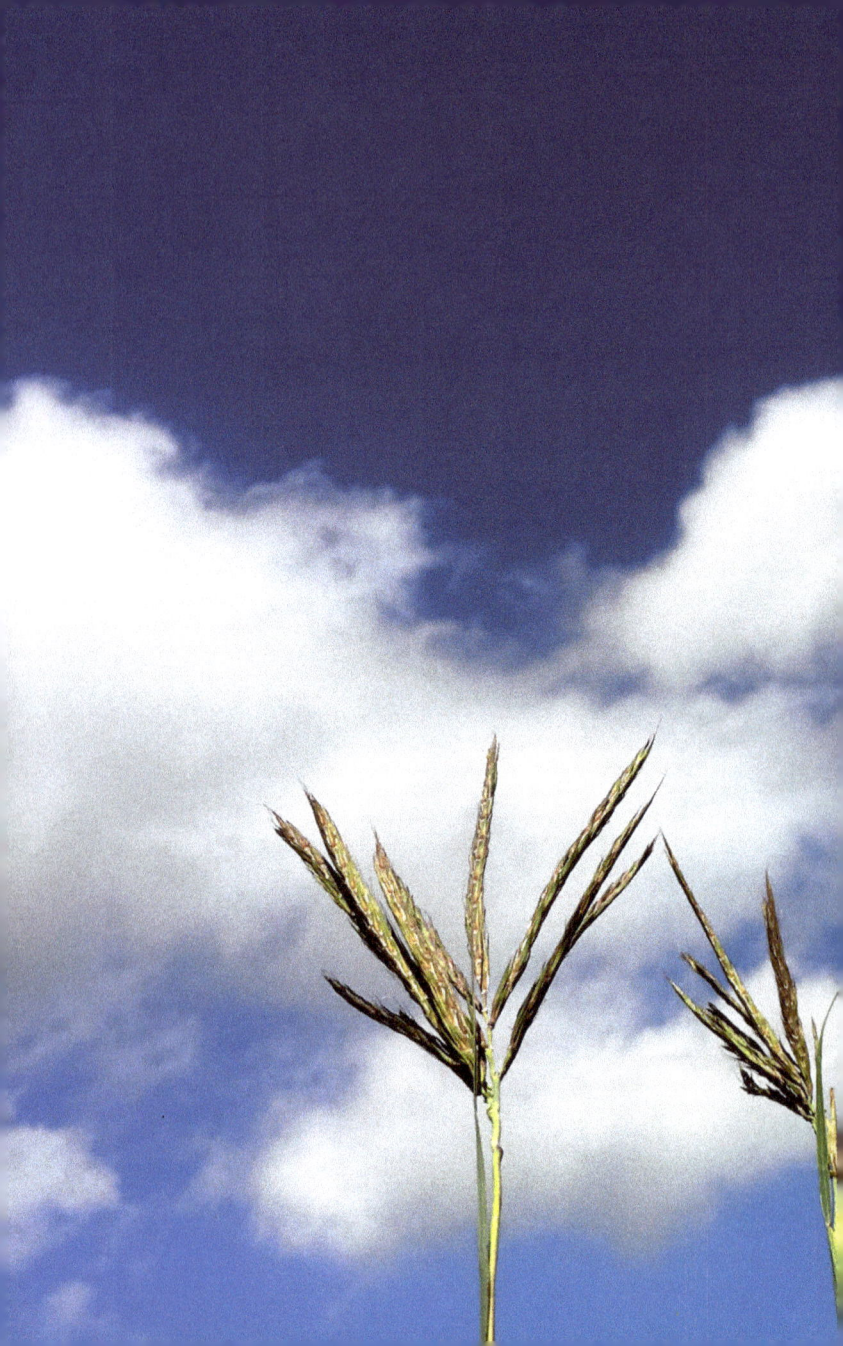

liberating to the soul
11 August
"You will realize your best destiny through the exercise of courage which means taking whatever action is most liberating to the soul even when you are afraid." -Martha Beck

the i am
12 August
"Ignore every bit of information that's directed at you if it in any way contradicts the I am you've placed in your imagination." -Wayne Dyer

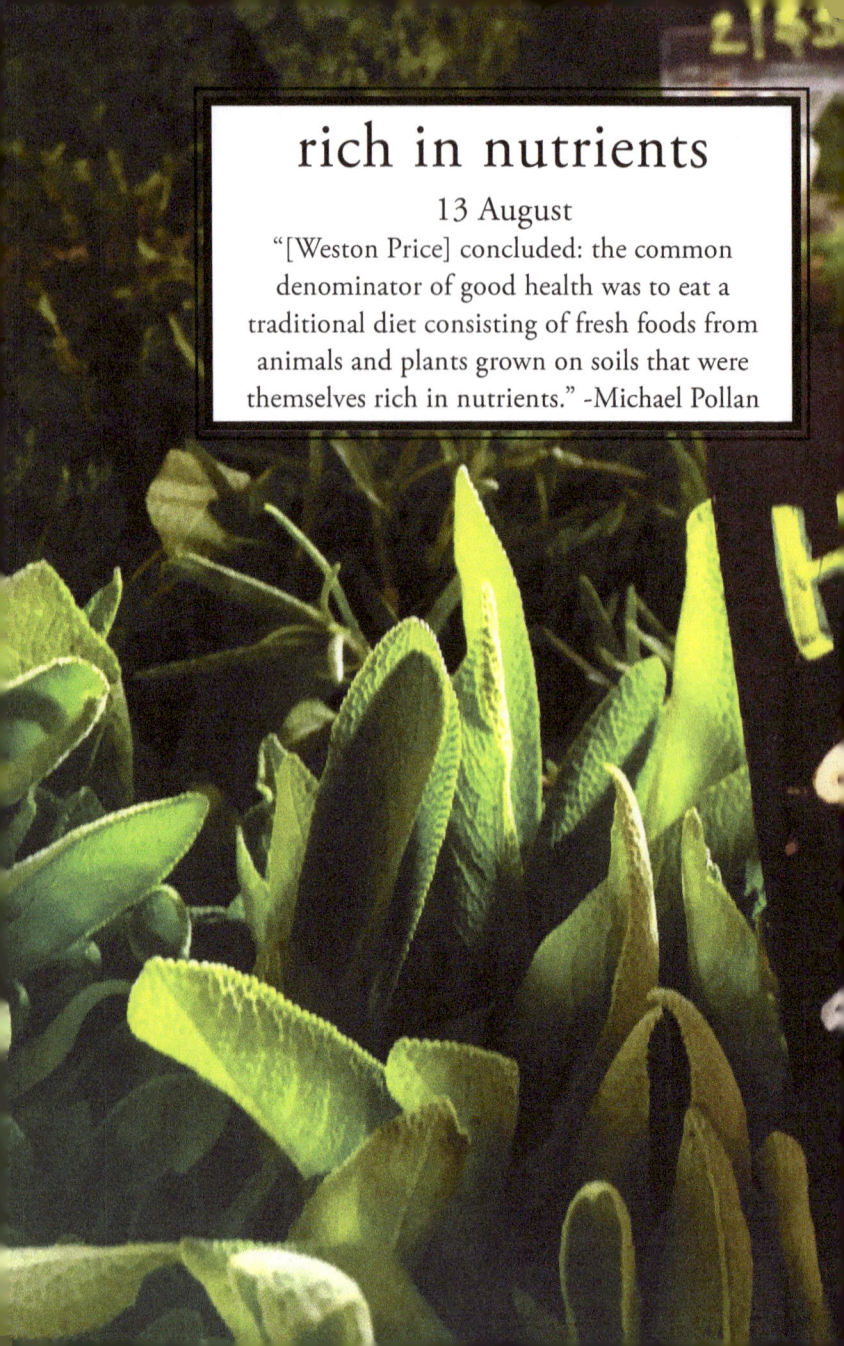

rich in nutrients

13 August

"[Weston Price] concluded: the common denominator of good health was to eat a traditional diet consisting of fresh foods from animals and plants grown on soils that were themselves rich in nutrients." -Michael Pollan

foncer, marquer

14 August
"Foncer, marquer to line a stew-pan or braising-pan with pork fat, vegetables, herbs and so on before putting in the meat."
-Elizabeth David

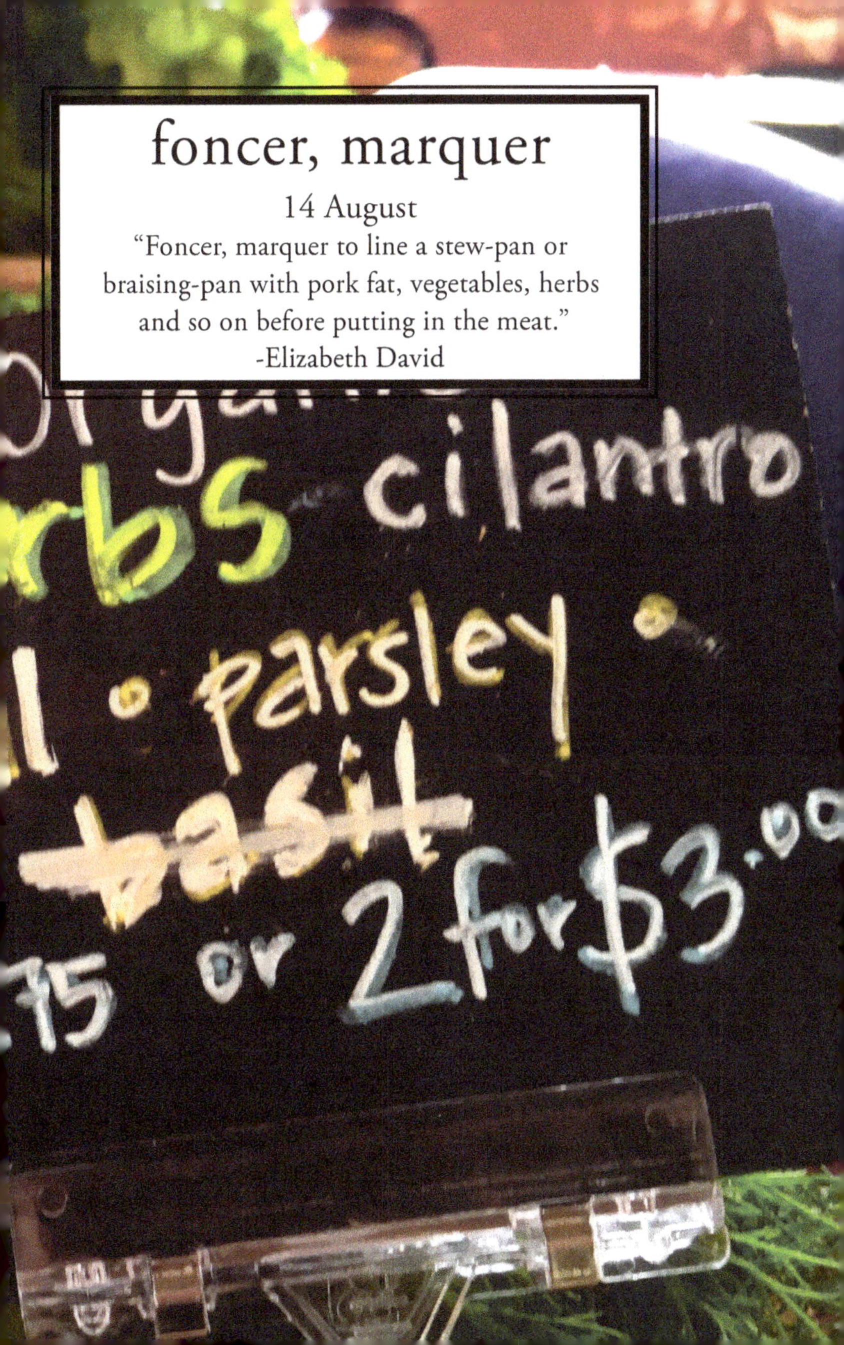

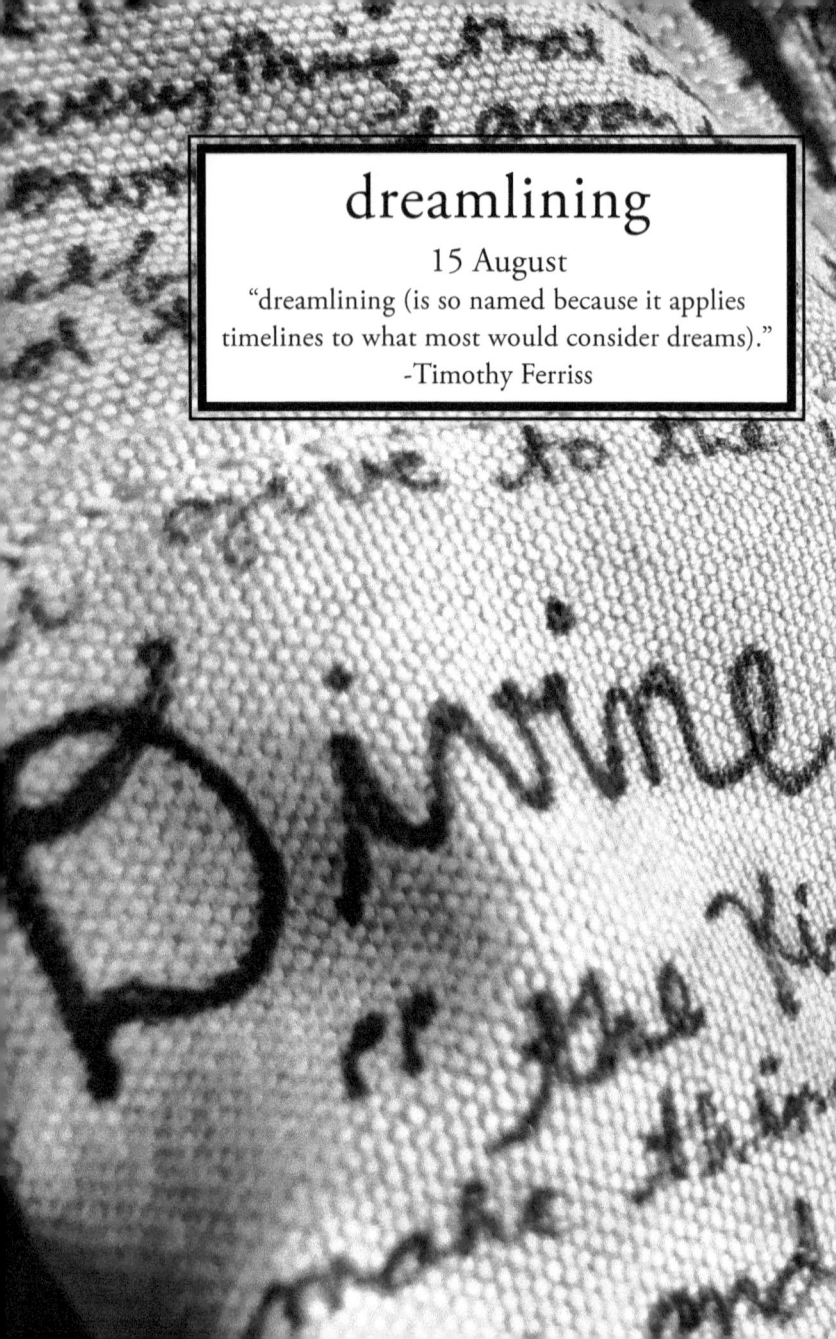

dreamlining

15 August

"dreamlining (is so named because it applies timelines to what most would consider dreams)."
-Timothy Ferriss

calm & happy

16 August

"Plato: he who is of calm and happy nature will hardly feel the pressure of age, but to him who is of an opposite disposition youth and age are equally a burden." -Paul Chek

walk with nature

17 August
"In every walk with Nature
one receives far more than he seeks."
-John Muir

liberation

18 August
"Liberation from the need to possess. And
liberation from conforming to a society built on
consumerism. This is the promise of minimalism:
to rejoice at the sight of all the things we do not
need. And to have our lives finally freed to pursue
the things we want to do." -Joshua Becker

ct Lake
E AREA

RIVER

l Forest

design

19 August

"Human beings are not designed to sit in the same place for hours on end. Research shows that sitting causes irreversible damage. In fact, sitting has even been labelled the new smoking."
-Anup Kanodia

upliftedness

20 August

"Eating and dressing well are ways of perking ourselves up and developing confidence in our basic goodness. It's a fine line, however, between taking pride in our appearance and being obsessed with it. Upliftedness is a way of expressing our human dignity; obsession is a way of wasting our life. Gradually, we get clear about this difference."
-Wayne Dyer

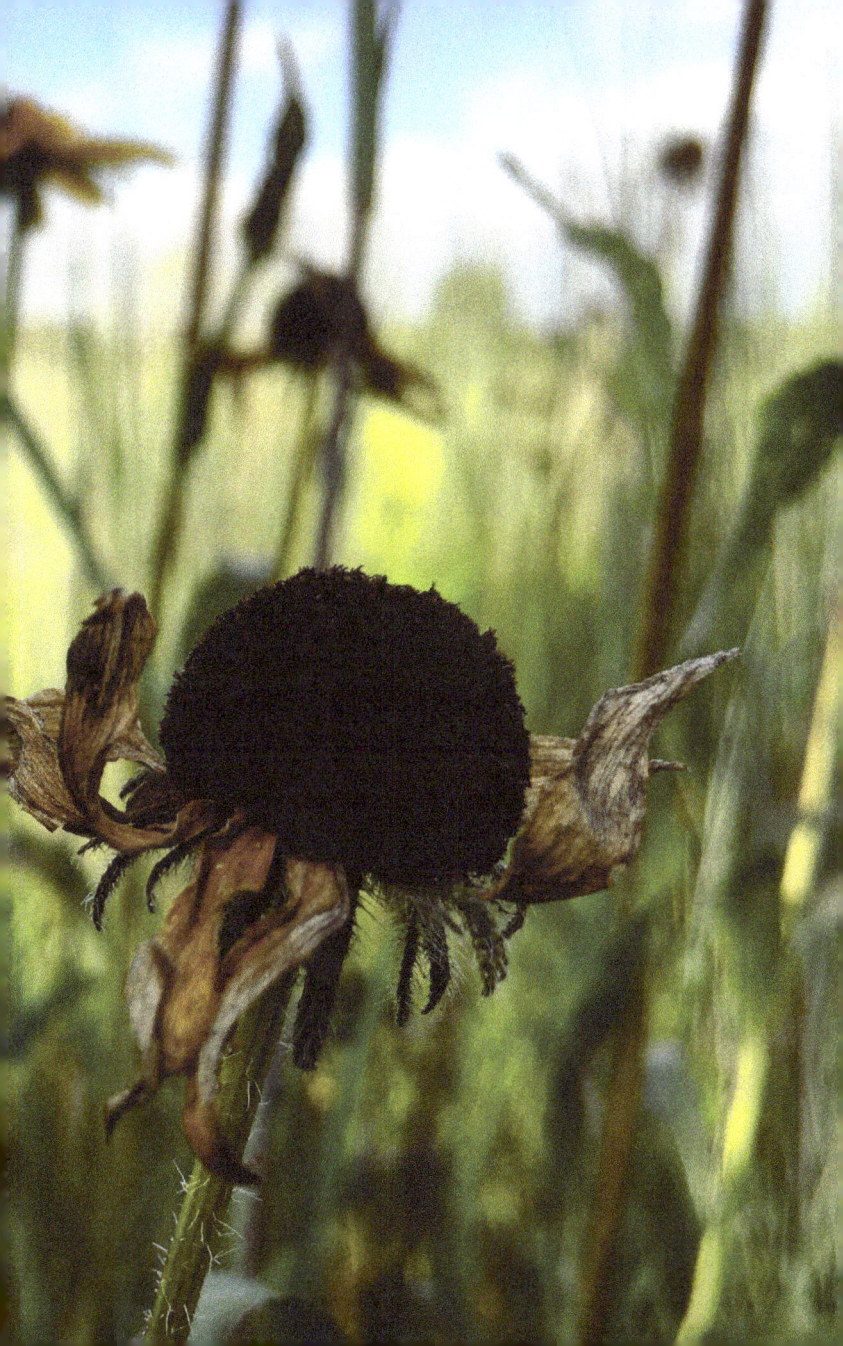

culinary transformations
21 August

"Fermentation happens...Yeast and bacteria are everywhere, in every breath we take and every bite we eat. Try as you might to eradicate them with antibacterial soaps and antibiotic drugs, there is no escaping them...Without them life could not be sustained. Certain microbial organisms can be harnessed to manifest extraordinary culinary transformations." -Sandor Ellix Katz

wild fermentation
22 August

"Live, unpasteurized, fermented foods have extraordinary nutritional value. They feed the bacteria which broke them down directly into your digestive system, where they keep breaking down food, aiding digestion and nutritional absorption." -Sandor Ellix Katz

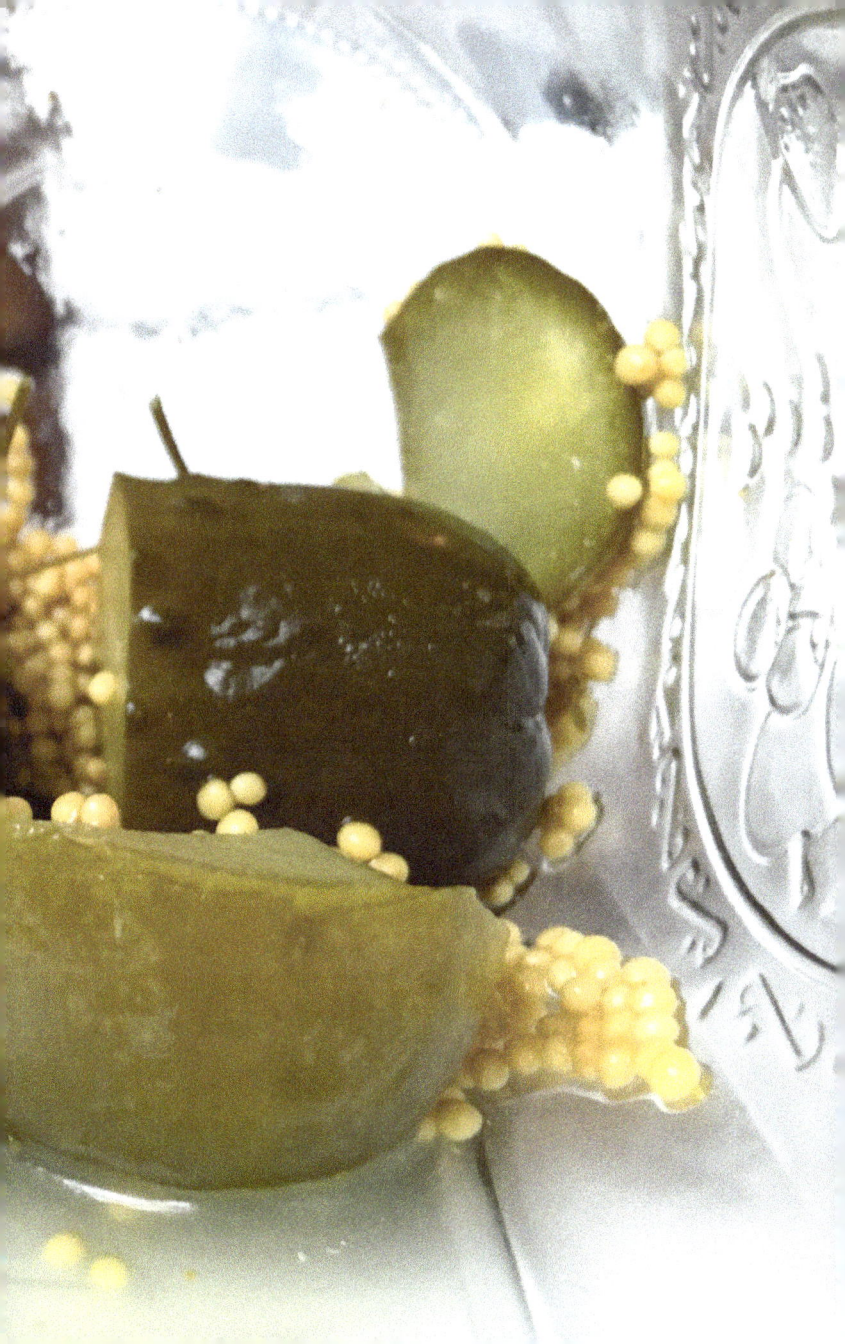

walking
23 August
"In places like rural Galacia, walking is an integral part of life…exercise for exercise's sake can be seen as rather ridiculous." -unknown

'work'
24 August
"It is us challenging the expectation that 'work' means sitting in front of a computer 9 to 5, 5 days a week." -Anup Kanodia

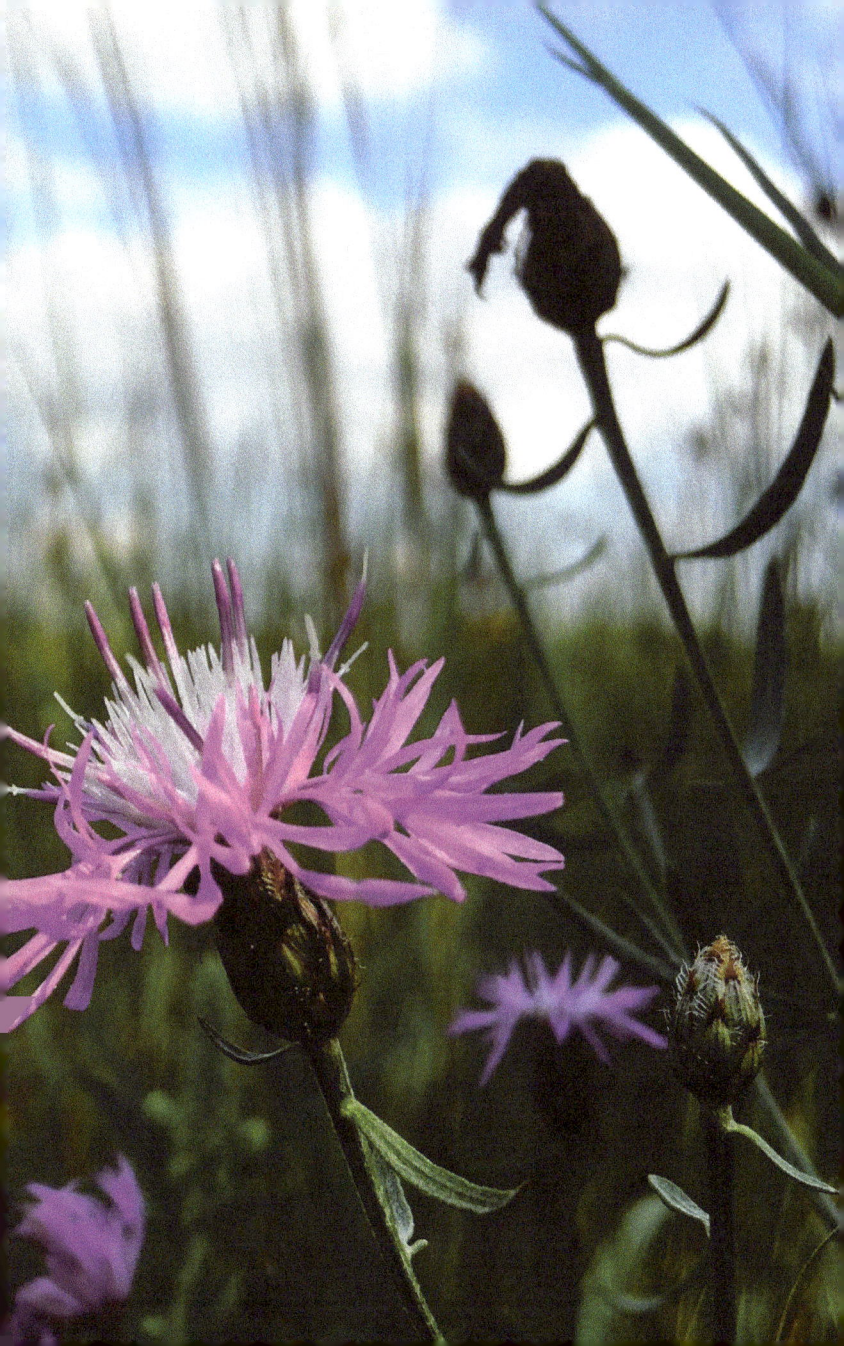

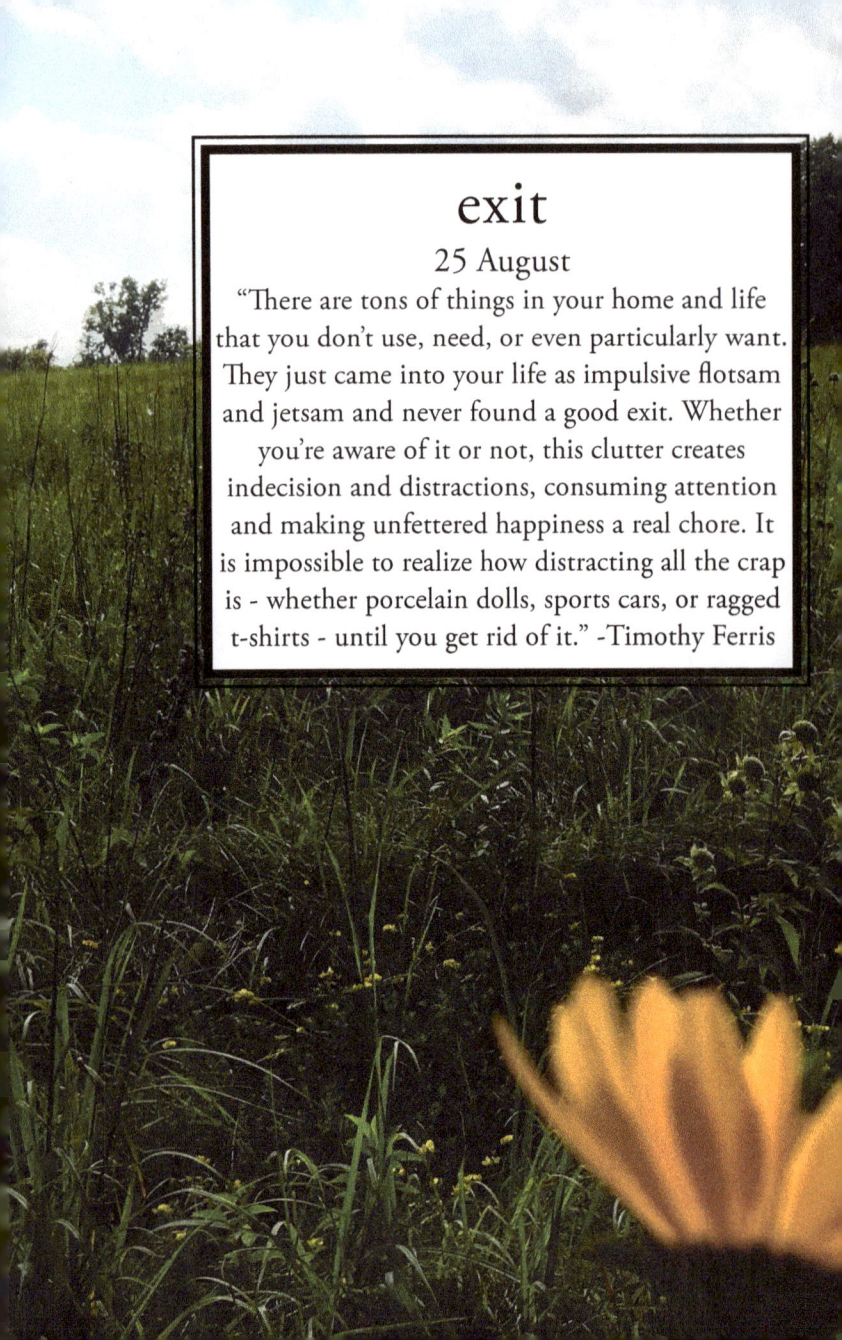

exit

25 August

"There are tons of things in your home and life that you don't use, need, or even particularly want. They just came into your life as impulsive flotsam and jetsam and never found a good exit. Whether you're aware of it or not, this clutter creates indecision and distractions, consuming attention and making unfettered happiness a real chore. It is impossible to realize how distracting all the crap is - whether porcelain dolls, sports cars, or ragged t-shirts - until you get rid of it." -Timothy Ferris

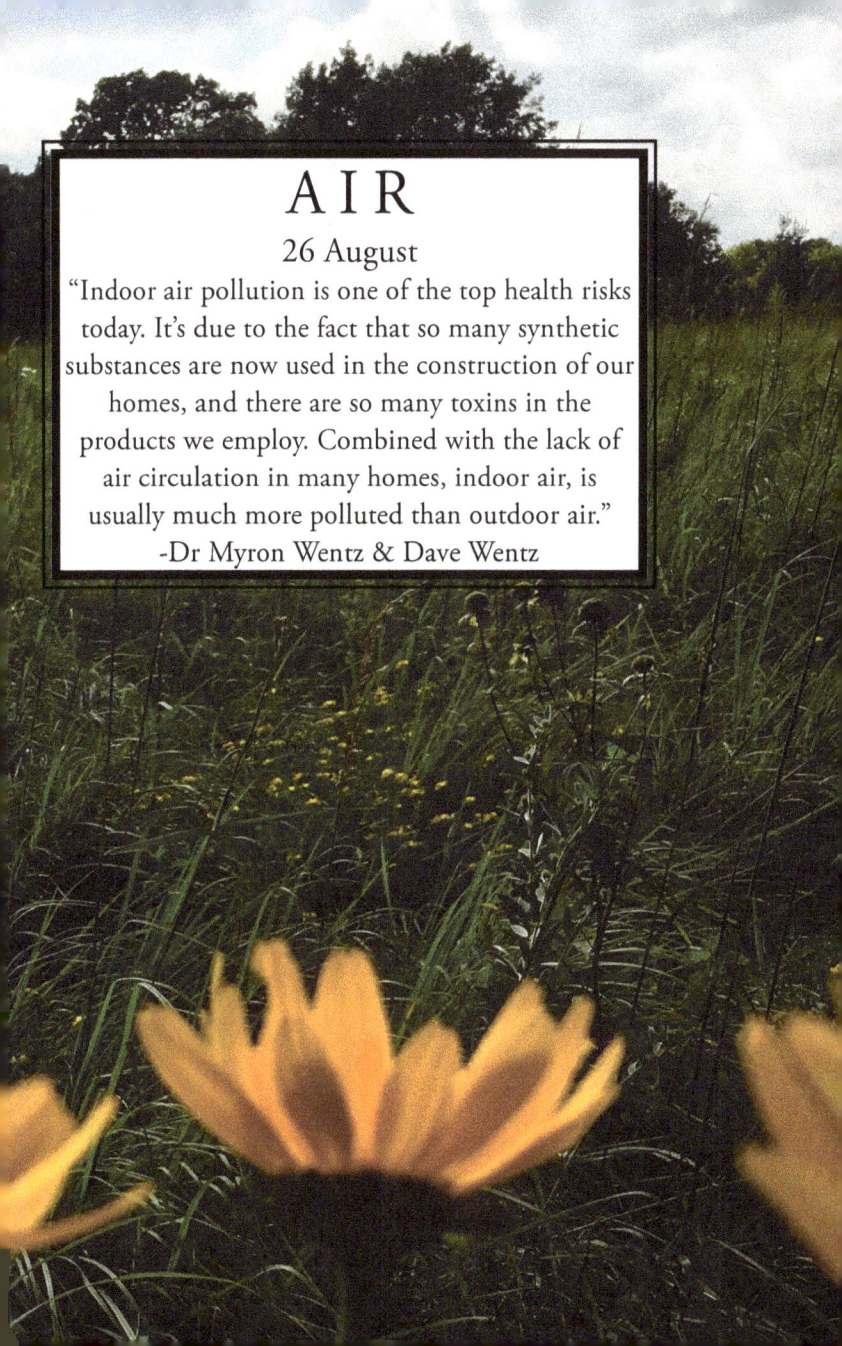

AIR
26 August
"Indoor air pollution is one of the top health risks today. It's due to the fact that so many synthetic substances are now used in the construction of our homes, and there are so many toxins in the products we employ. Combined with the lack of air circulation in many homes, indoor air, is usually much more polluted than outdoor air."
-Dr Myron Wentz & Dave Wentz

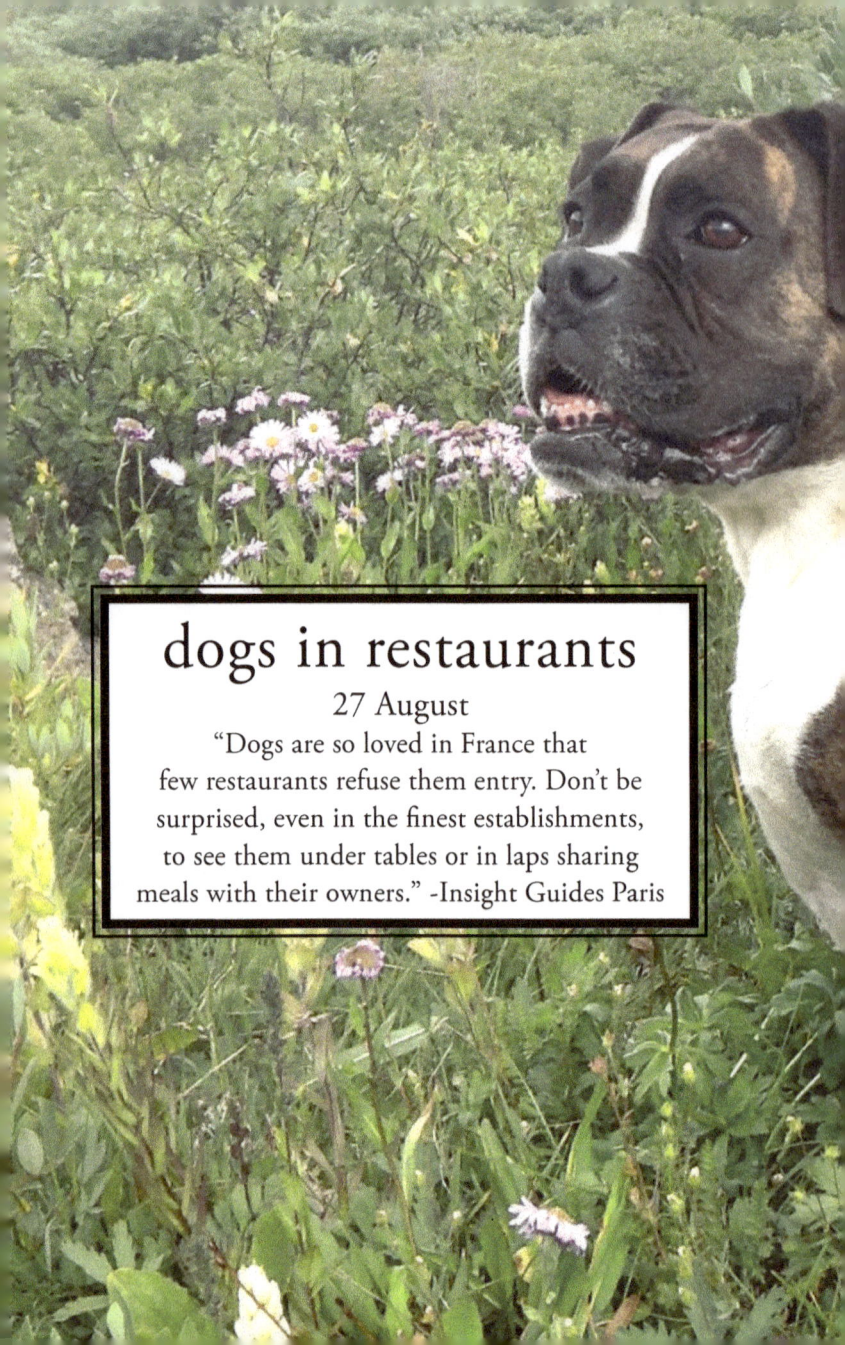

dogs in restaurants
27 August
"Dogs are so loved in France that few restaurants refuse them entry. Don't be surprised, even in the finest establishments, to see them under tables or in laps sharing meals with their owners." -Insight Guides Paris

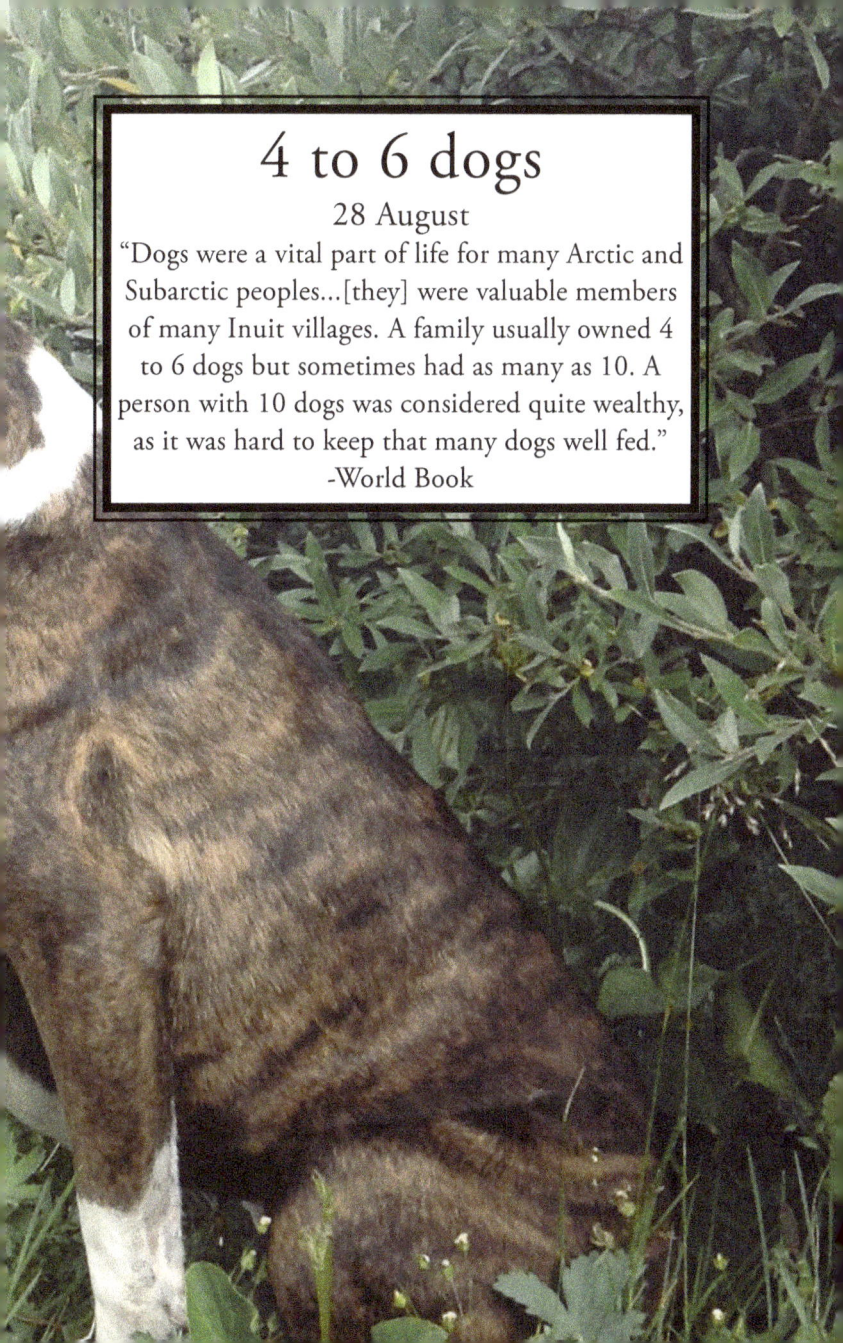

4 to 6 dogs
28 August

"Dogs were a vital part of life for many Arctic and Subarctic peoples...[they] were valuable members of many Inuit villages. A family usually owned 4 to 6 dogs but sometimes had as many as 10. A person with 10 dogs was considered quite wealthy, as it was hard to keep that many dogs well fed."
-World Book

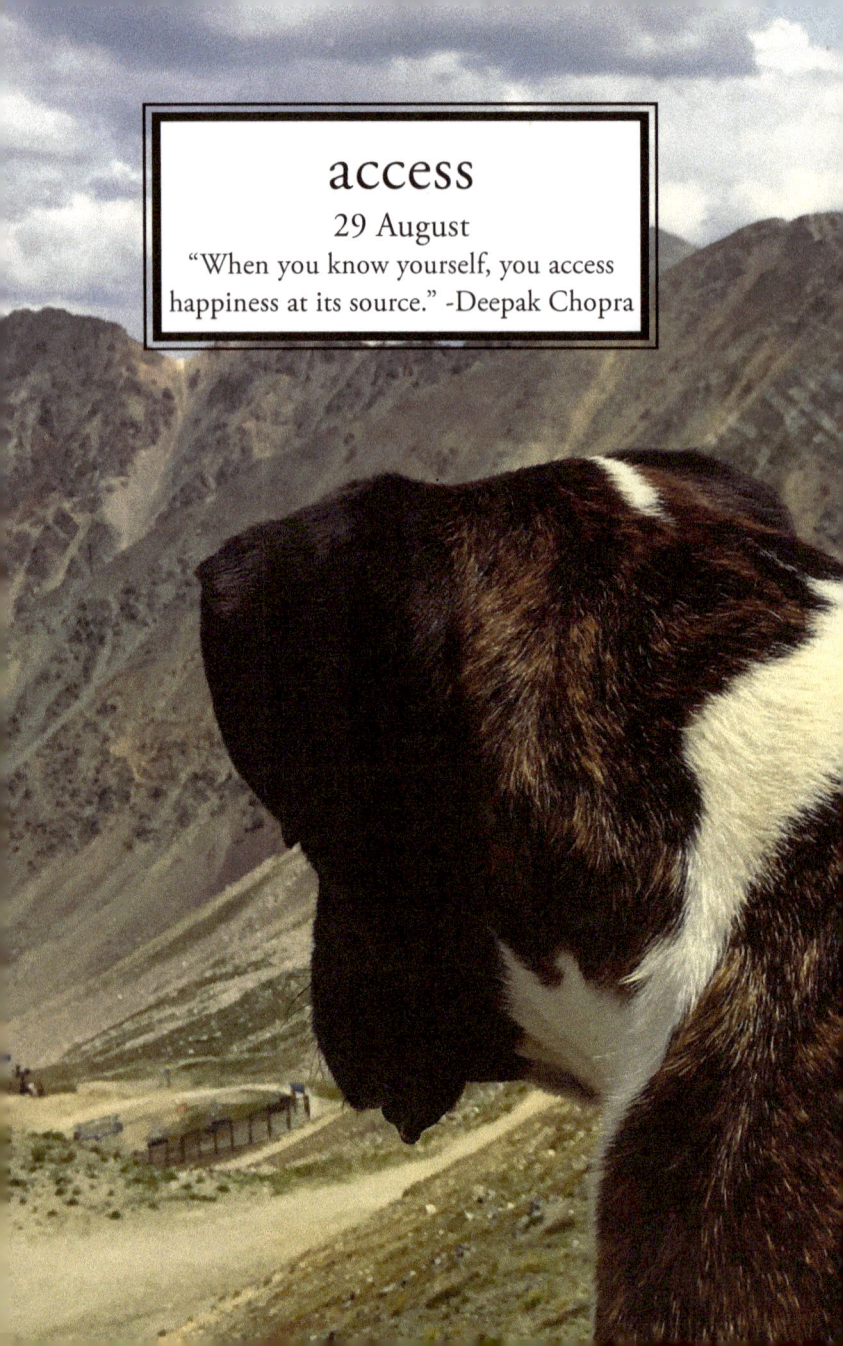

access

29 August

"When you know yourself, you access happiness at its source." -Deepak Chopra

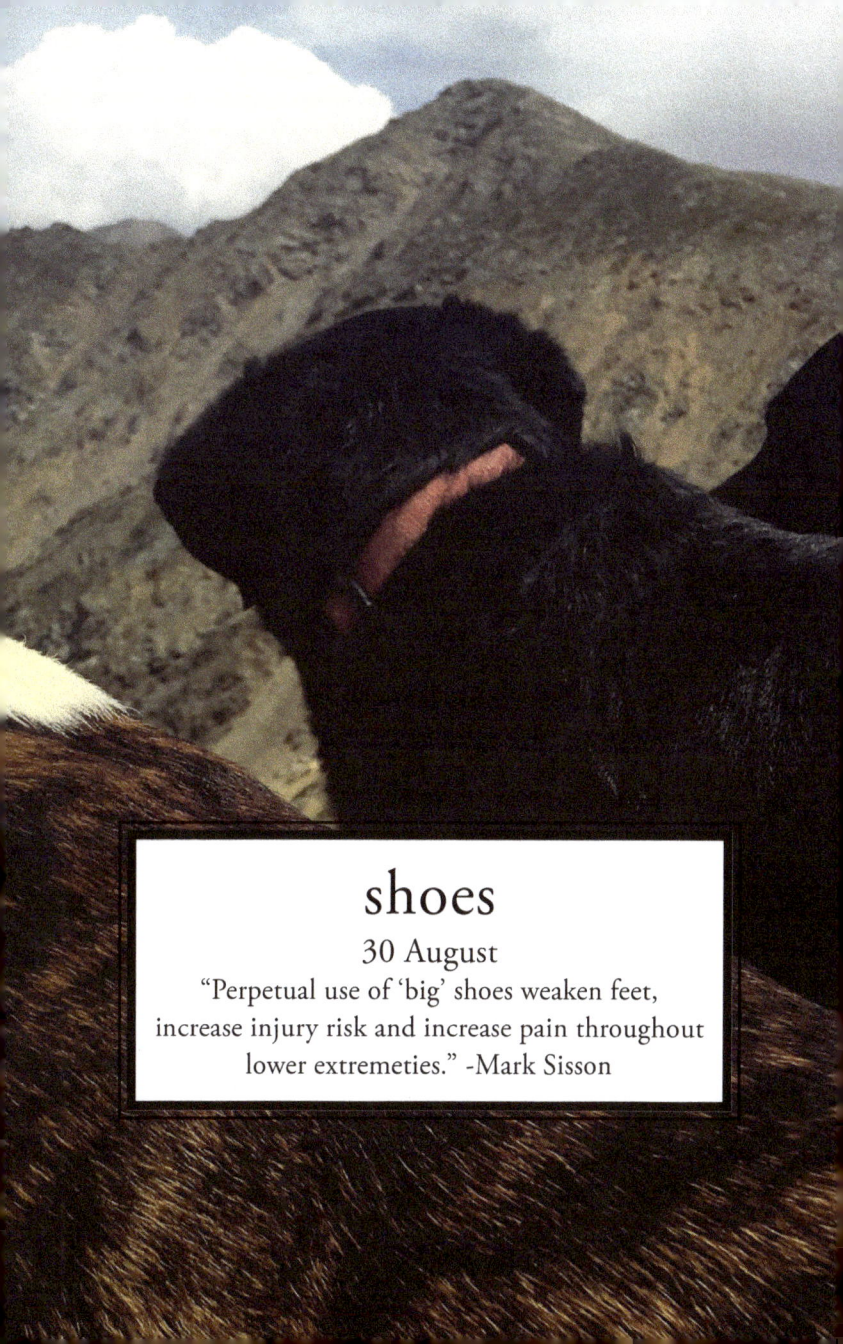

shoes
30 August
"Perpetual use of 'big' shoes weaken feet, increase injury risk and increase pain throughout lower extremeties." -Mark Sisson

test results

31 August

She would like to see how her lipids are doing on her current diet (mainly meat and fat).

component results:

cholesterol, total: 247 (H)

triglycerides: 24 (L)

HDL cholesterol: 135

LDL cholesterol: 107

chol/hdl ratio: 1.83

"I've never seen test results like these!" ob gyn

"I've never seen test results like these!" md

eating

1 September

usually once a day - mornings

+60% fat made by nature (pork fat, butter, raw cheese, olive oil, coconut oil, duck fat, beef fat)

+15% protein made by nature (grass-fed meat, liver, bone broth, soy-free eggs, raw cheese, fish, seafood)

+10% carbohydrates made by nature (herbs, pickles, lemon, lime, raw cheese, avocado, microgreens...)

health: impeccable

happiness: 300%!!!!!

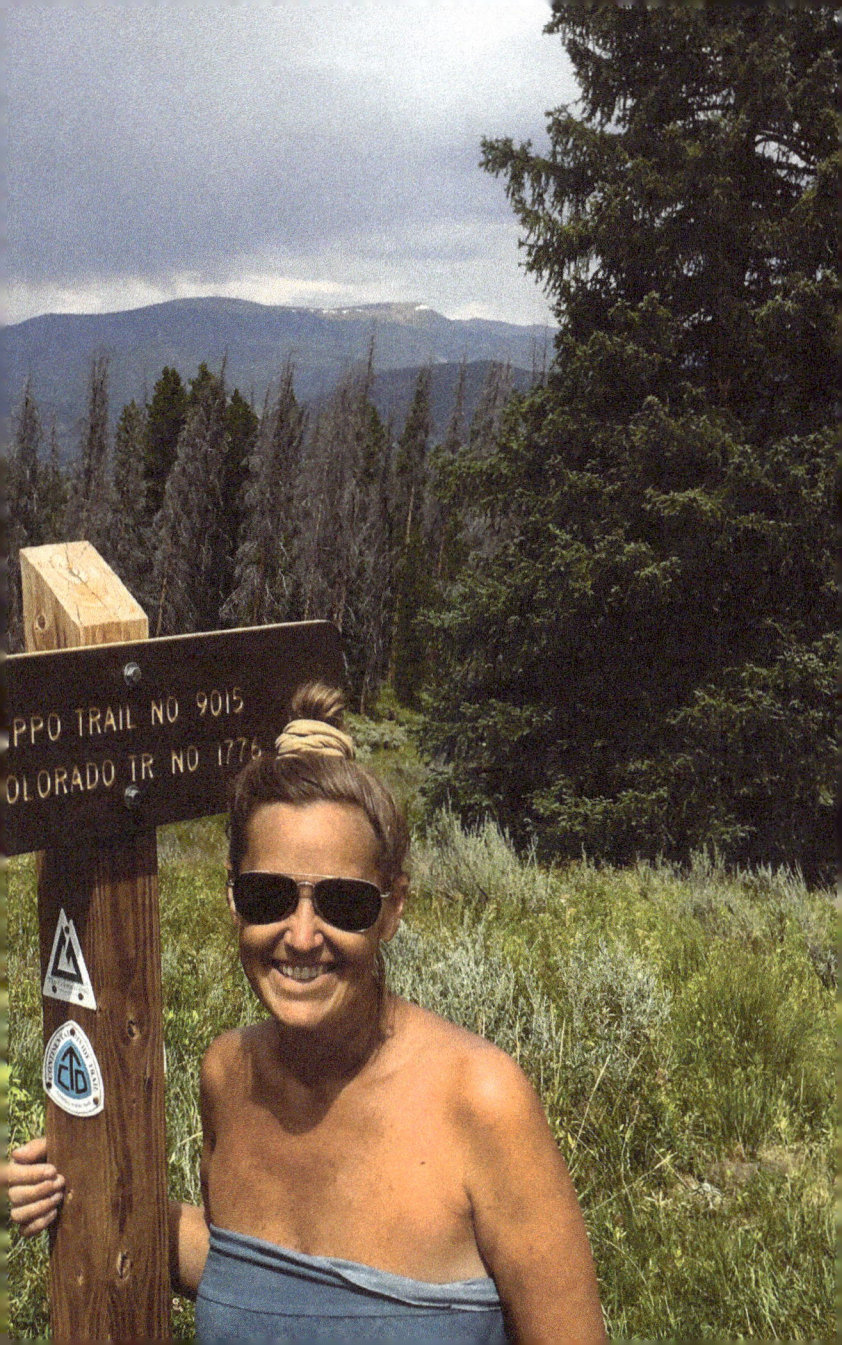

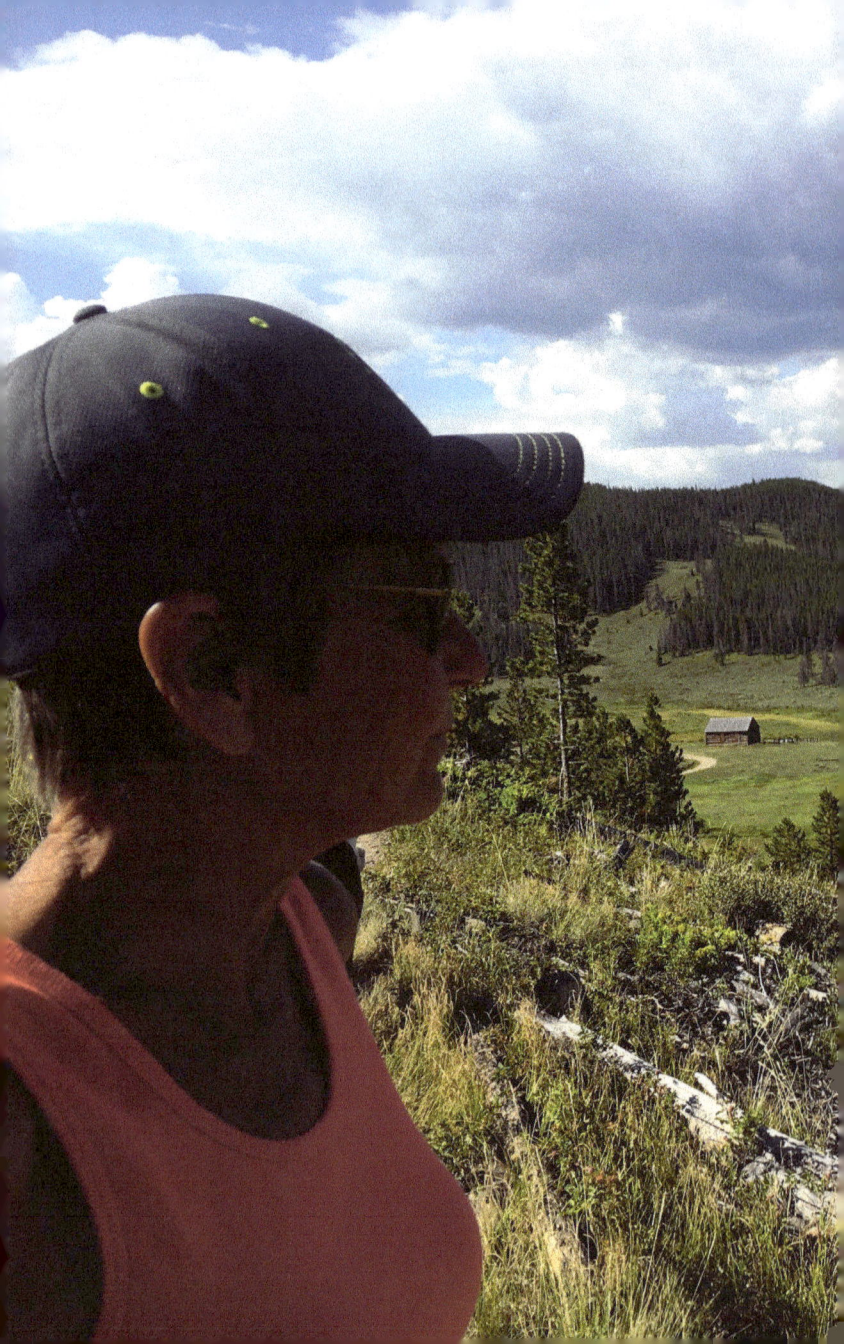

awareness
2 September
"Aching, longing, hungering and thirsting are the signals by which our authentic selves call us toward our Destiny. To eradicate our awareness of these sensations is to lose our place in the universe." -Martha Beck

magic
3 September
"Doing what you want as opposed to what you feel obligated to do." -Timothy Ferriss

lovestars
4 September
"The story of your best destiny is already written in the stars." -Martha Beck

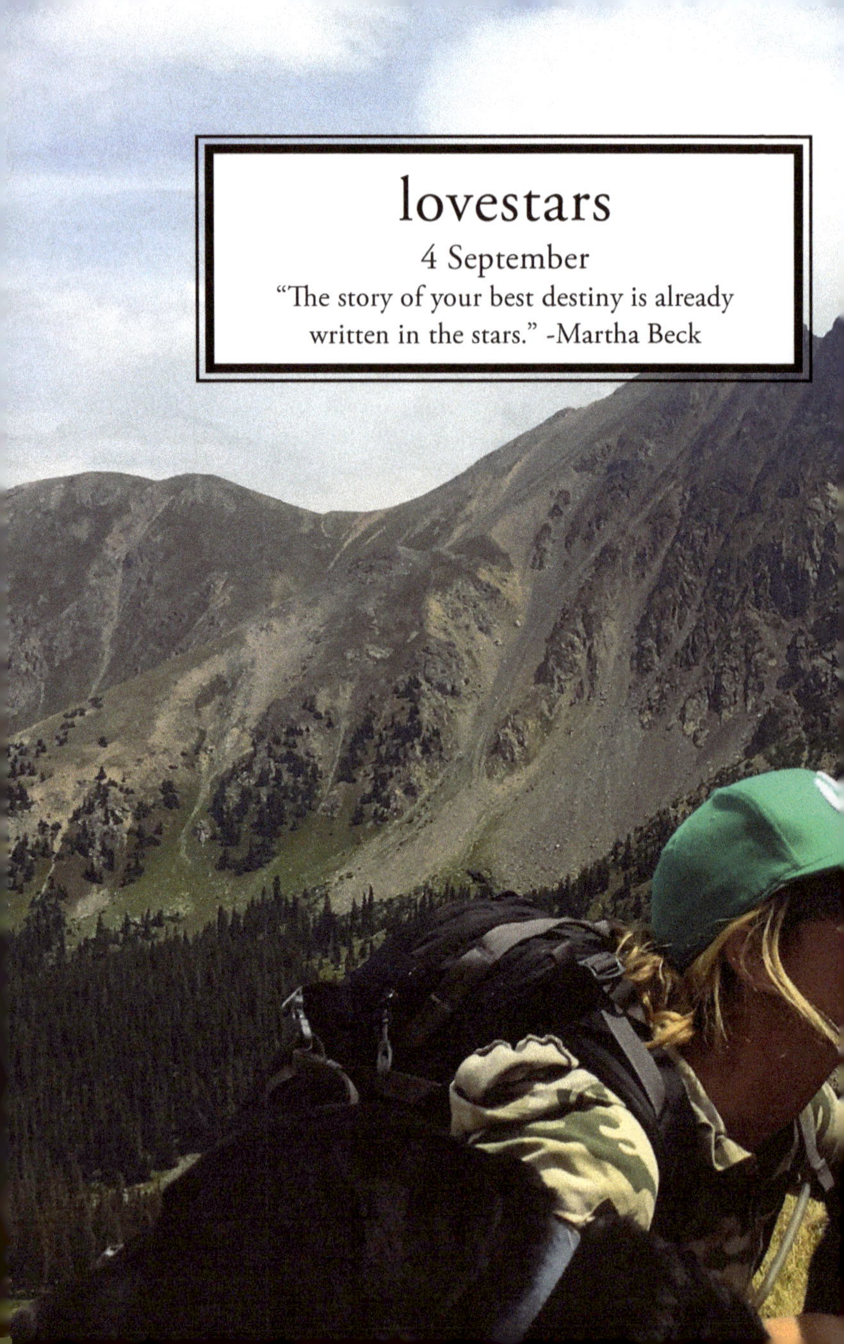

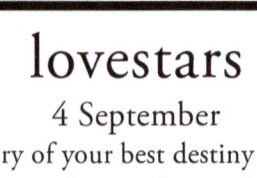

LoveFinder

5 September

"Be a LoveFinder! (There are no ordinary moments) kicking a ball around with a child, watching the shape of the clouds, hearing the sounds of the seasons, saying goodnight to a loved one - every single experience of life is an opportunity to experience gratitude."
-Wayne Dyer

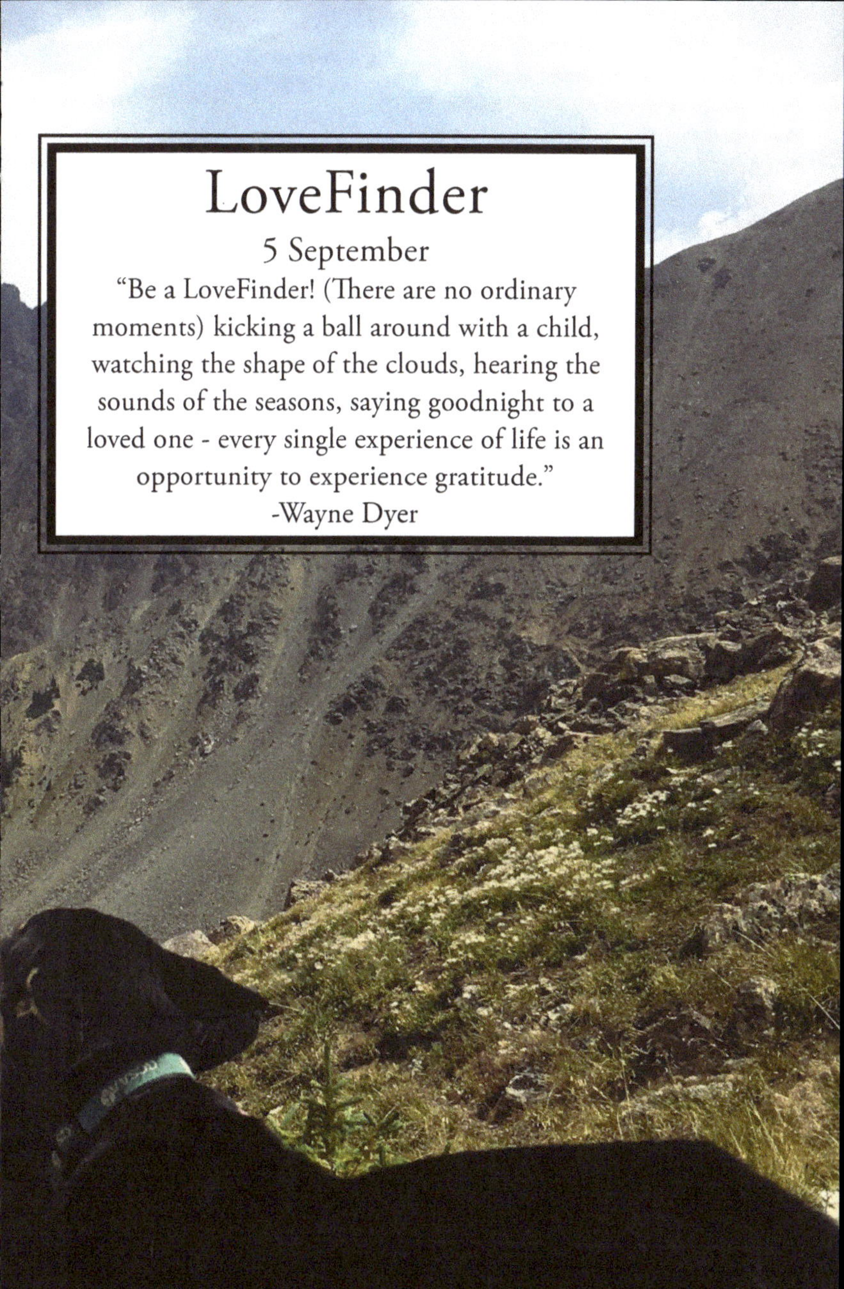

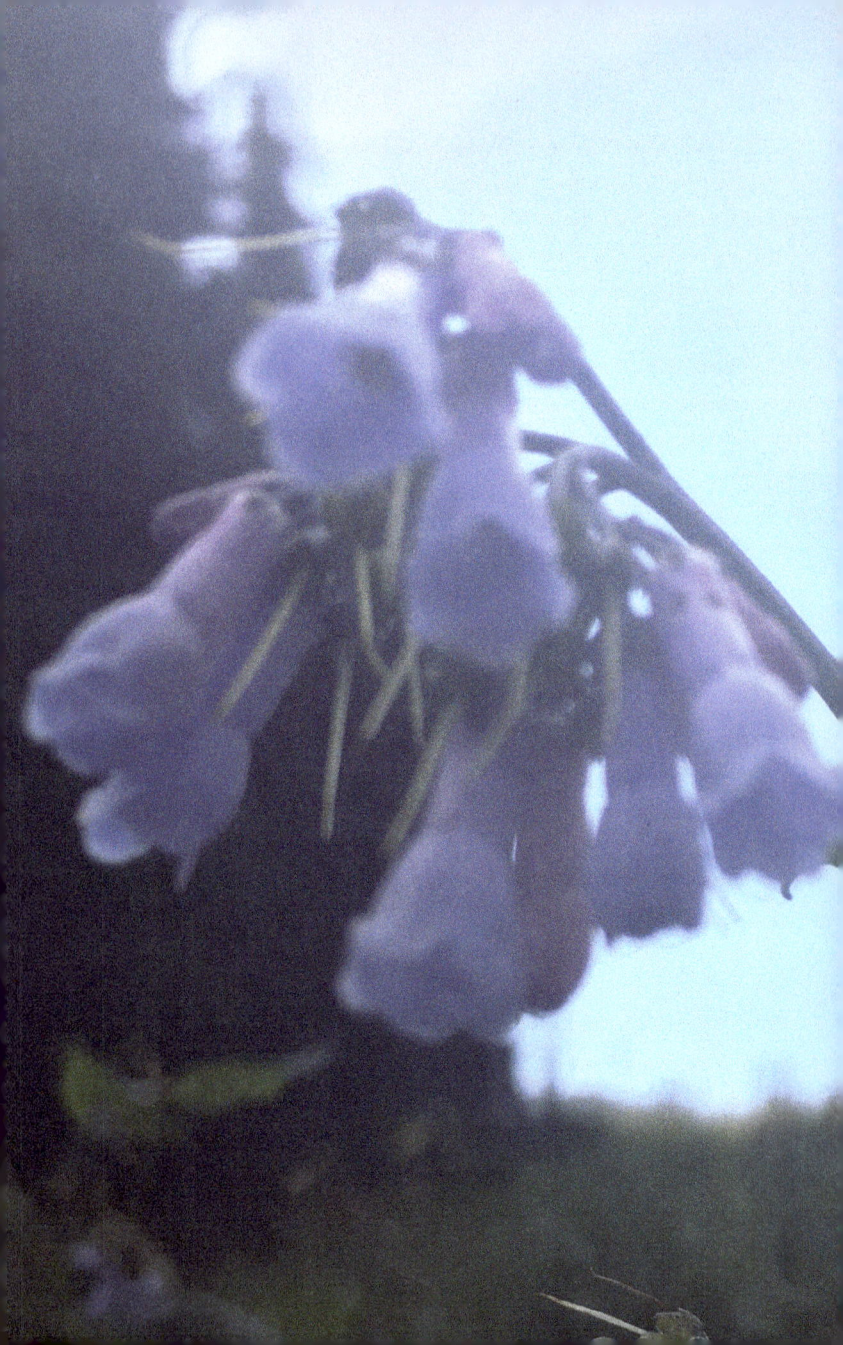

space
6 September
"Although not large, the space I live in is graced only with those things that speak to my heart. My lifestyle brings me joy." -Marie Kondo

useful & beautiful
7 September
"Have nothing in your house that you do not know to be useful, or believe to be beautiful."
-William Morris

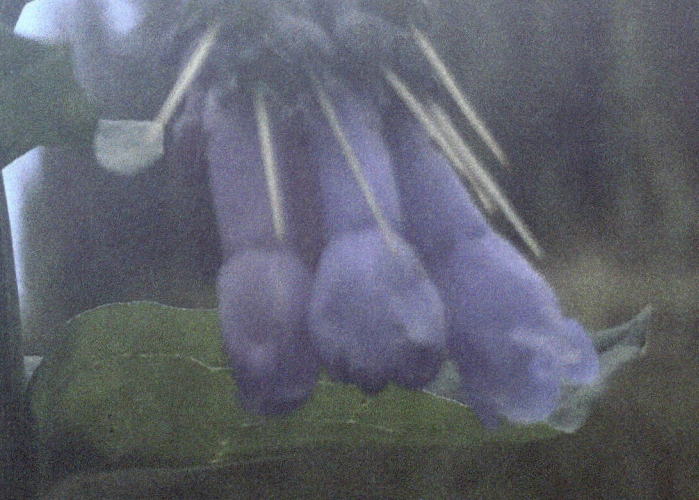

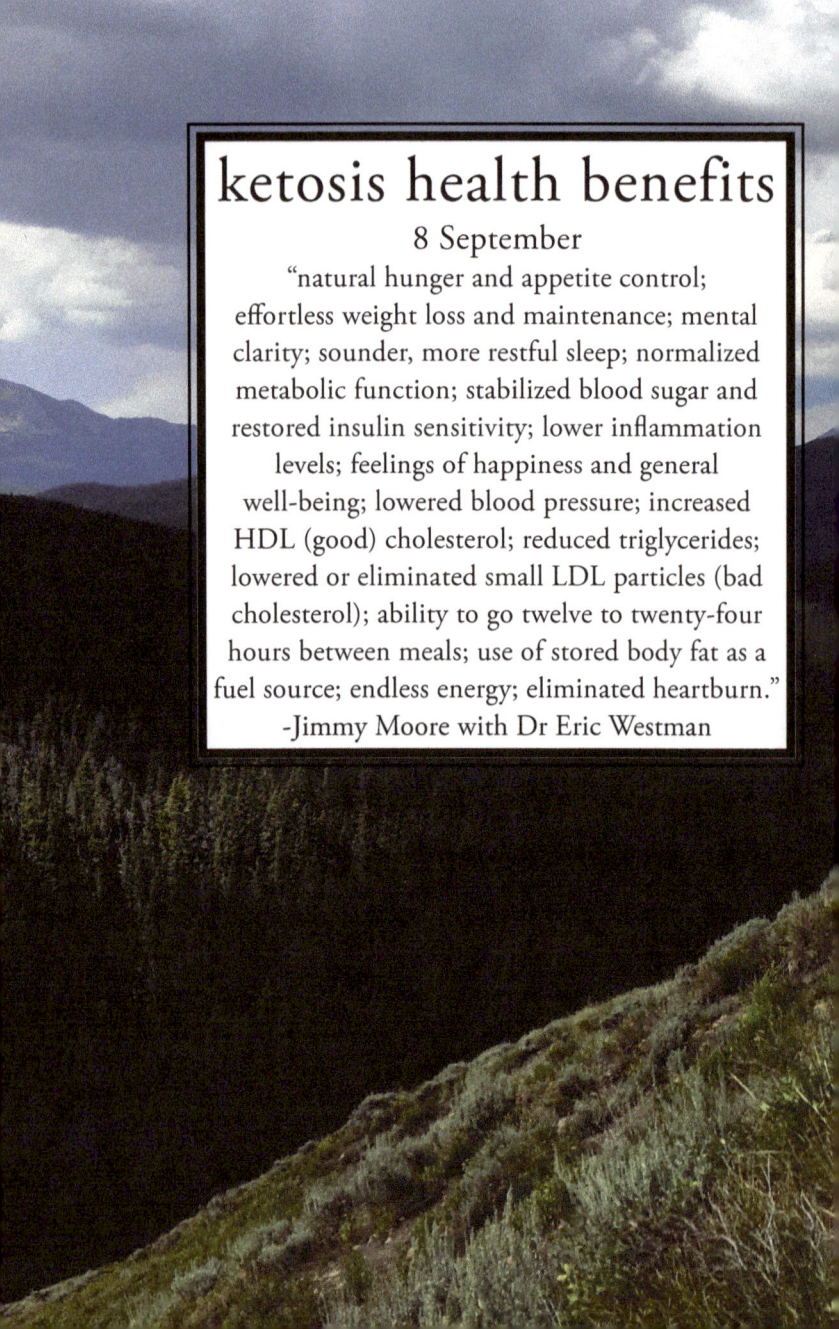

ketosis health benefits
8 September

"natural hunger and appetite control; effortless weight loss and maintenance; mental clarity; sounder, more restful sleep; normalized metabolic function; stabilized blood sugar and restored insulin sensitivity; lower inflammation levels; feelings of happiness and general well-being; lowered blood pressure; increased HDL (good) cholesterol; reduced triglycerides; lowered or eliminated small LDL particles (bad cholesterol); ability to go twelve to twenty-four hours between meals; use of stored body fat as a fuel source; endless energy; eliminated heartburn."

-Jimmy Moore with Dr Eric Westman

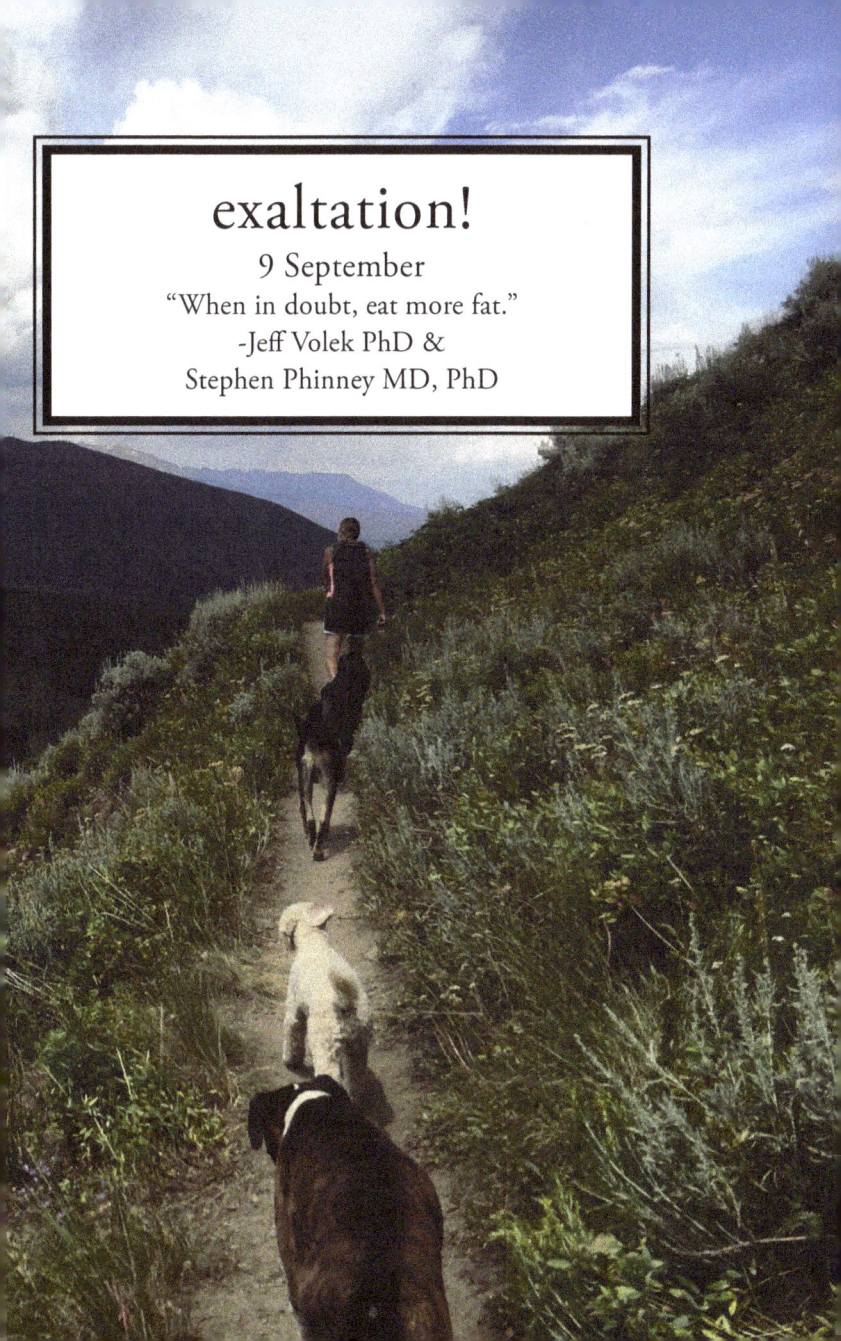
exaltation!
9 September
"When in doubt, eat more fat."
-Jeff Volek PhD &
Stephen Phinney MD, PhD

more keto benefits
10 September
"better fertility; prevention of traumatic brain injury; increased sex drive; improved immune system; slowed aging due to reduction in free radical production; improvements in blood chemistry; optimized cognitive function and improved memory; reduced acne breakouts and other skin conditions; heightened understanding of how foods affect your body; improvements in metabolic health markers; faster and better recovery from exercise; decreased anxiety and mood swings."
-Jimmy Moore with Dr Eric Westman

genius
11 September
"When you're in my house you shall do as I do and believe who I believe in. So Bart, butter your bacon." -Homer Simpson

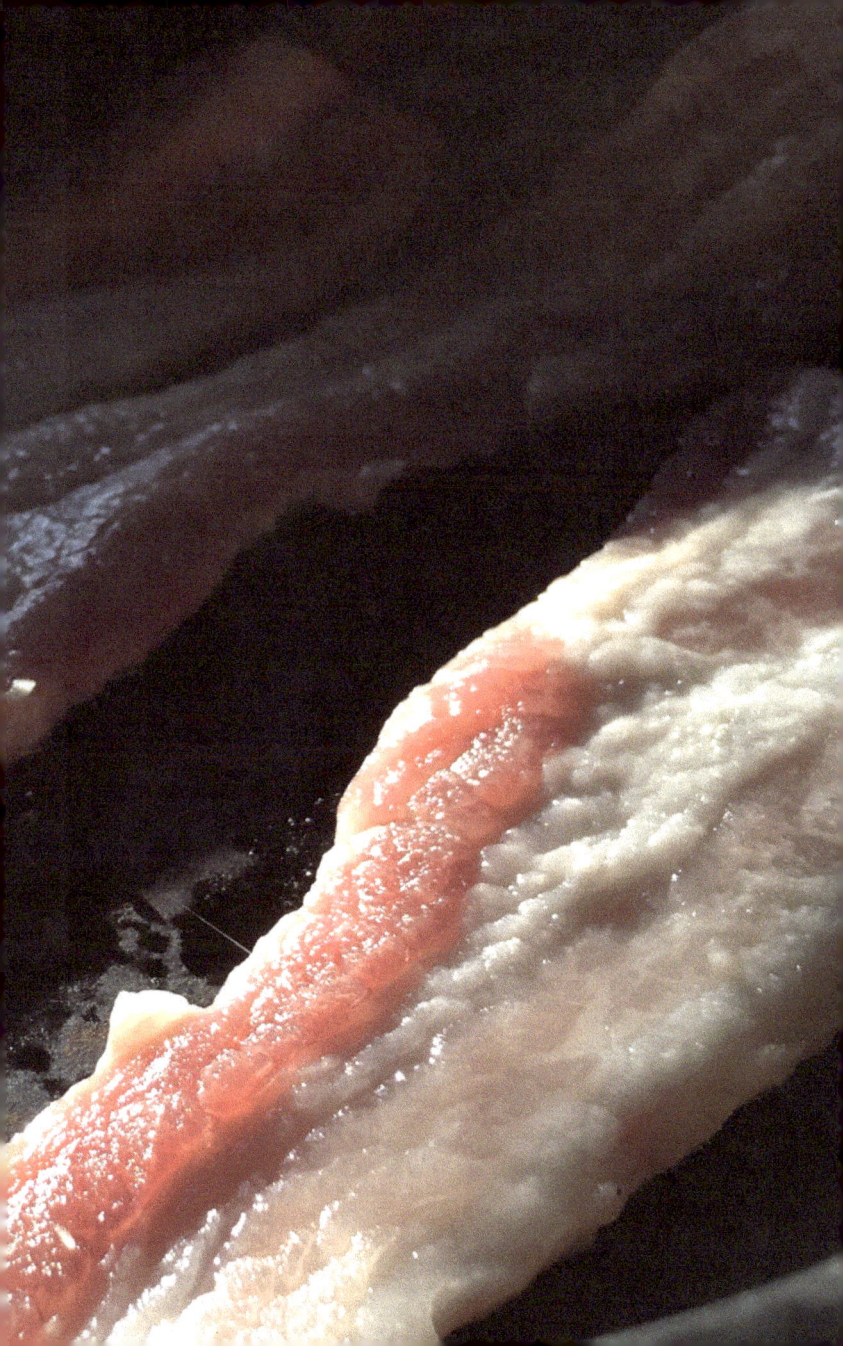

spark joy
12 September

"Are you happy wearing clothes that don't give you pleasure? Do you feel joy when surrounded by piles of unread books that don't touch your heart? Do you think that owning accessories you know you'll never use will ever bring you happiness? Imagine living in a space that contains only things that spark joy. Isn't this the lifestyle you dream of? Keep only those things that speak to your heart. Then take the plunge and discard all the rest. By doing this, you can reset your life and embark on a new lifestyle." -Marie Kondo

no exceptions
13 September

"We should only wear clothes because we love them, they look good on us, and they speak to who we are as people. No exceptions."
-Jennifer L. Scott

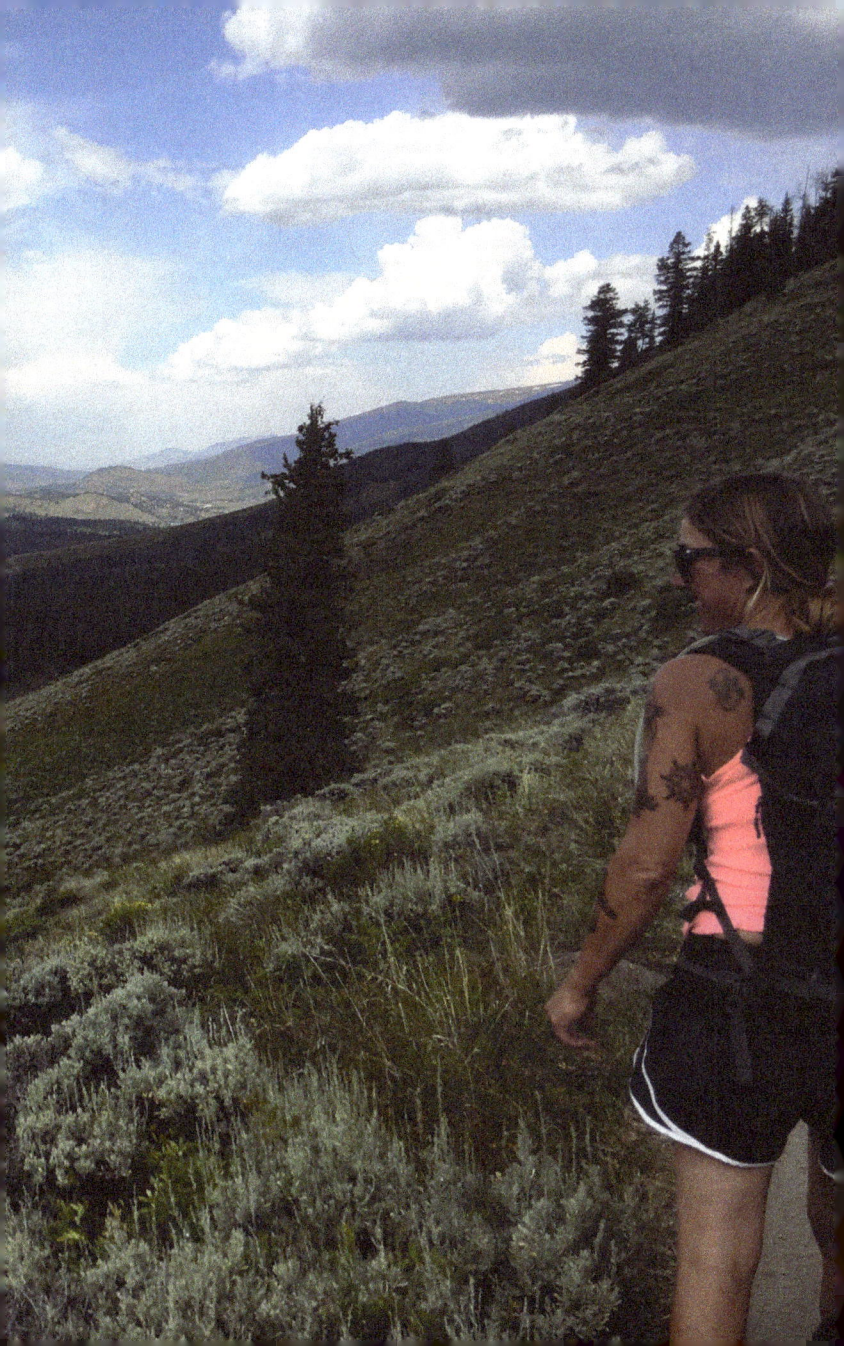

producing ketones

14 September

"When you start to burn fat for fuel and produce ketones, it's very possible to feel completely satisfied and energized on one, maybe two meals a day." -Jimmy Moore

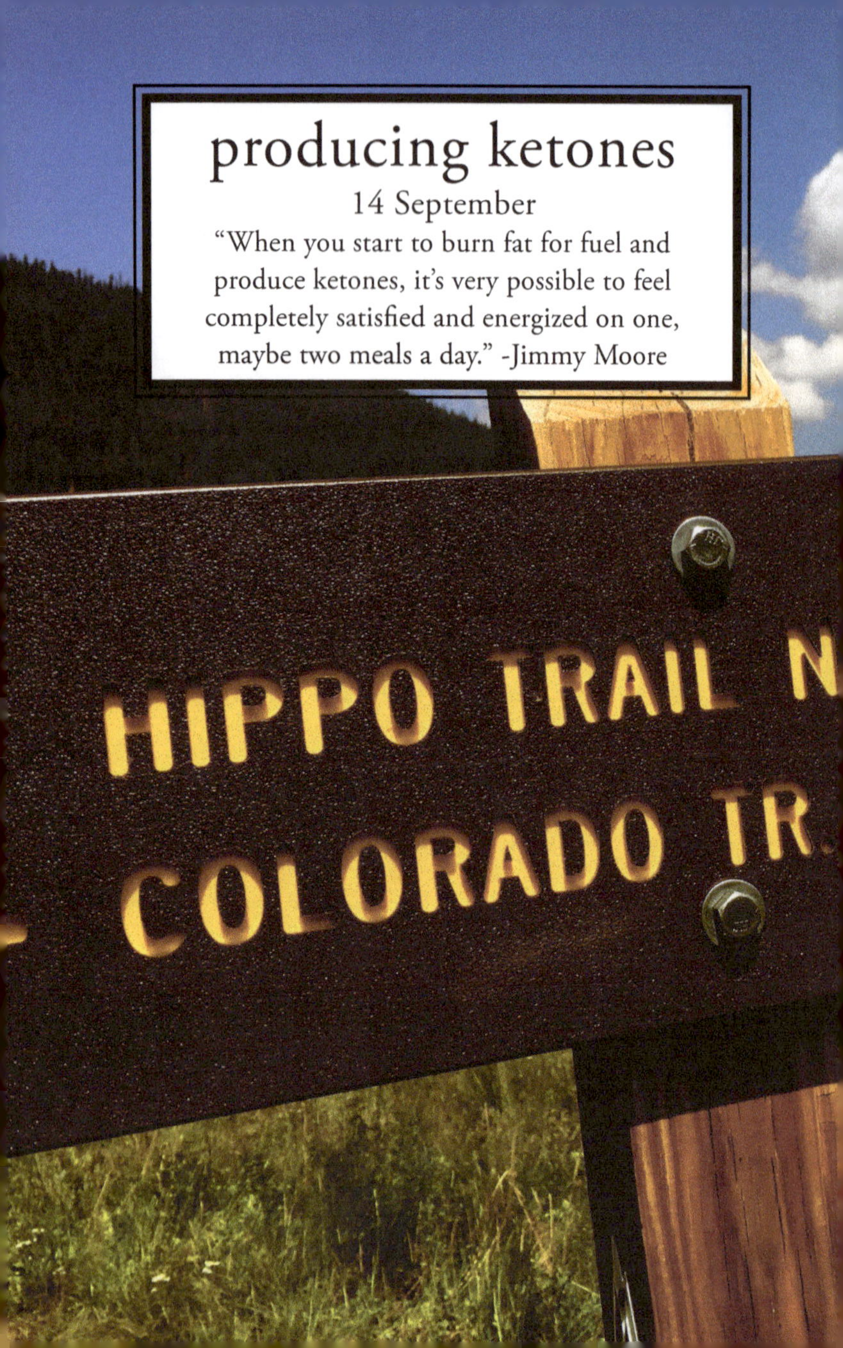

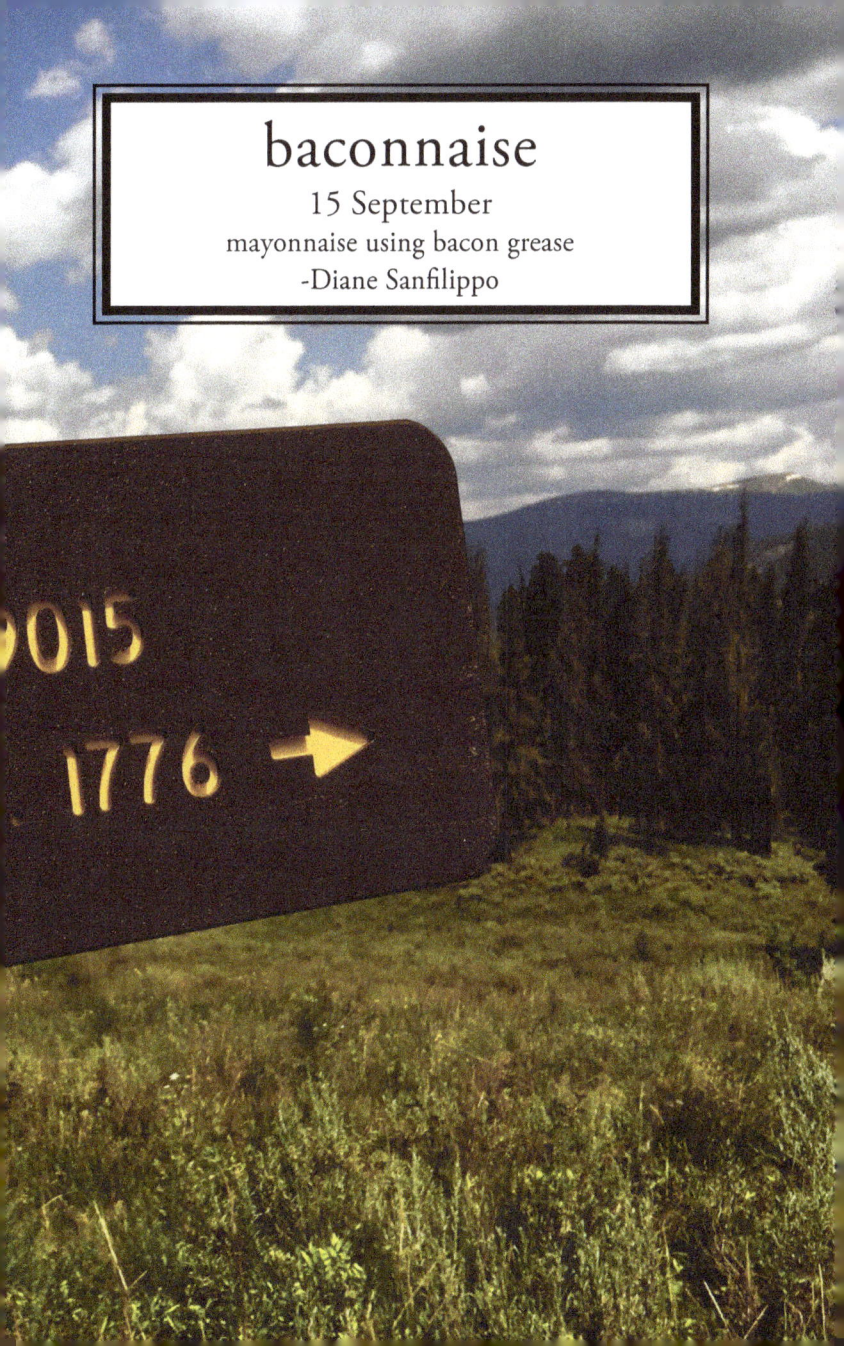

baconnaise

15 September
mayonnaise using bacon grease
-Diane Sanfilippo

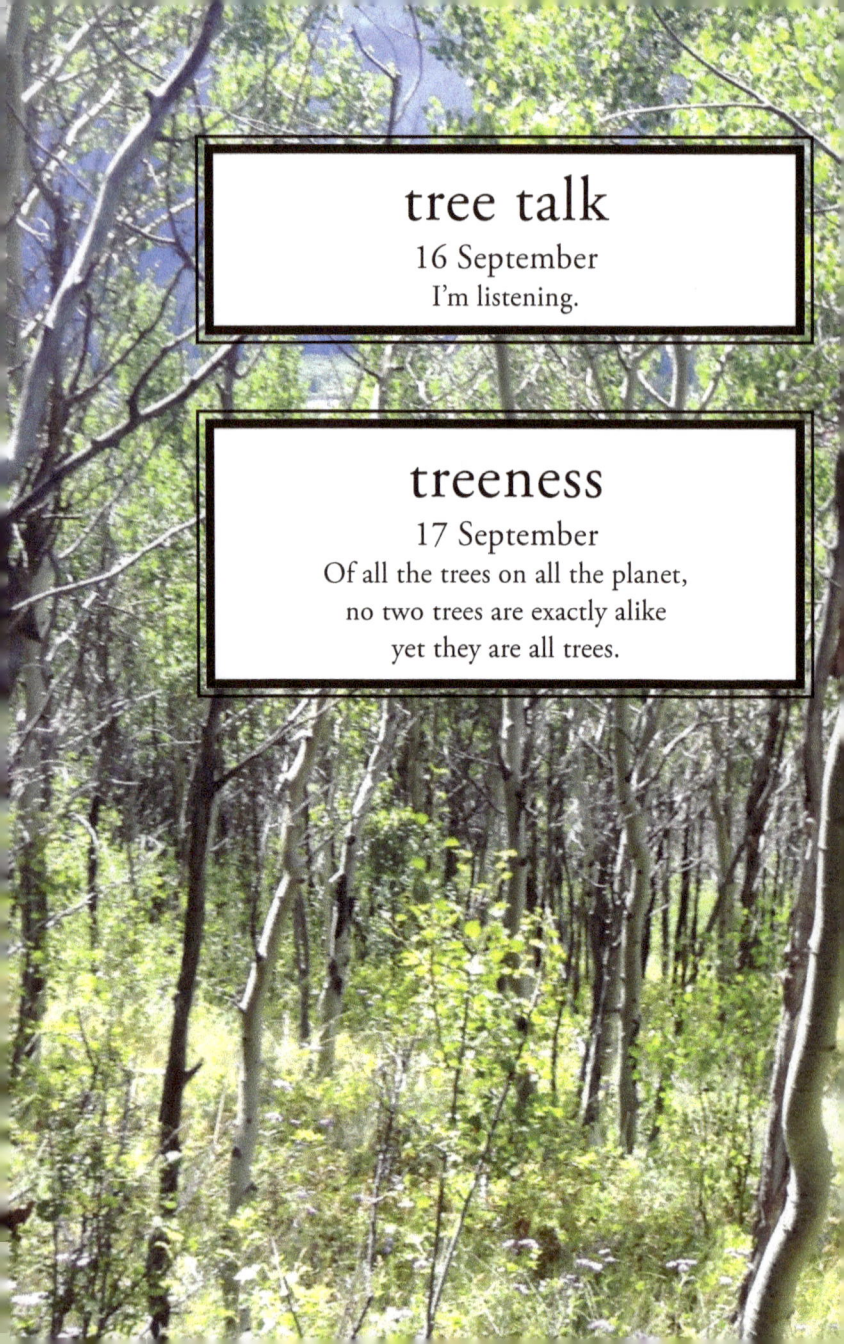

tree talk
16 September
I'm listening.

treeness
17 September
Of all the trees on all the planet,
no two trees are exactly alike
yet they are all trees.

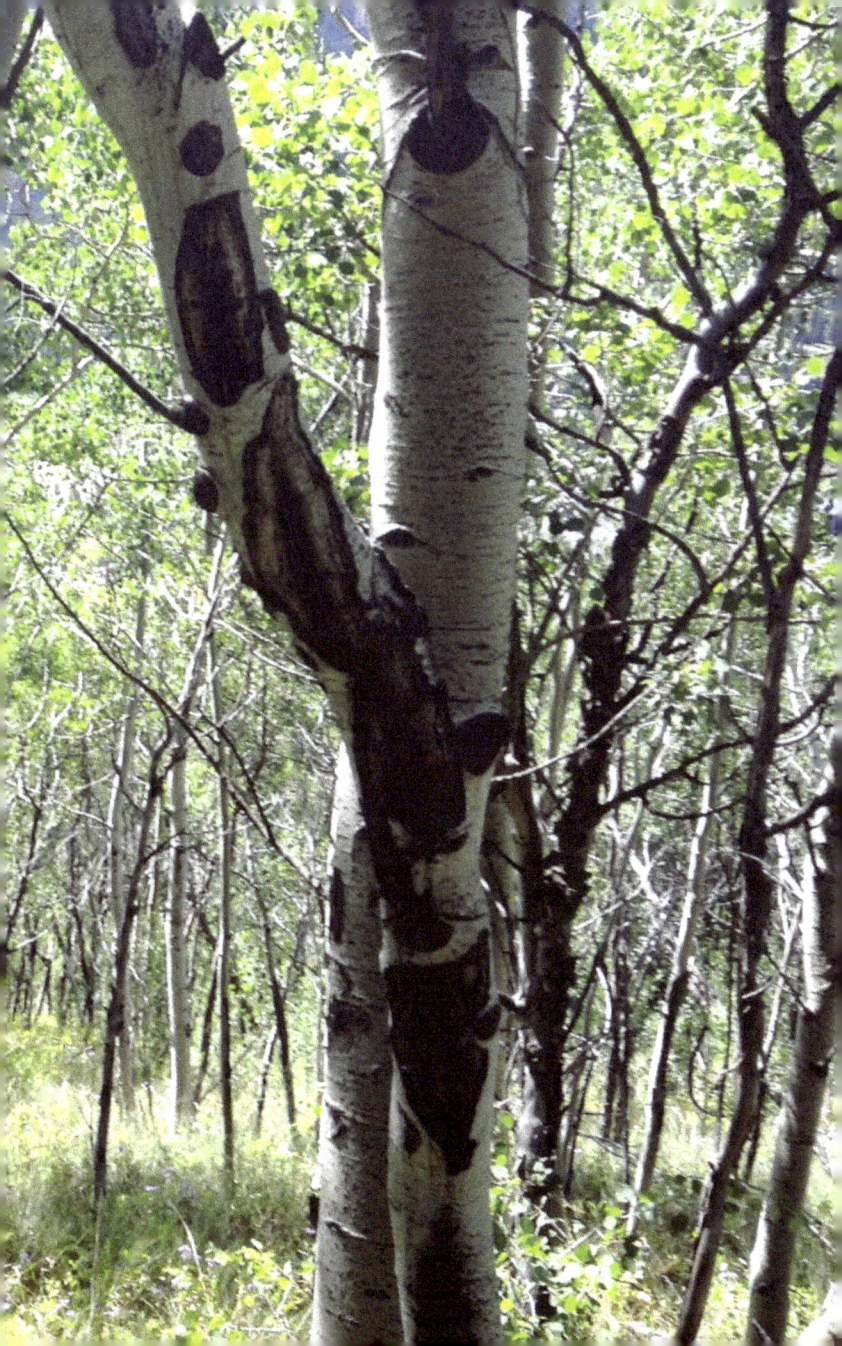

choose well
18 September
"Buy less, choose well, make it last...we are moving from a culture of appearances to a culture of values, and everything we do, wear and eat will reflect that." -Johanna Björk

design by Nature
19 September
"Every time you spend money, you're casting a vote for the kind of world you want."
-Anne Lappé

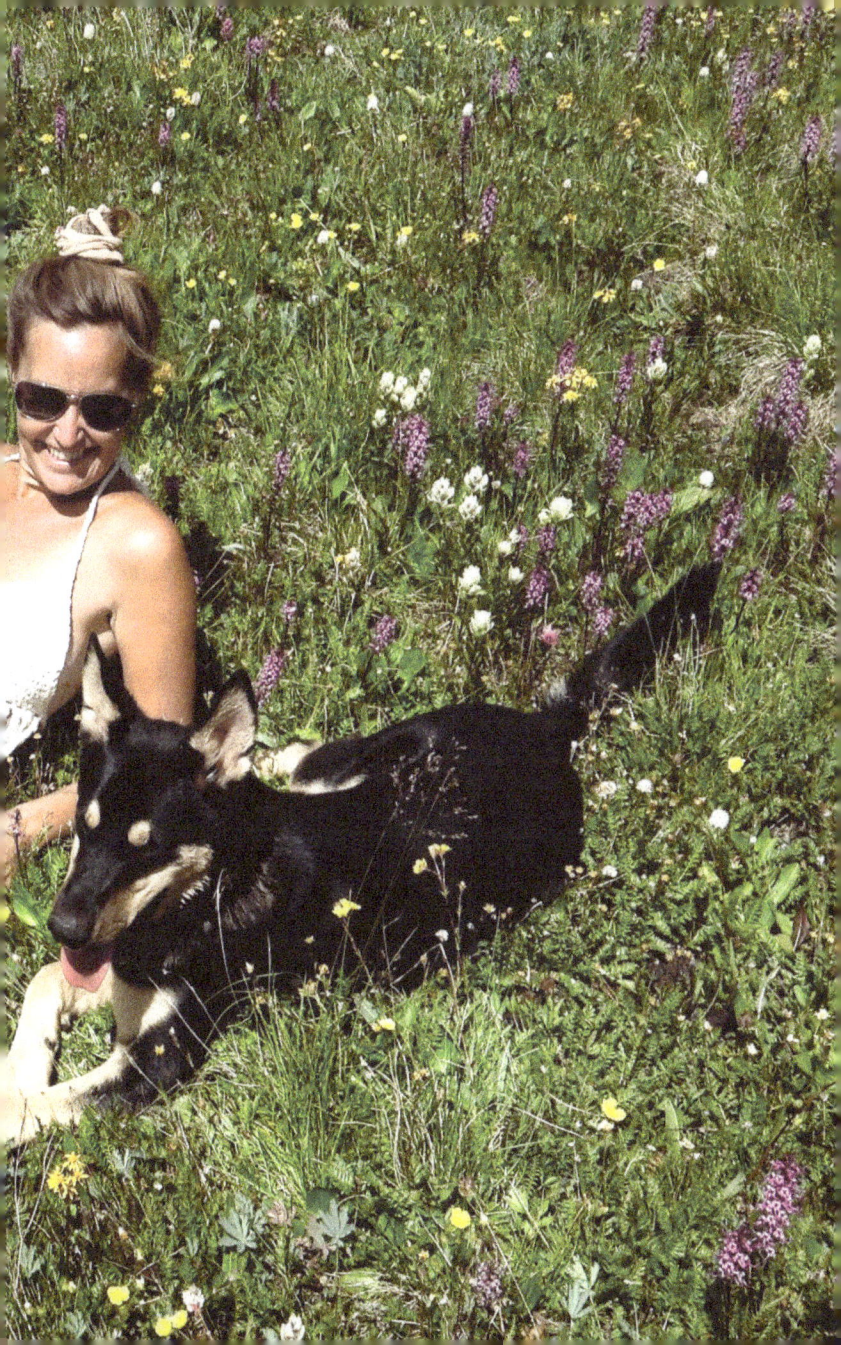

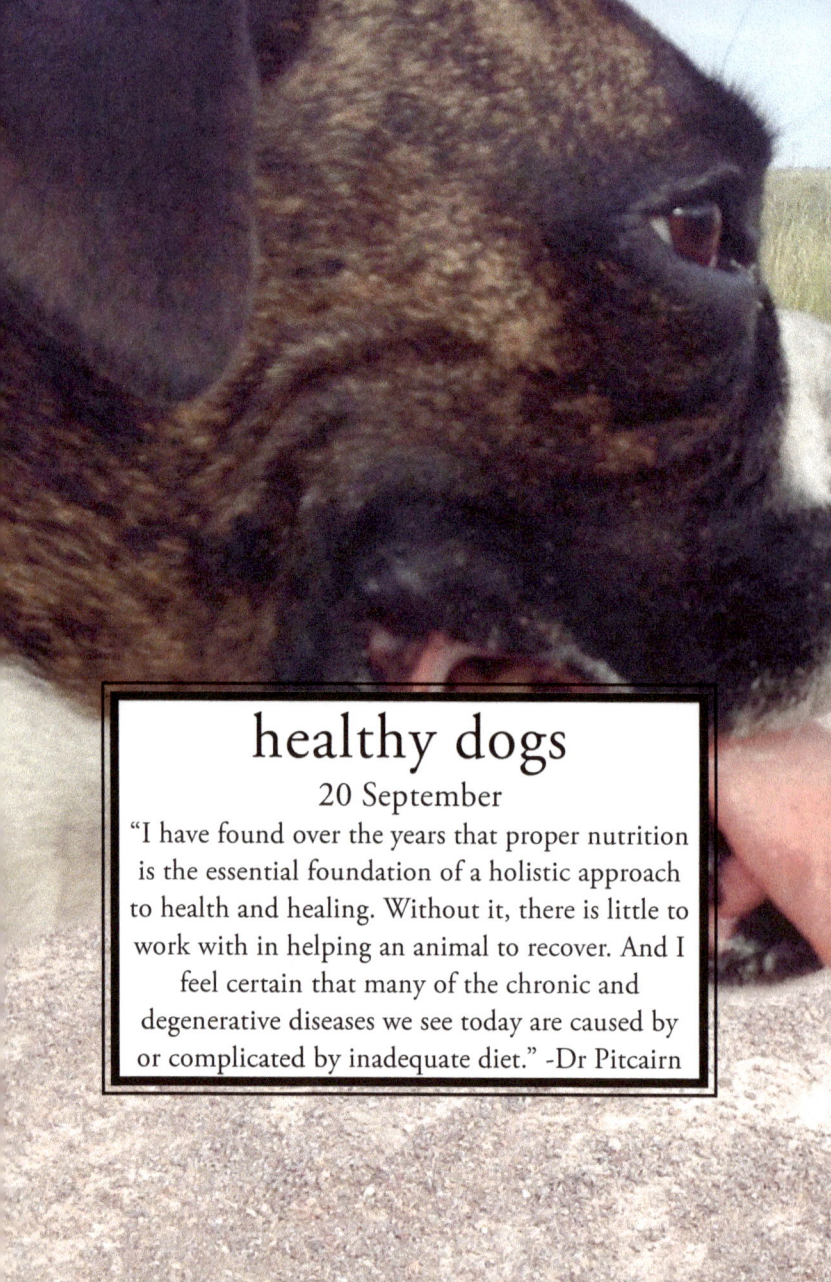

healthy dogs
20 September

"I have found over the years that proper nutrition is the essential foundation of a holistic approach to health and healing. Without it, there is little to work with in helping an animal to recover. And I feel certain that many of the chronic and degenerative diseases we see today are caused by or complicated by inadequate diet." -Dr Pitcairn

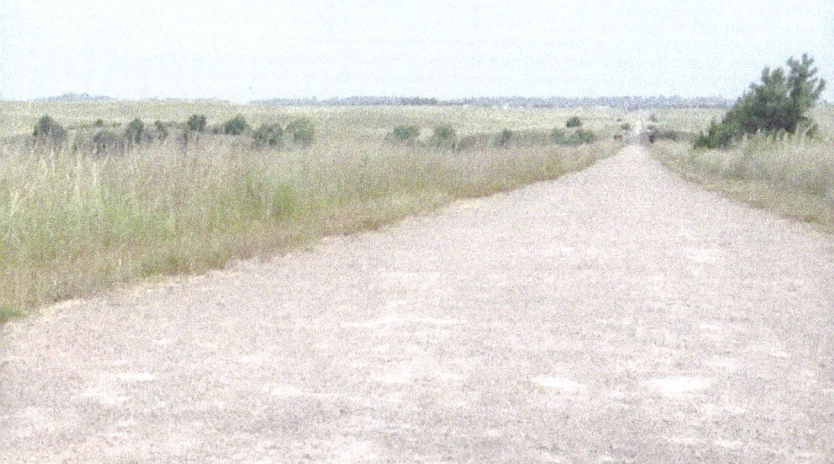

European dogs
21 September

"All of us - humans and animals - should have a variety of fresh, wholesome, unprocessed food... Europeans feed their dogs much more naturally... Many breeders have commented...that such European dogs are far healthier than American dogs. No diet that we can formulate from least-cost products and process for convenience and long storage can ever rival those mysteriously complex fresh-food diets offered for eons by Nature herself." -Dr Pitcairn

wings
22 September
"Evolution is written on the wings of butterflies."
-Charles Darwin

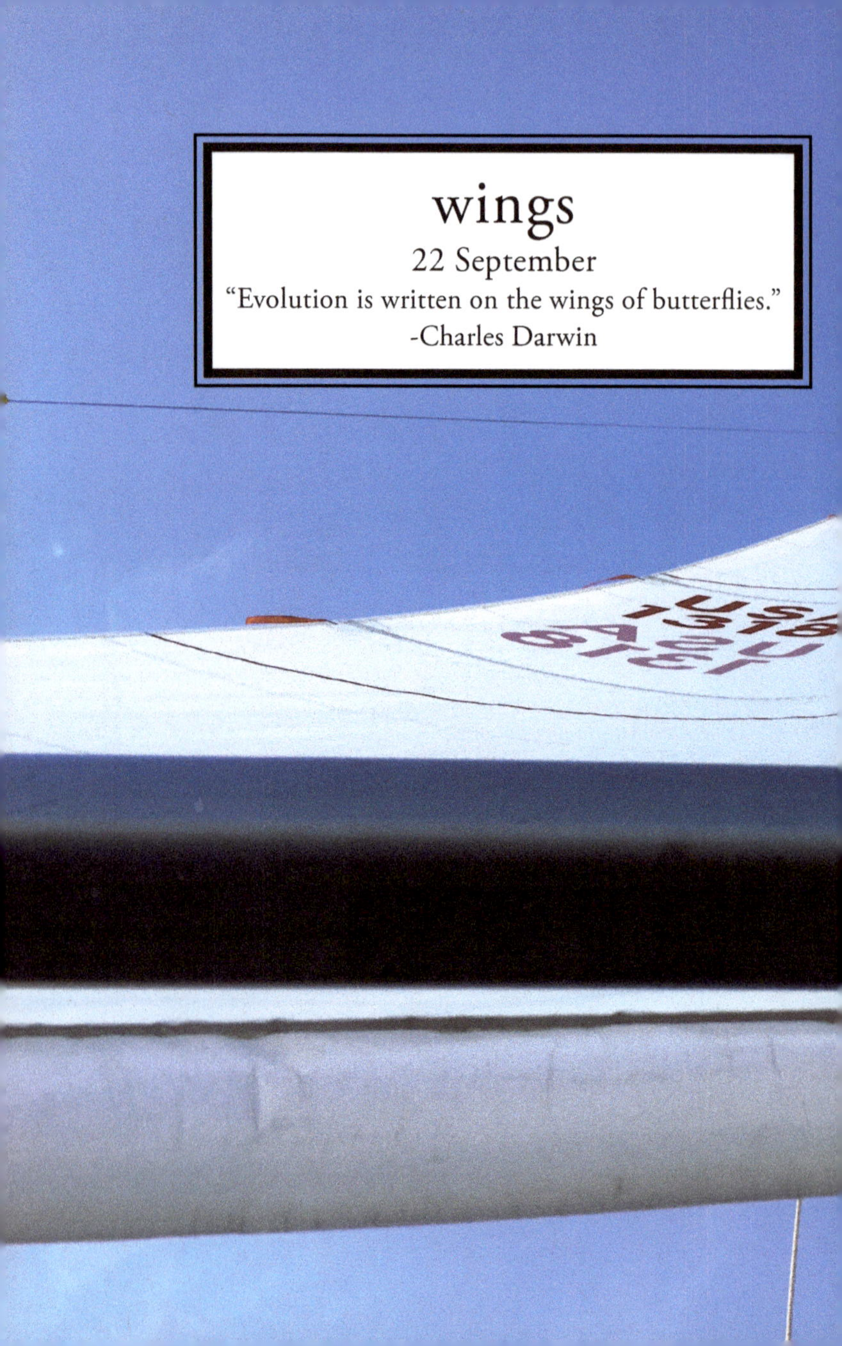

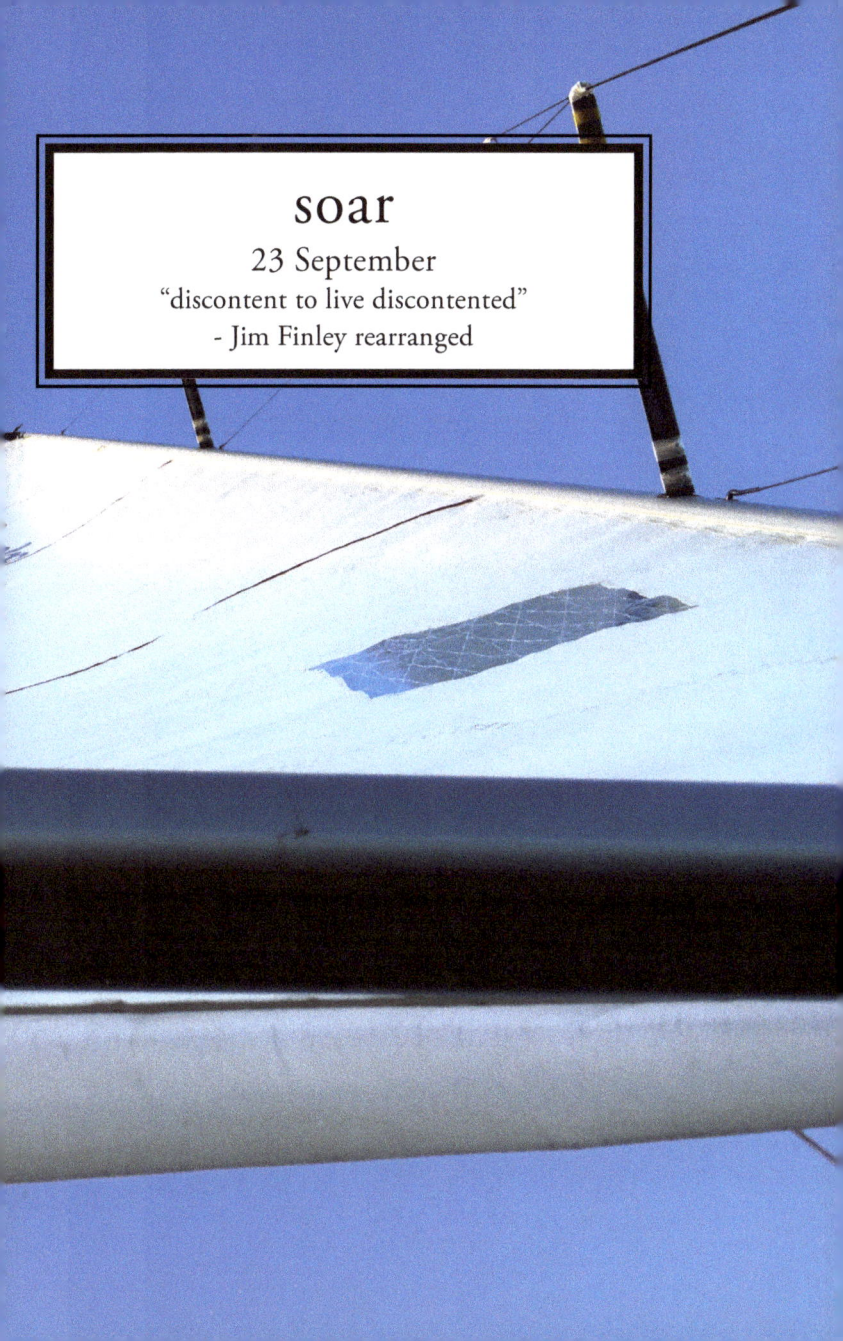

soar

23 September
"discontent to live discontented"
- Jim Finley rearranged

habitat

24 September

"When species live inside their natural habitat they have 'normal' (species-typical) health and longevity." -John Durant

our tissues
25 September

"Marc Lappé: Sensitive assays have detected residues of over a hundred different foreign chemicals and metals in our tissues - compounds and substances that were virtually absent from the environments of our predecessors." -Dr Pitcairn

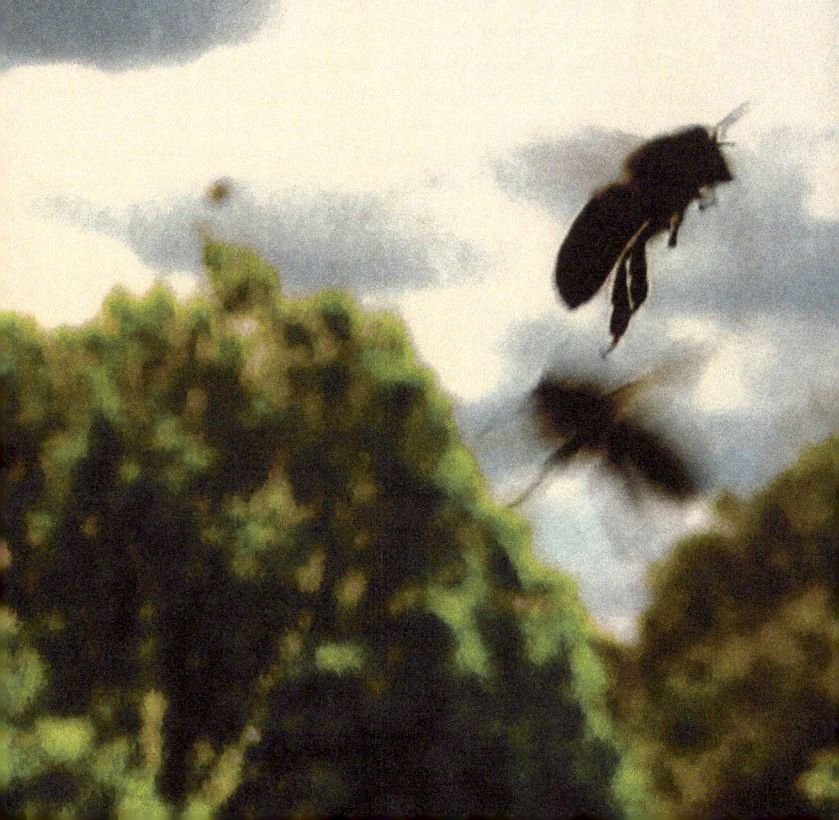

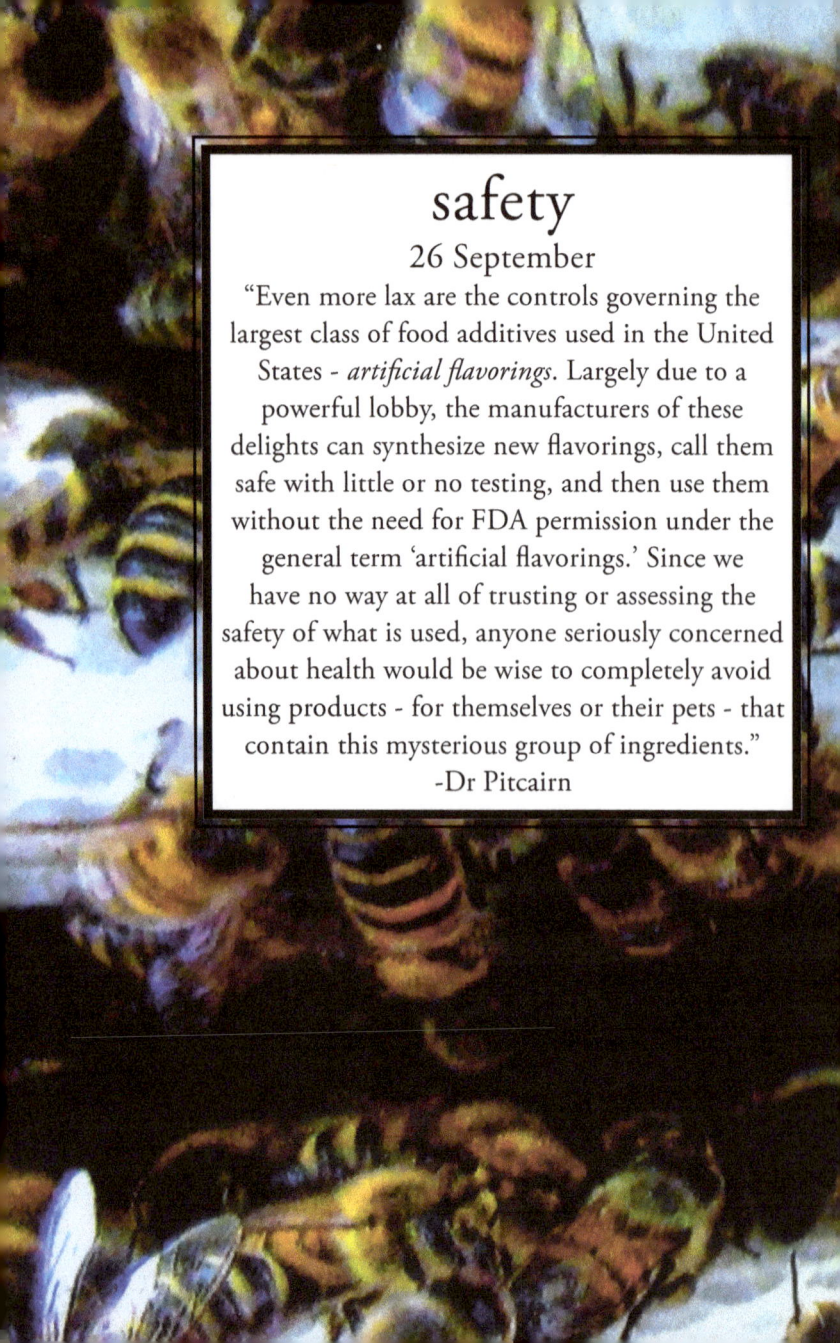

safety
26 September

"Even more lax are the controls governing the largest class of food additives used in the United States - *artificial flavorings*. Largely due to a powerful lobby, the manufacturers of these delights can synthesize new flavorings, call them safe with little or no testing, and then use them without the need for FDA permission under the general term 'artificial flavorings.' Since we have no way at all of trusting or assessing the safety of what is used, anyone seriously concerned about health would be wise to completely avoid using products - for themselves or their pets - that contain this mysterious group of ingredients."

-Dr Pitcairn

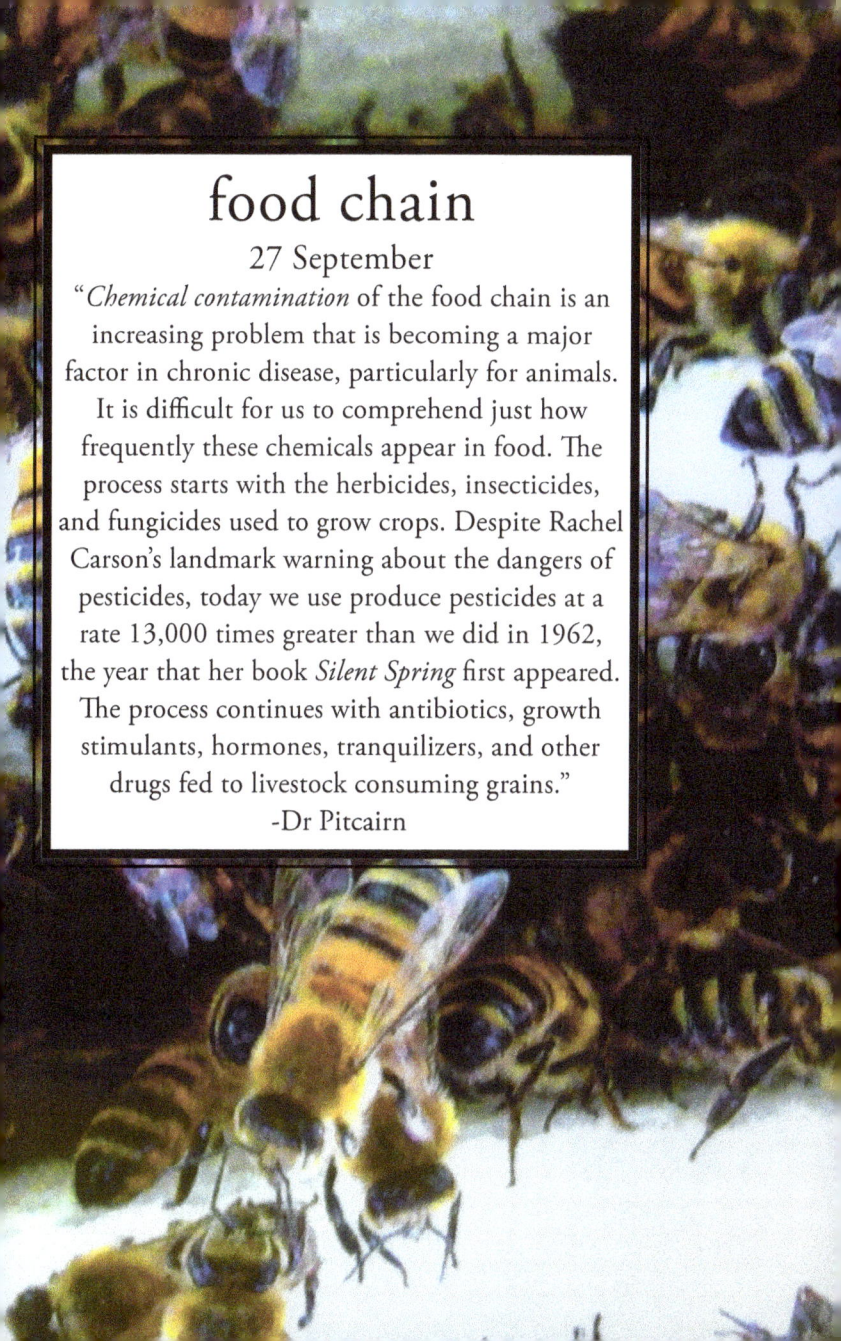

food chain
27 September

"*Chemical contamination* of the food chain is an increasing problem that is becoming a major factor in chronic disease, particularly for animals. It is difficult for us to comprehend just how frequently these chemicals appear in food. The process starts with the herbicides, insecticides, and fungicides used to grow crops. Despite Rachel Carson's landmark warning about the dangers of pesticides, today we use produce pesticides at a rate 13,000 times greater than we did in 1962, the year that her book *Silent Spring* first appeared. The process continues with antibiotics, growth stimulants, hormones, tranquilizers, and other drugs fed to livestock consuming grains."

-Dr Pitcairn

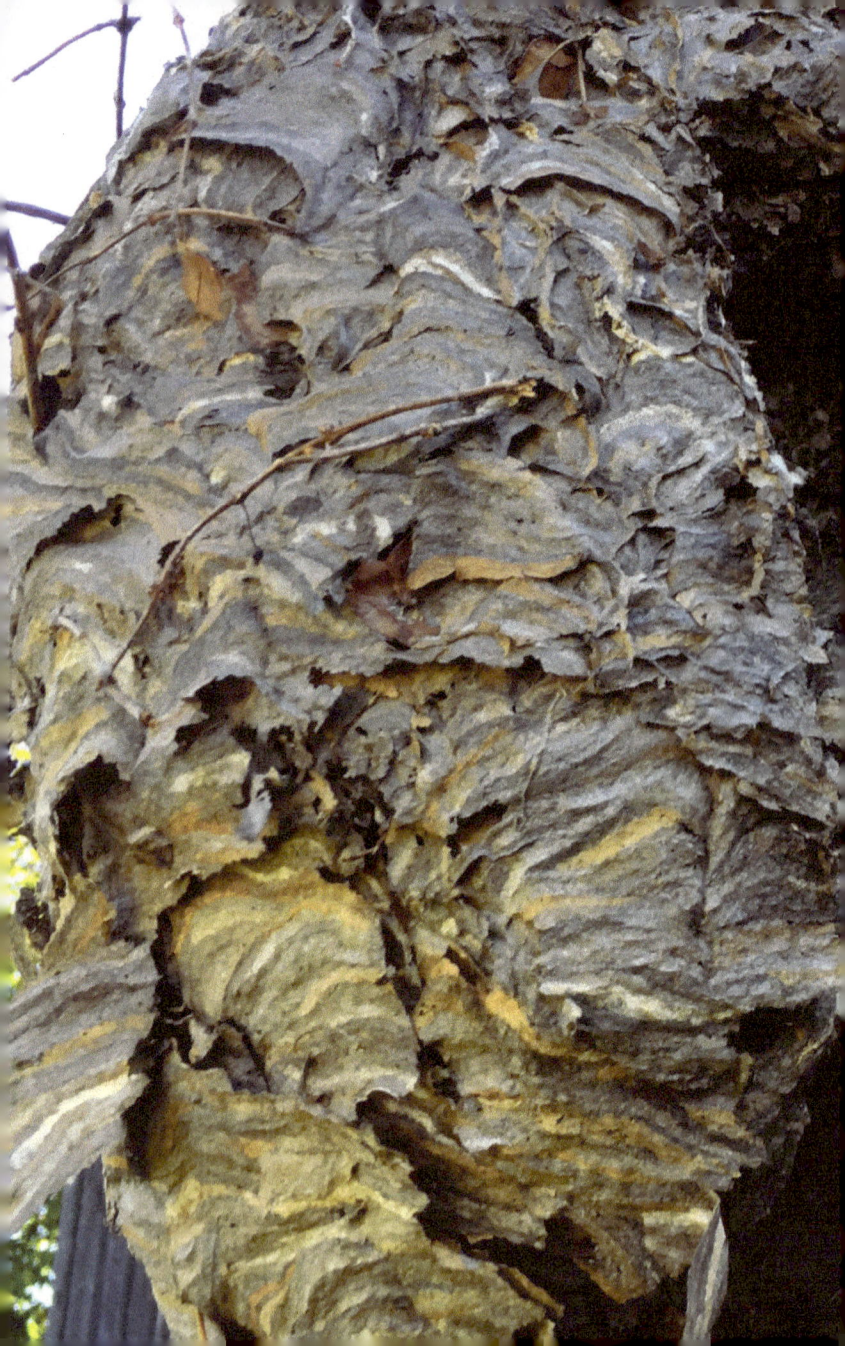

minerals

28 September

"Minerals are lost in the treatment of drinking water. Water was the largest source of calcium and magnesium in Paleolithic diets, but modern water treatment removes most dissolved minerals."
Paul Jaminet PhD &
Shou-Ching Jaminet PhD

environment

29 September

"Crops (and livestock) are products of their environment, and how they are raised determines what nutrition they ultimately provide. It is well known that there can be considerable variation in protein content, vitamins, and minerals, for example, depending on the soil, the amount of irrigation, the time of harvesting, and the storage period." -Dr Pitcairn

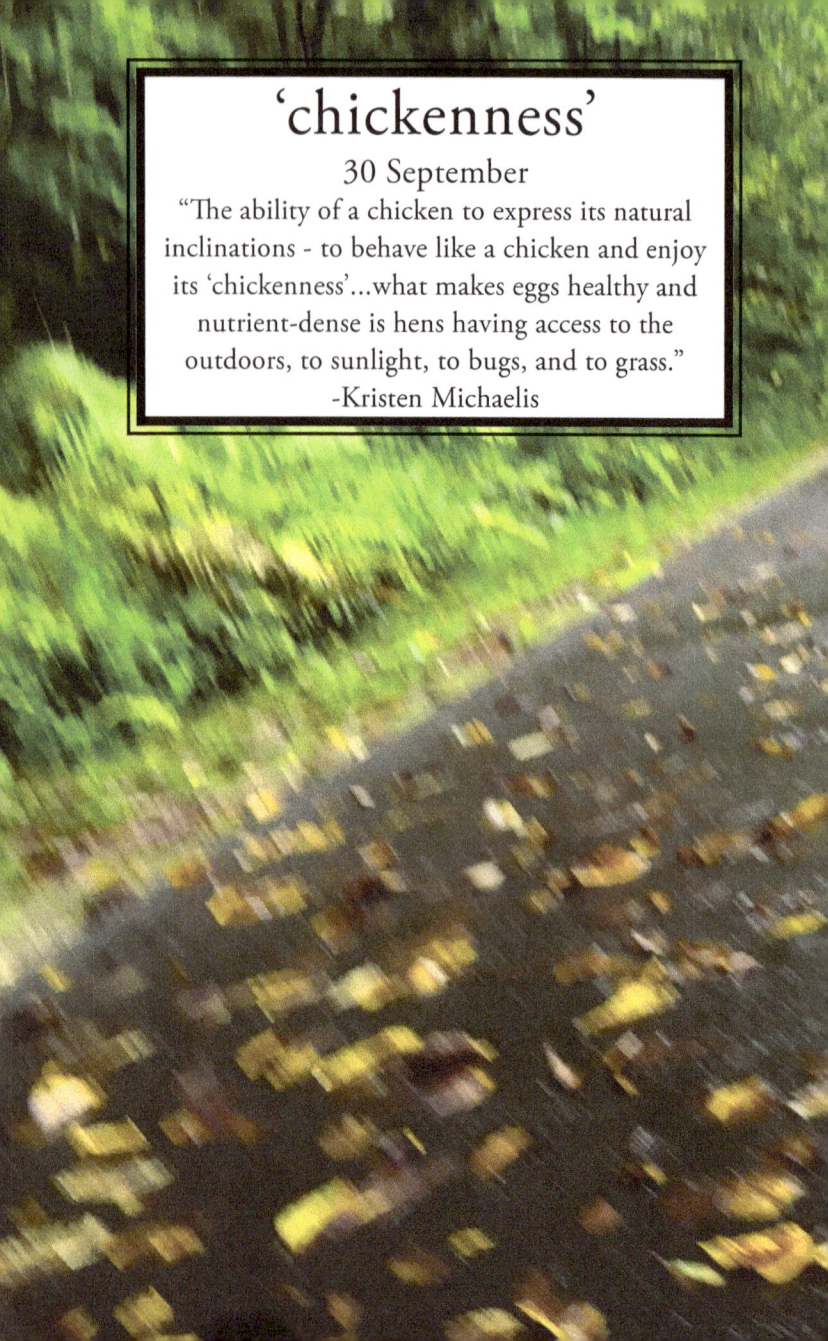

'chickenness'
30 September

"The ability of a chicken to express its natural inclinations - to behave like a chicken and enjoy its 'chickenness'...what makes eggs healthy and nutrient-dense is hens having access to the outdoors, to sunlight, to bugs, and to grass."
-Kristen Michaelis

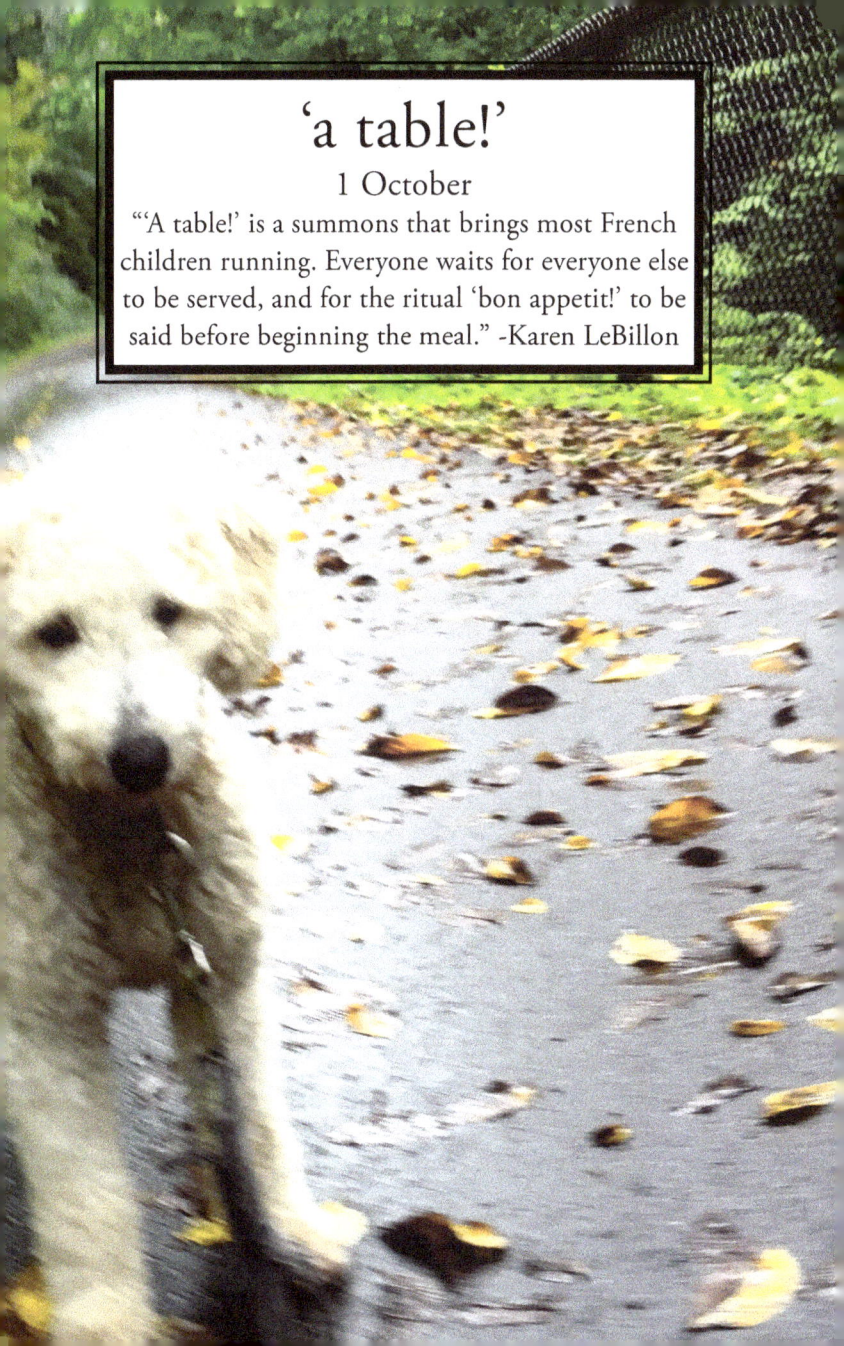

'a table!'
1 October

"'A table!' is a summons that brings most French children running. Everyone waits for everyone else to be served, and for the ritual 'bon appetit!' to be said before beginning the meal." -Karen LeBillon

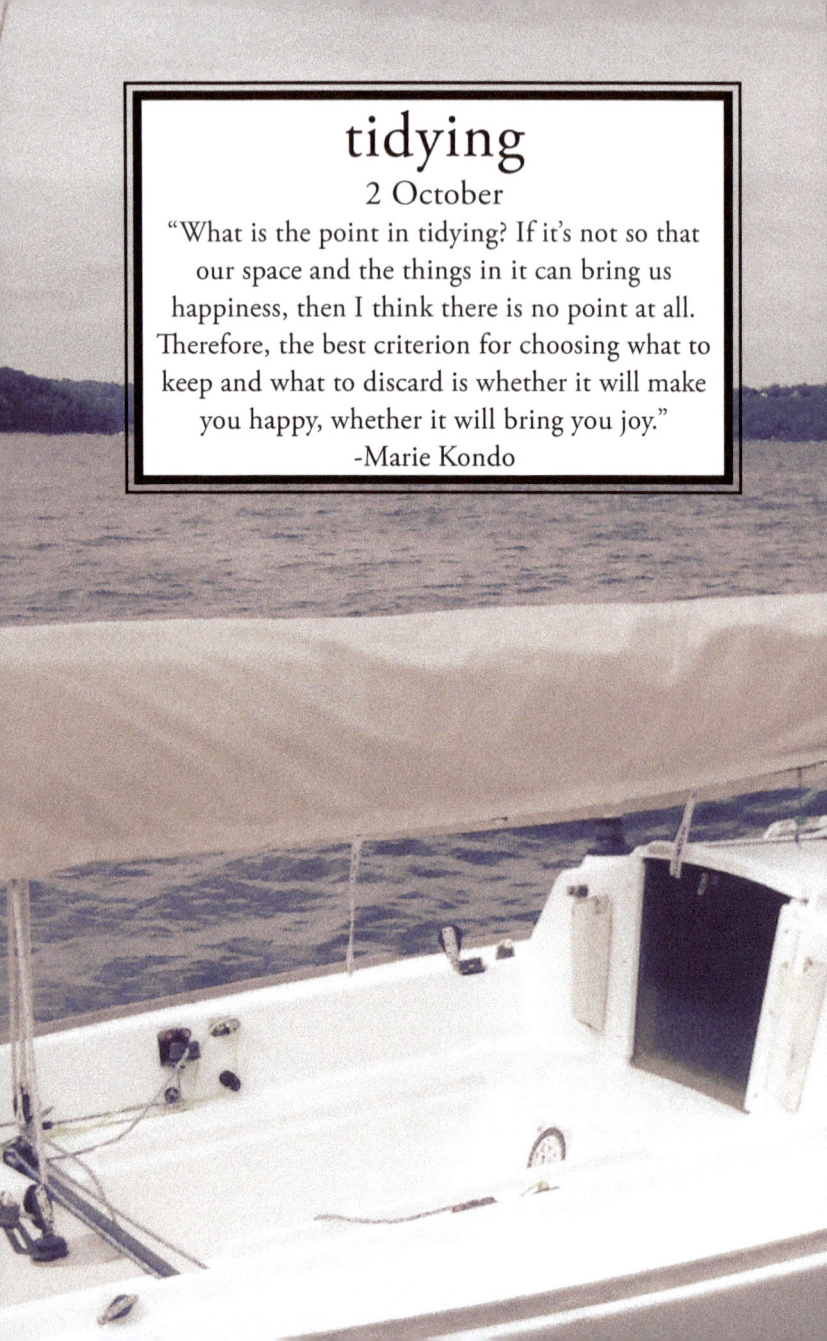

tidying

2 October

"What is the point in tidying? If it's not so that our space and the things in it can bring us happiness, then I think there is no point at all. Therefore, the best criterion for choosing what to keep and what to discard is whether it will make you happy, whether it will bring you joy."
-Marie Kondo

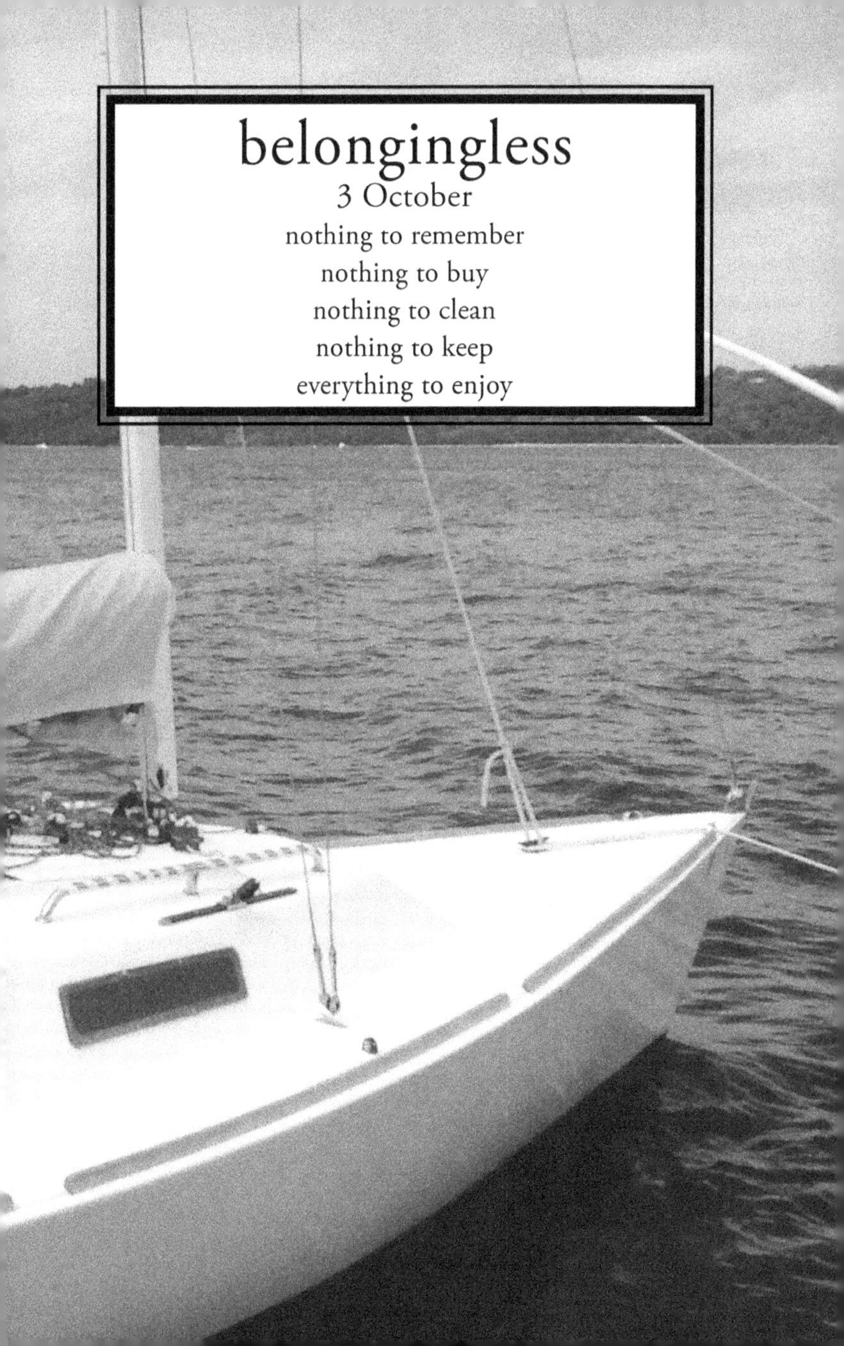

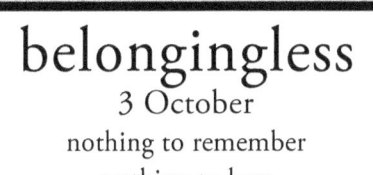

belongingless
3 October
nothing to remember
nothing to buy
nothing to clean
nothing to keep
everything to enjoy

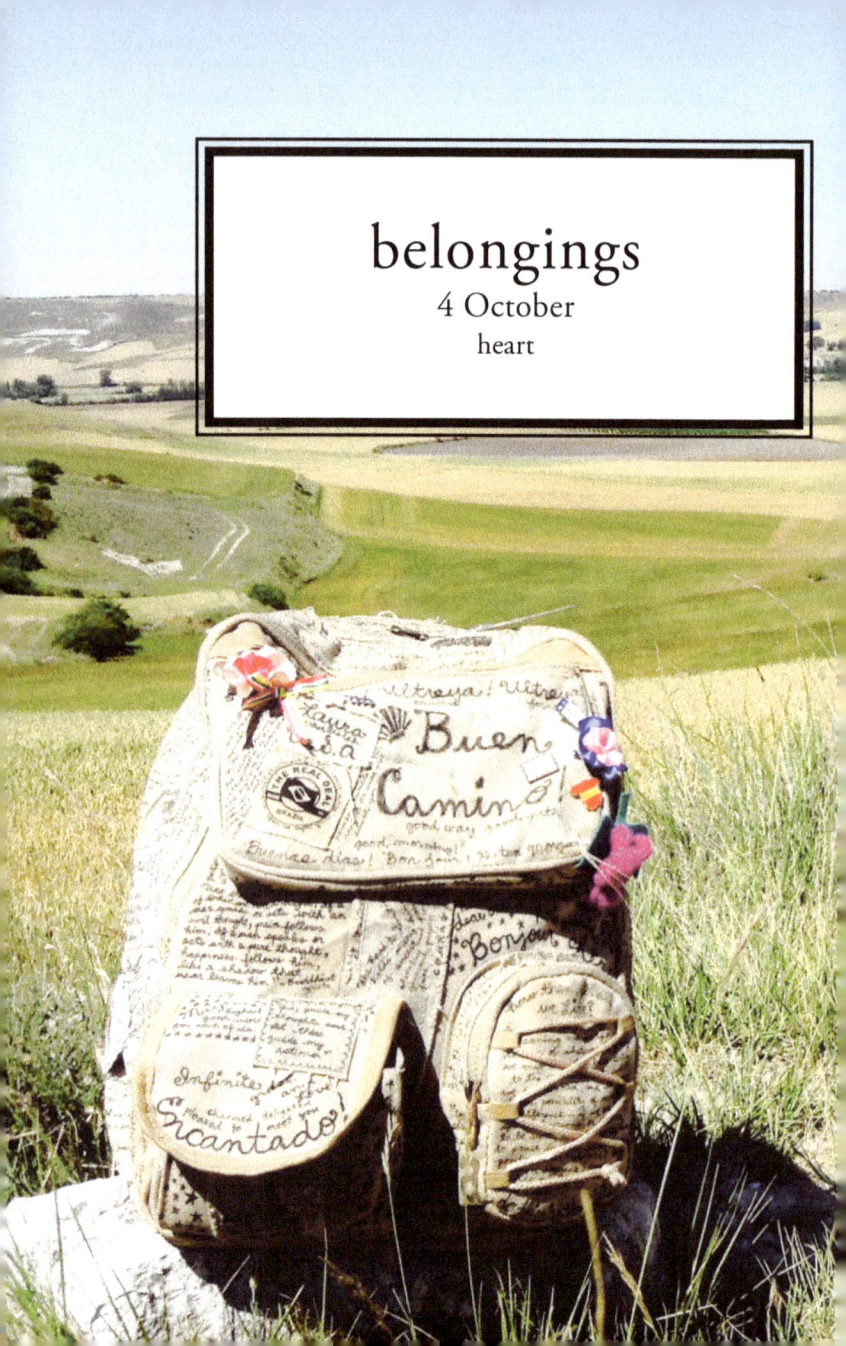

belongings
4 October
heart

simplicity
5 October

"Richard Foster's principles for simplicity: Buy things for their usefulness rather than their status or prestige. Learn the difference between a real need and an addiction. Develop a habit of giving things away. Avoid unnecessary and short-lived technological gadgets that promise to "save time." Enjoy things without owning them (public libraries and state parks). Nurture awe and appreciation for nature. Spend more time outdoors! Get out -and stay out- of debt. Use plain, honest speech. Say what you mean and keep your commitments. Reject anything that oppresses others (buy Fair Trade products). Live simply so that others may simply live." -Richard Rohr

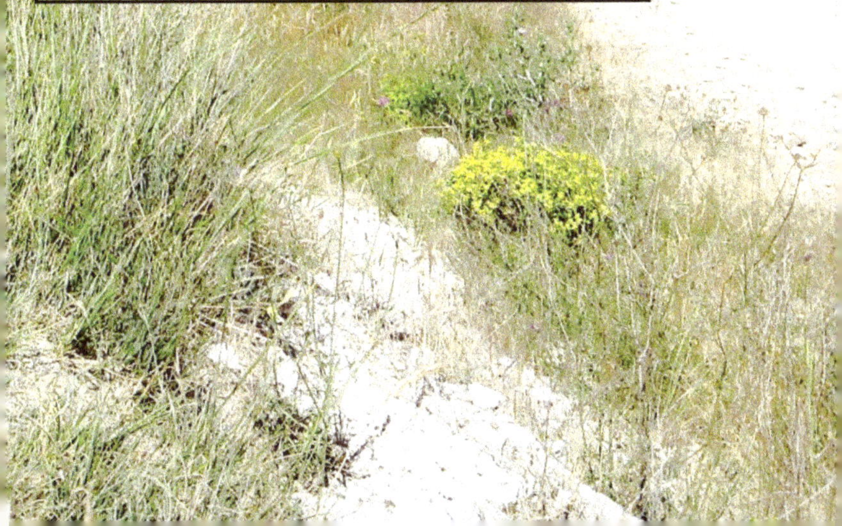

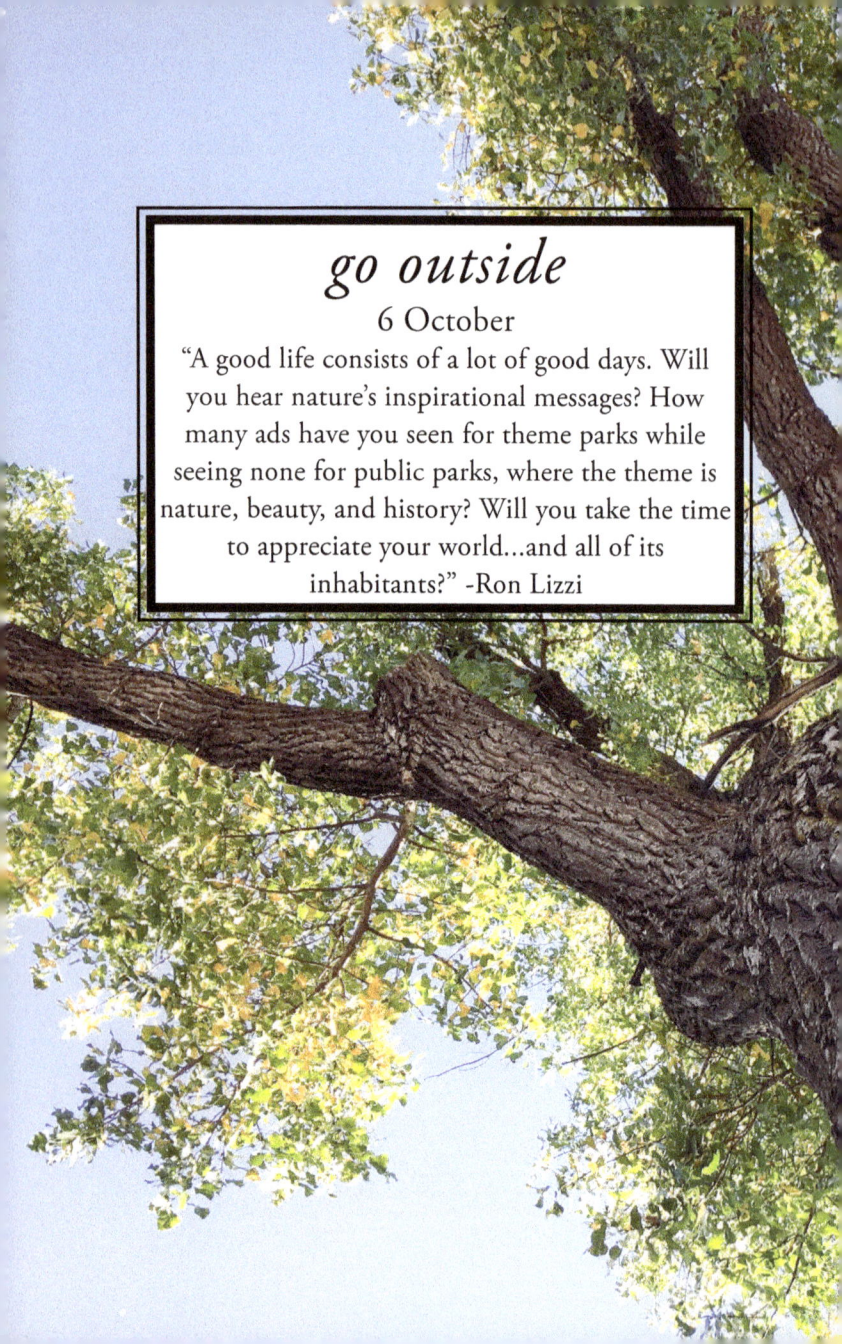

go outside
6 October

"A good life consists of a lot of good days. Will you hear nature's inspirational messages? How many ads have you seen for theme parks while seeing none for public parks, where the theme is nature, beauty, and history? Will you take the time to appreciate your world...and all of its inhabitants?" -Ron Lizzi

be

7 October

Be still and know that I am God.
Be still and know that I am.
Be still and know.
Be still.
Be.

-Richard Rohr

come with love

8 October

"Let no one enter your kingdom unless they come with love. All others, you simply stand back and witness them and yourself in this little drama that is unfolding. Once you stop the false identification of yourself, you are free. Being the witness is your ticket to freedom." -Wayne Dyer

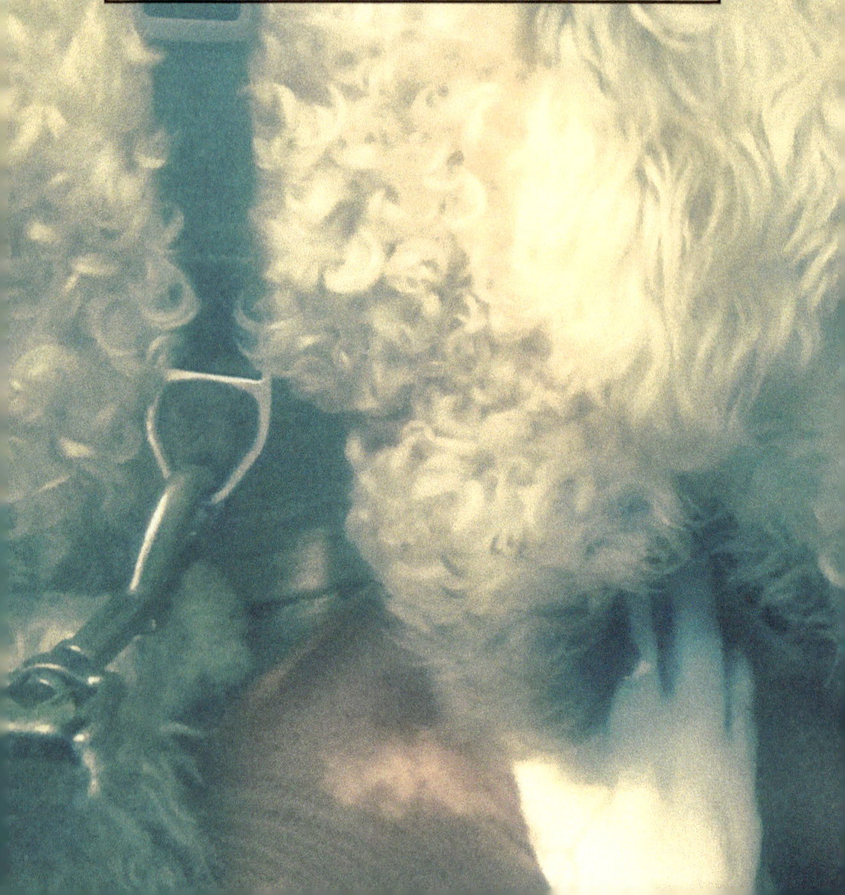

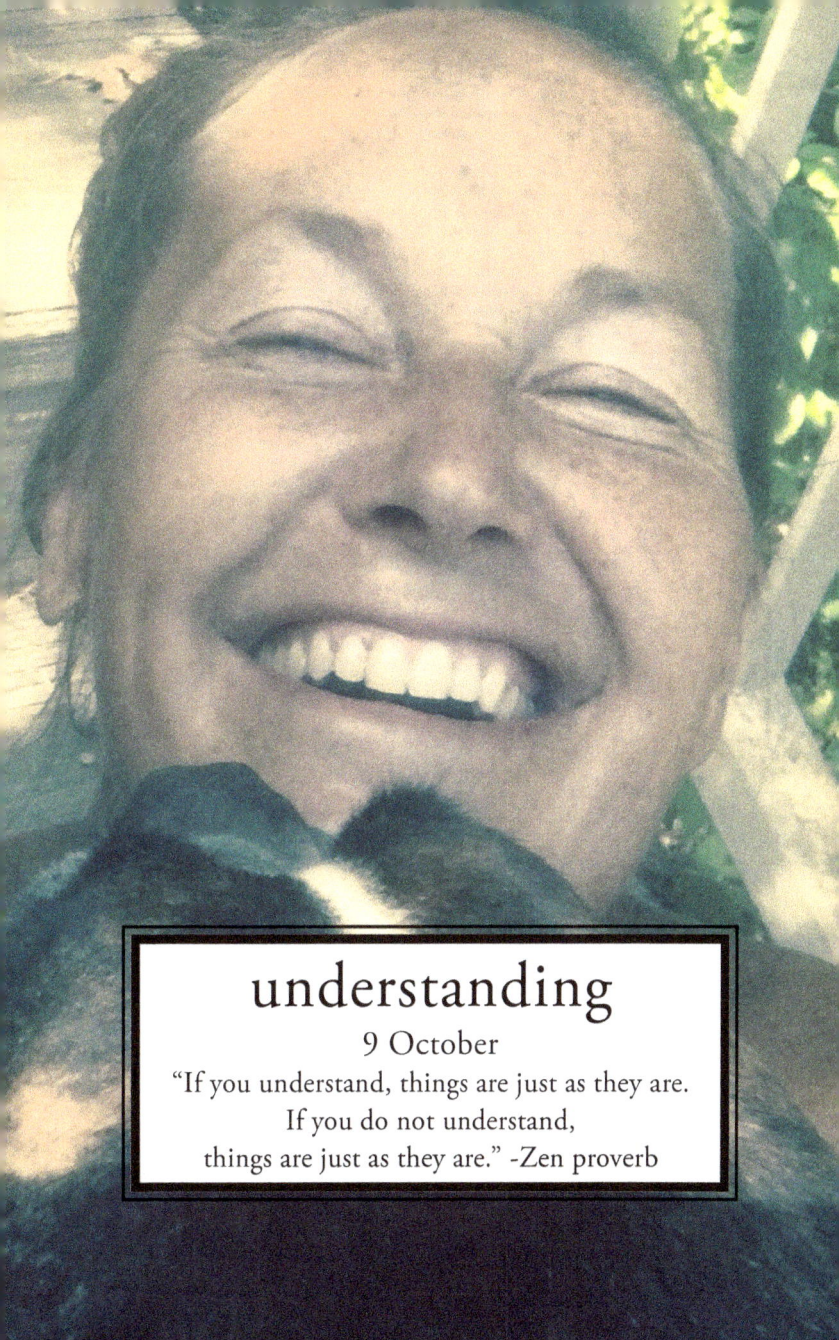

understanding

9 October

"If you understand, things are just as they are.
If you do not understand,
things are just as they are." -Zen proverb

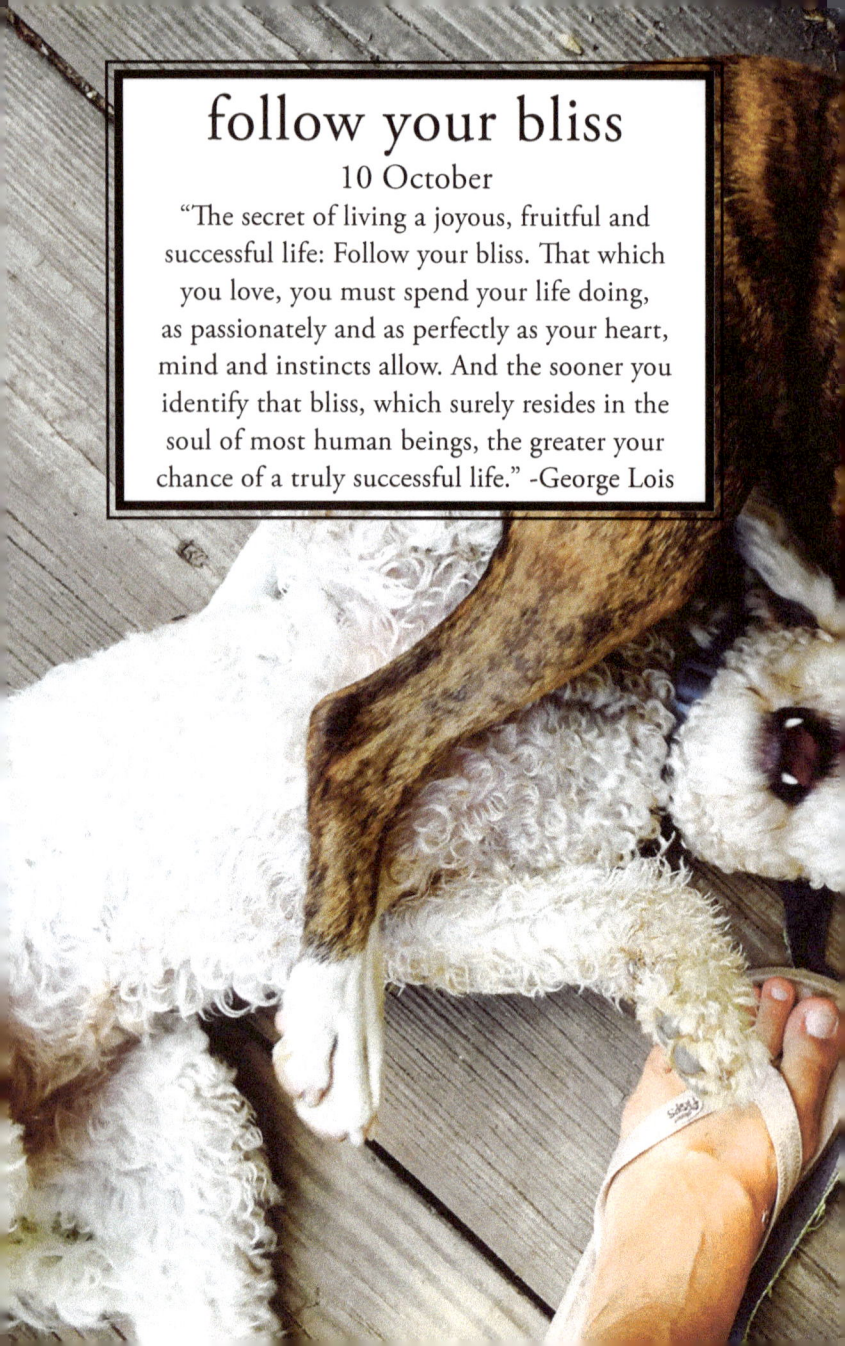

follow your bliss

10 October

"The secret of living a joyous, fruitful and successful life: Follow your bliss. That which you love, you must spend your life doing, as passionately and as perfectly as your heart, mind and instincts allow. And the sooner you identify that bliss, which surely resides in the soul of most human beings, the greater your chance of a truly successful life." -George Lois

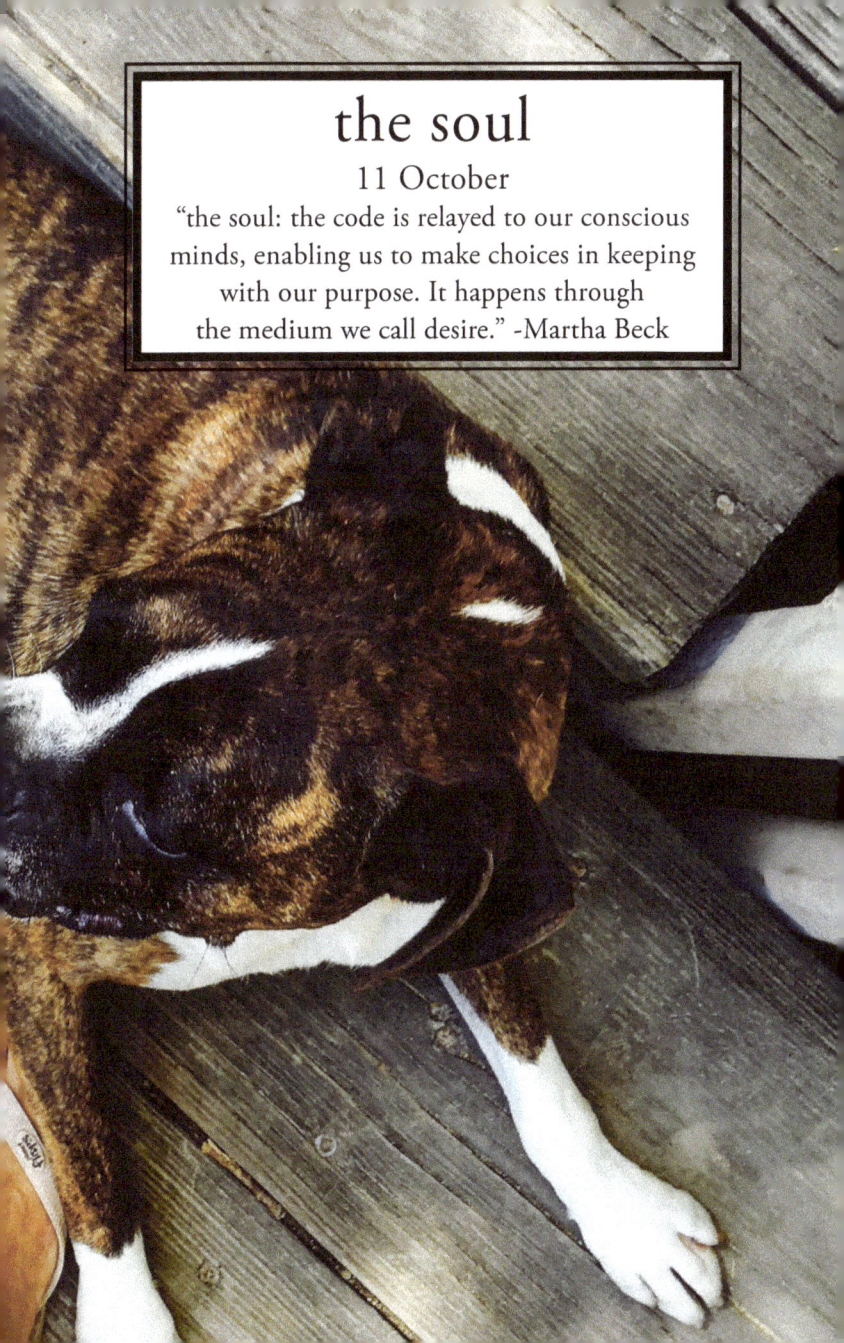

the soul
11 October
"the soul: the code is relayed to our conscious minds, enabling us to make choices in keeping with our purpose. It happens through the medium we call desire." -Martha Beck

gentle properties
12 October

"One of the ways I suggest my patients stay clean and use proper sanitation - yet not go overboard - is by choosing natural plant-based products such as essential oils. These aromatic compounds are extracted from plants that contain gentle antimicrobial properties. For example, tea tree oil, also known as melaleuca, has 327 medical studies to date proving its benefits as a gentle topical antimicrobial. A little tea tree oil mixed with water or coconut oil is a much safer hand sanitizer than the bottles of brightly colored gel you'll find at the drugstore." -Dr Josh Axe

everything we touch
13 October

"Remember, it's not only what we eat but also what we touch. Everything we press, tap, rub, or nudge sheds microbes or other molecules that are quickly absorbed through our pores and directly into the bloodstream. Our body's largest organ, the skin, is the first line of defense for our immune system - which leaves it vulnerable to the chemical onslaught as well... soap, deodorant, toothpaste, shampoo, hair conditioner, lip balm, sunscreen, body lotion, shaving products...makeup...dishwasher detergent, laundry detergent, floor cleaner, furniture polish, glass cleaner...your goal should be to minimize your exposure to potentially harmful toxins that are proven to not only damage your gut lining and create antibiotic resistance, but affect your body's endocrine system, leaving your thyroid, pancreas, and adrenal glands even more vulnerable than before." -Dr Josh Axe

eat money
14 October
"Only when the last tree has died and the last river been poisoned and the last fish been caught will we realize we cannot eat money." -Cree saying

whew!
15 October
I am not my name. I am not my body. I am not my mind. I am not my job. I am not my relationships. I am not my country/race/religion.

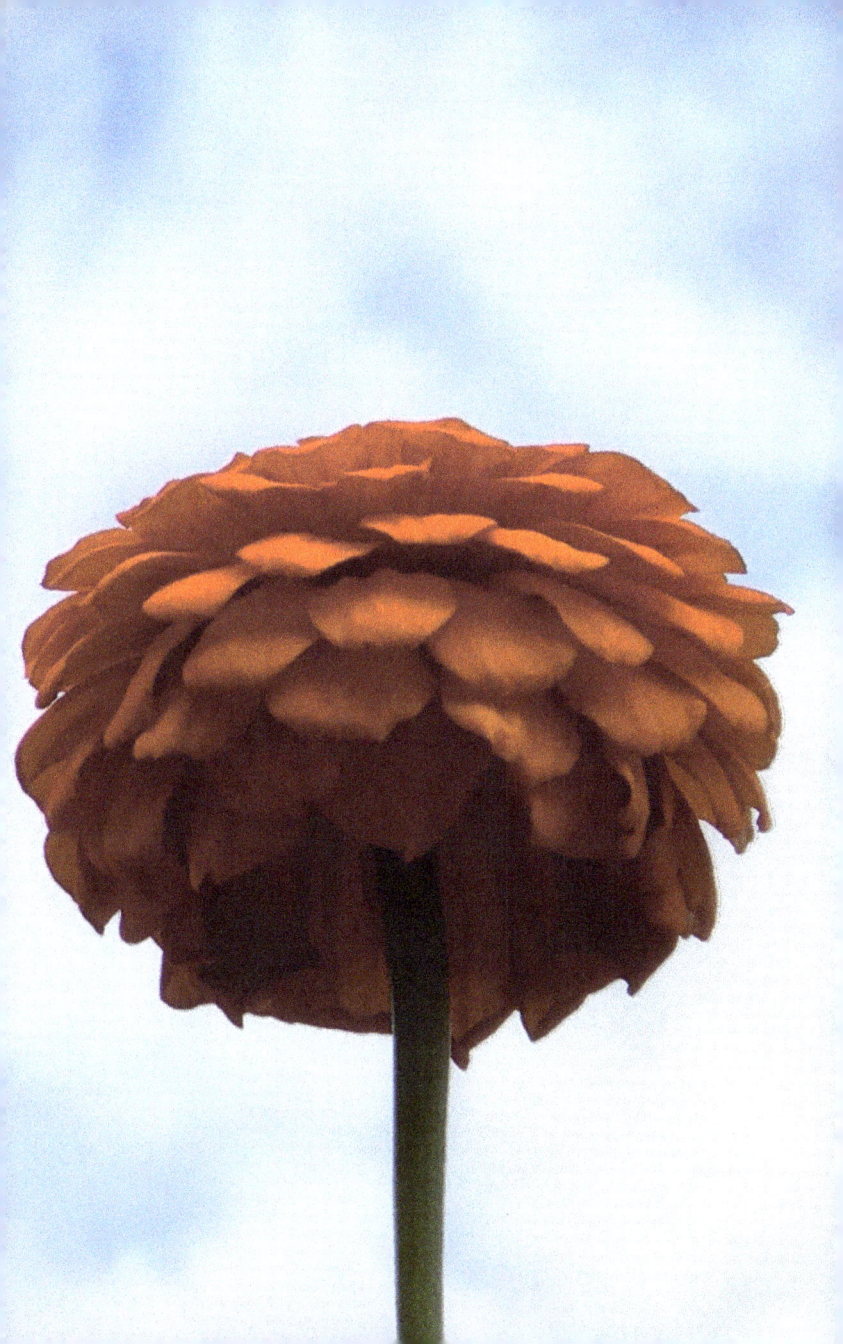

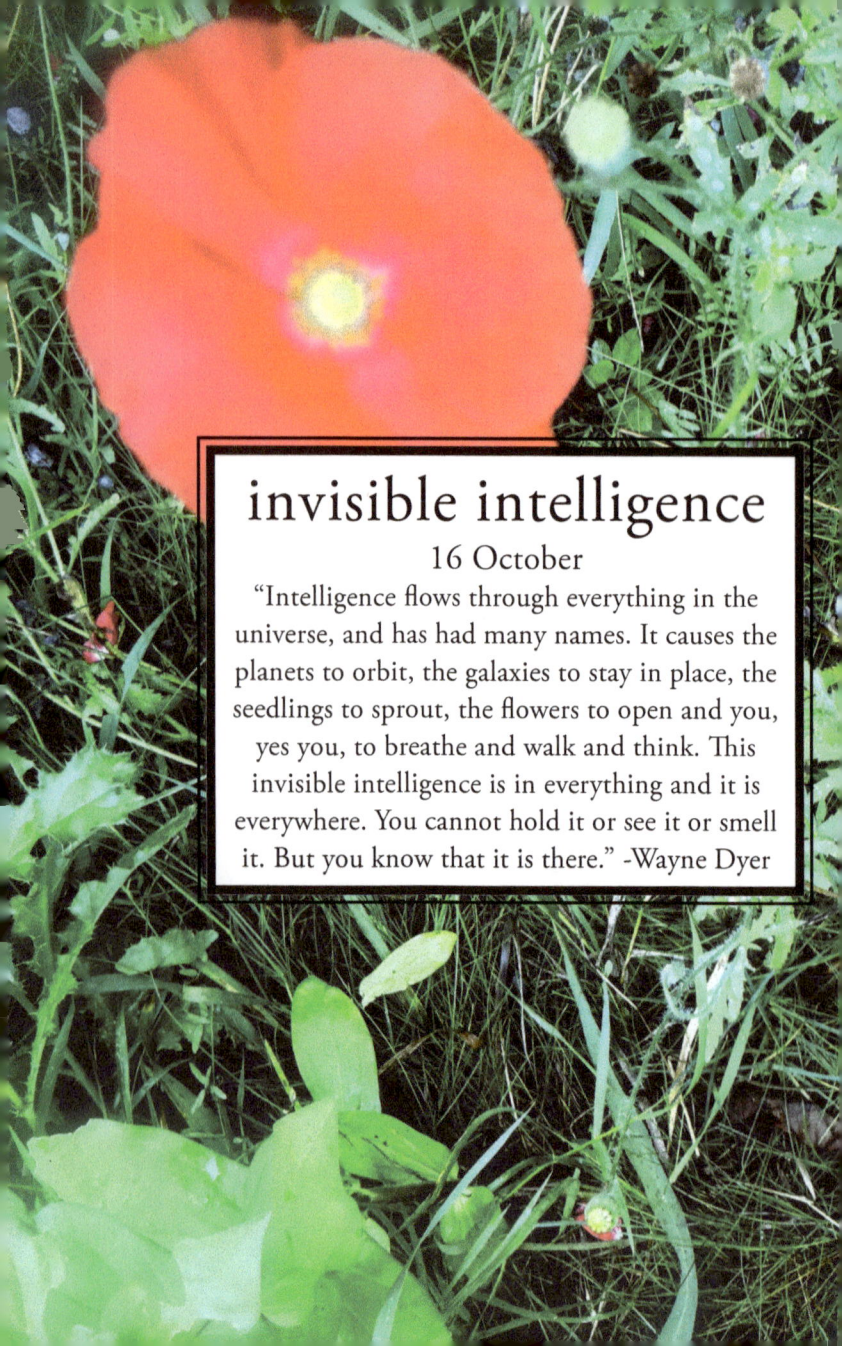

invisible intelligence
16 October

"Intelligence flows through everything in the universe, and has had many names. It causes the planets to orbit, the galaxies to stay in place, the seedlings to sprout, the flowers to open and you, yes you, to breathe and walk and think. This invisible intelligence is in everything and it is everywhere. You cannot hold it or see it or smell it. But you know that it is there." -Wayne Dyer

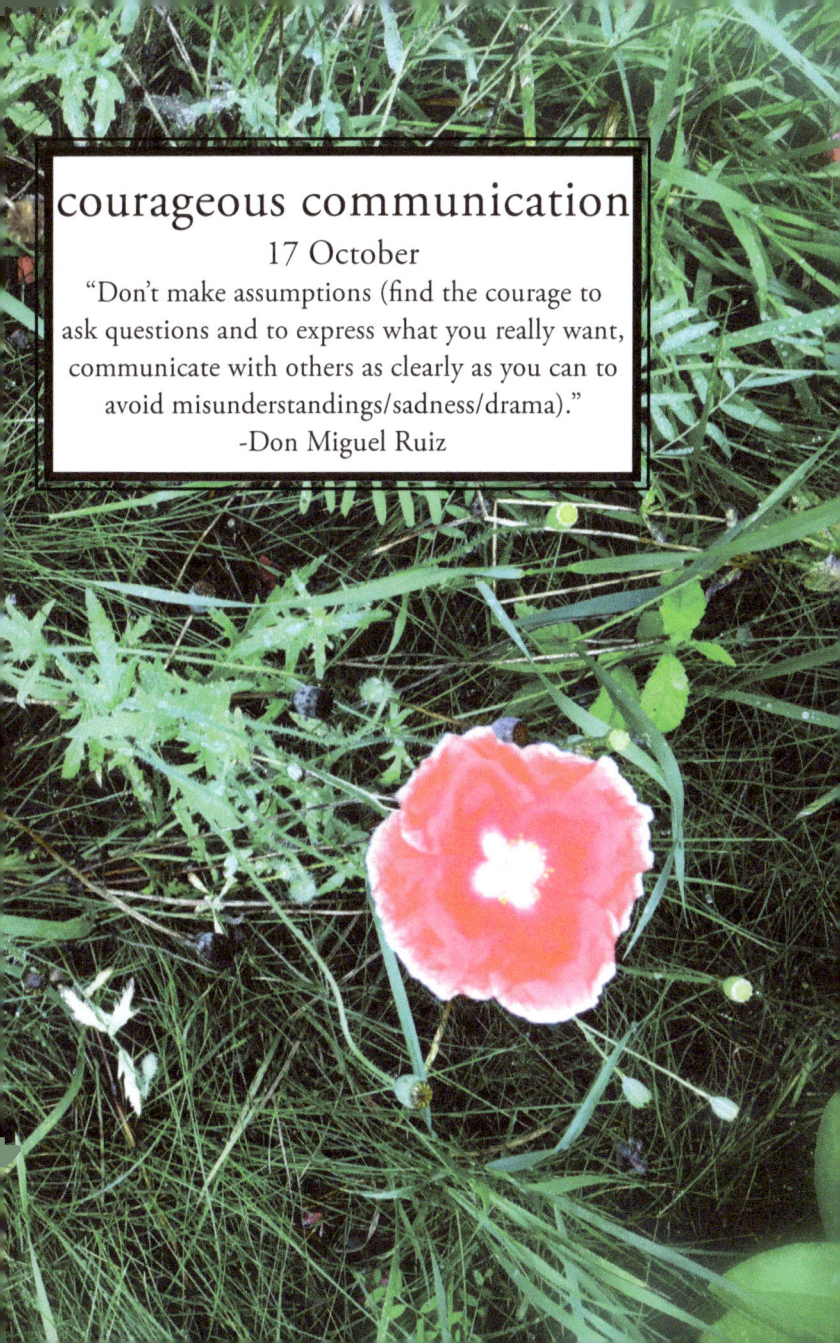

courageous communication
17 October
"Don't make assumptions (find the courage to ask questions and to express what you really want, communicate with others as clearly as you can to avoid misunderstandings/sadness/drama)."
-Don Miguel Ruiz

honor your genes

18 October

"Manage stress levels with plenty of sleep, play, sunlight, fresh air, and creative outlets and by avoiding trauma that often arises from stupid mistakes, rebel against the tremendous cultural movement toward sedentary lifestyles, excessive digital stimulation, and insufficient rest. Honor your primal genes by slowing down and simplifying your life. Your ancestors worked hard to survive, but their regular respites from stress gave them the peace of mind and body that are so highly coveted today." -Mark Sisson

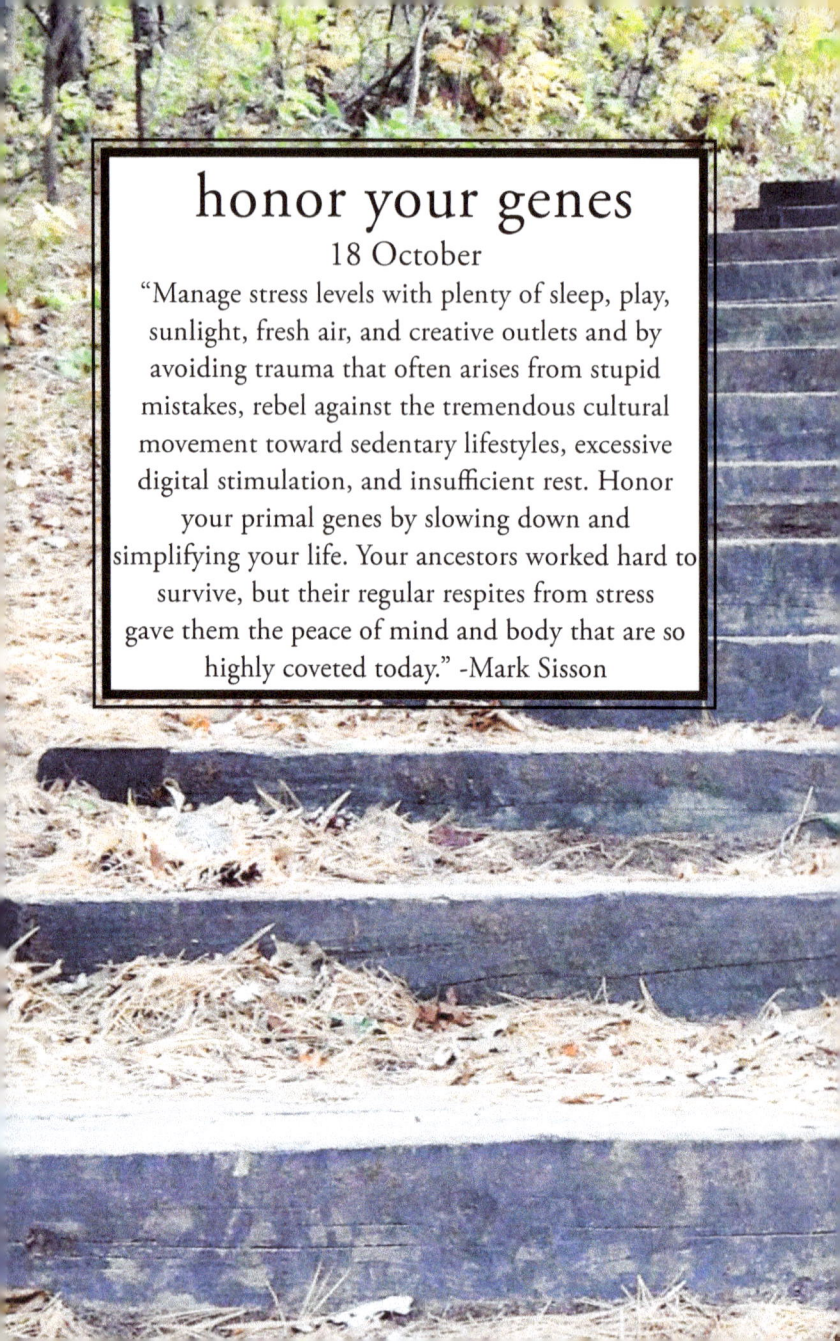

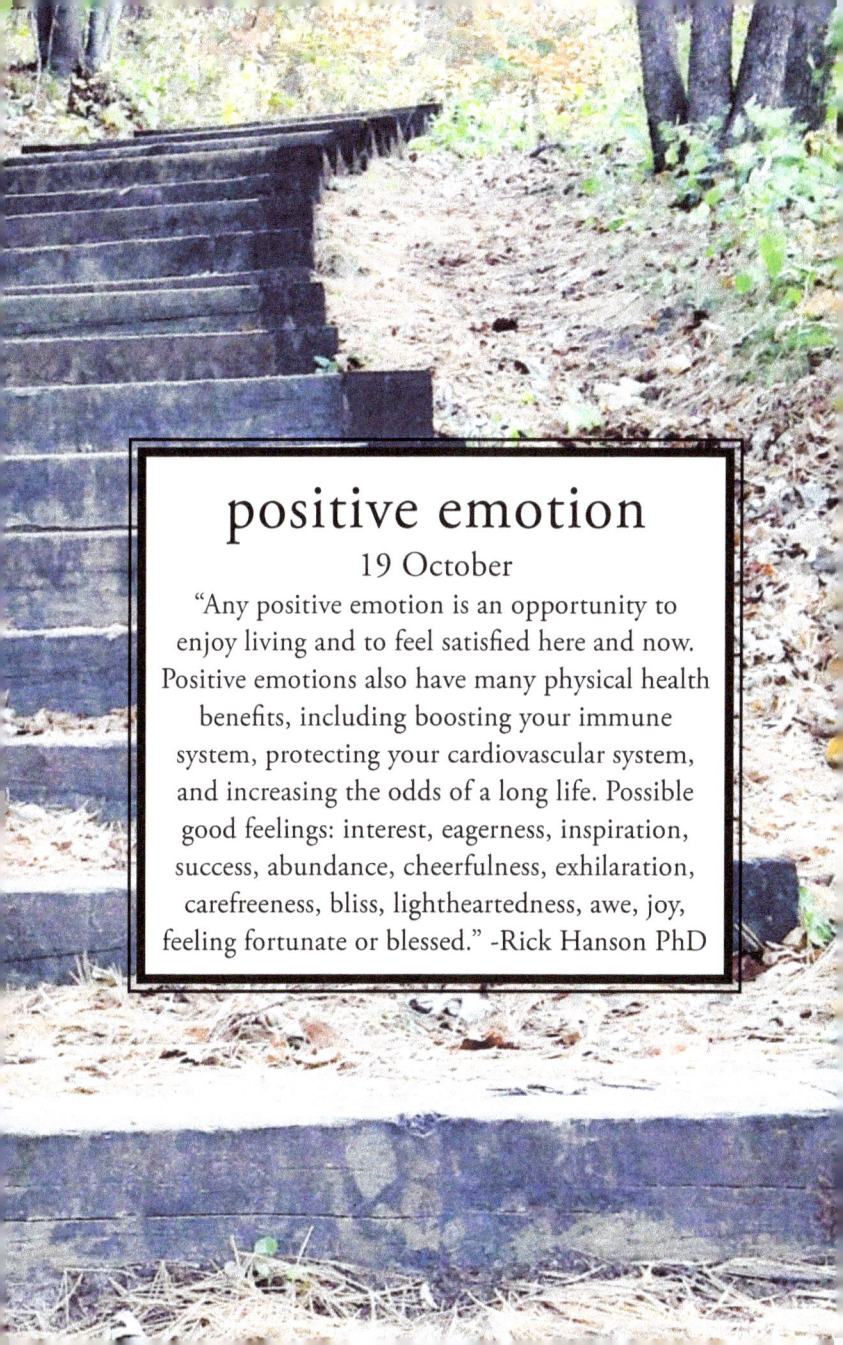

positive emotion
19 October

"Any positive emotion is an opportunity to enjoy living and to feel satisfied here and now. Positive emotions also have many physical health benefits, including boosting your immune system, protecting your cardiovascular system, and increasing the odds of a long life. Possible good feelings: interest, eagerness, inspiration, success, abundance, cheerfulness, exhilaration, carefreeness, bliss, lightheartedness, awe, joy, feeling fortunate or blessed." -Rick Hanson PhD

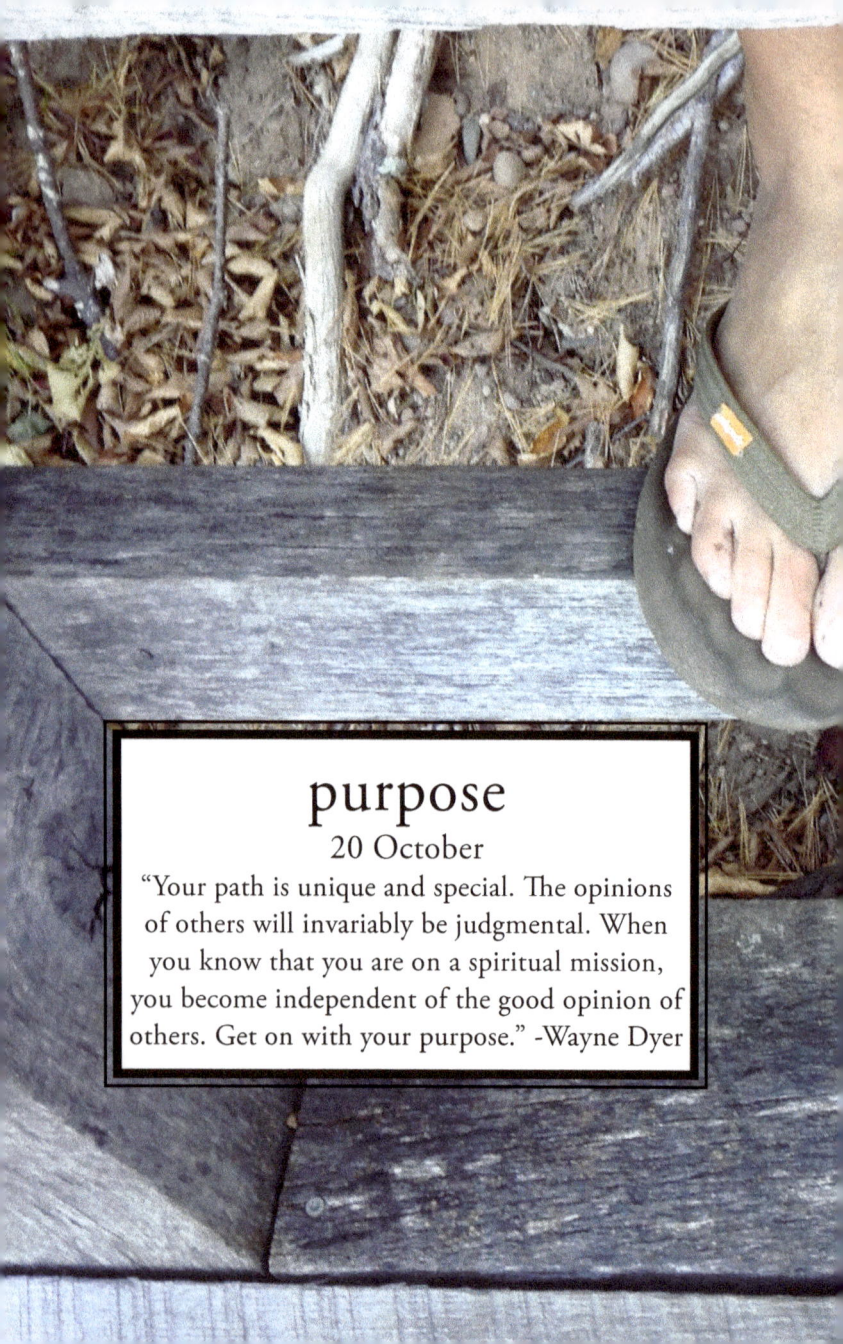

purpose
20 October

"Your path is unique and special. The opinions of others will invariably be judgmental. When you know that you are on a spiritual mission, you become independent of the good opinion of others. Get on with your purpose." -Wayne Dyer

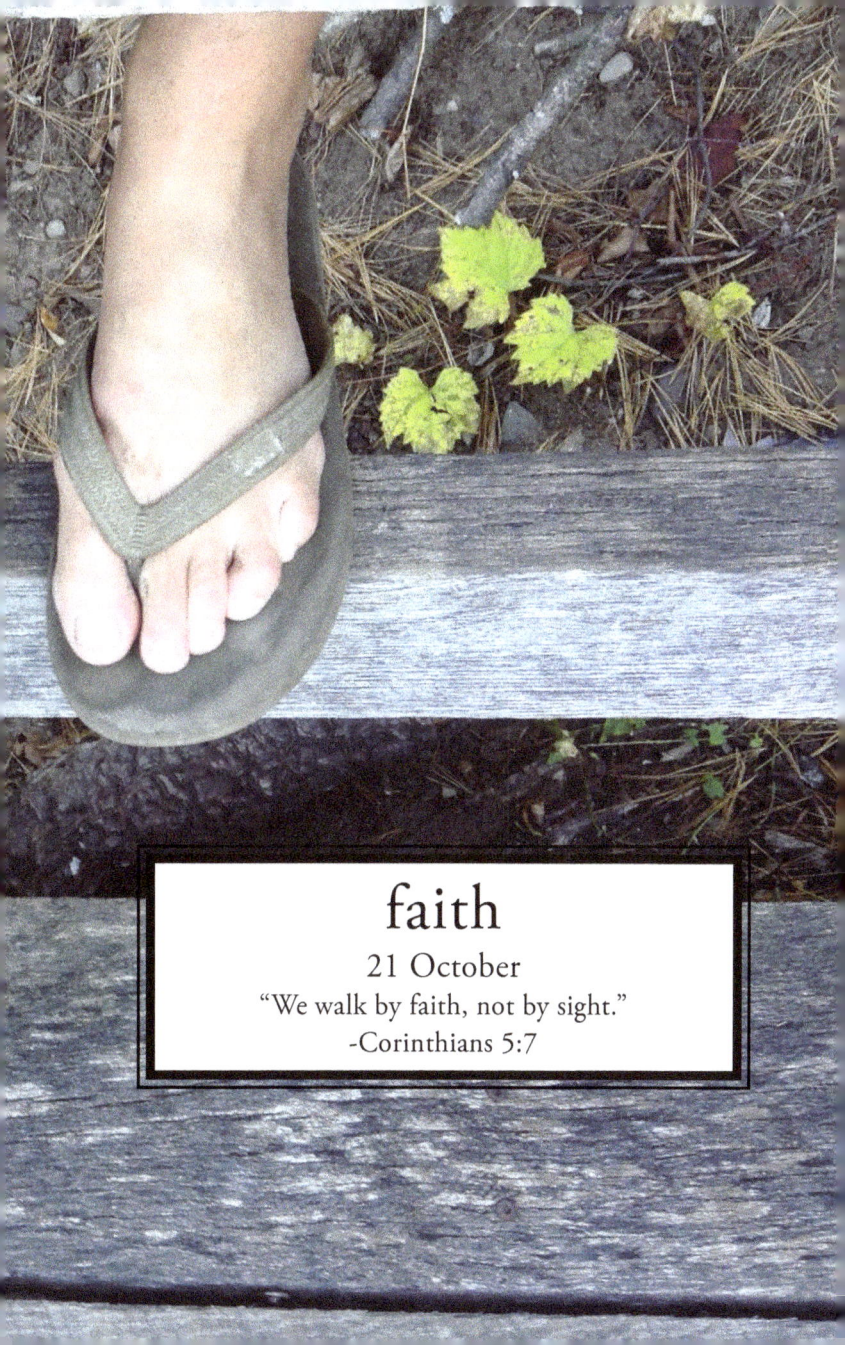

faith

21 October
"We walk by faith, not by sight."
-Corinthians 5:7

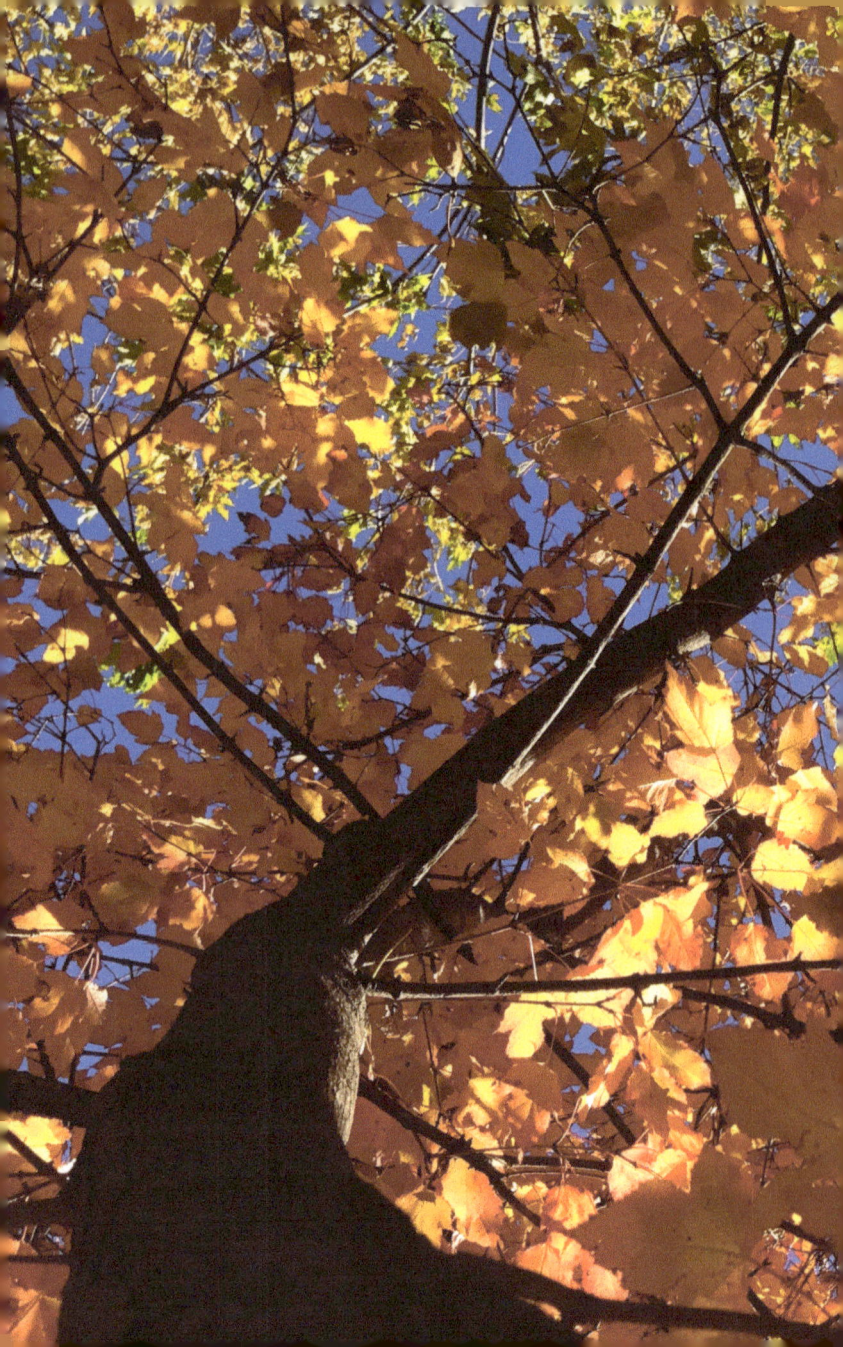

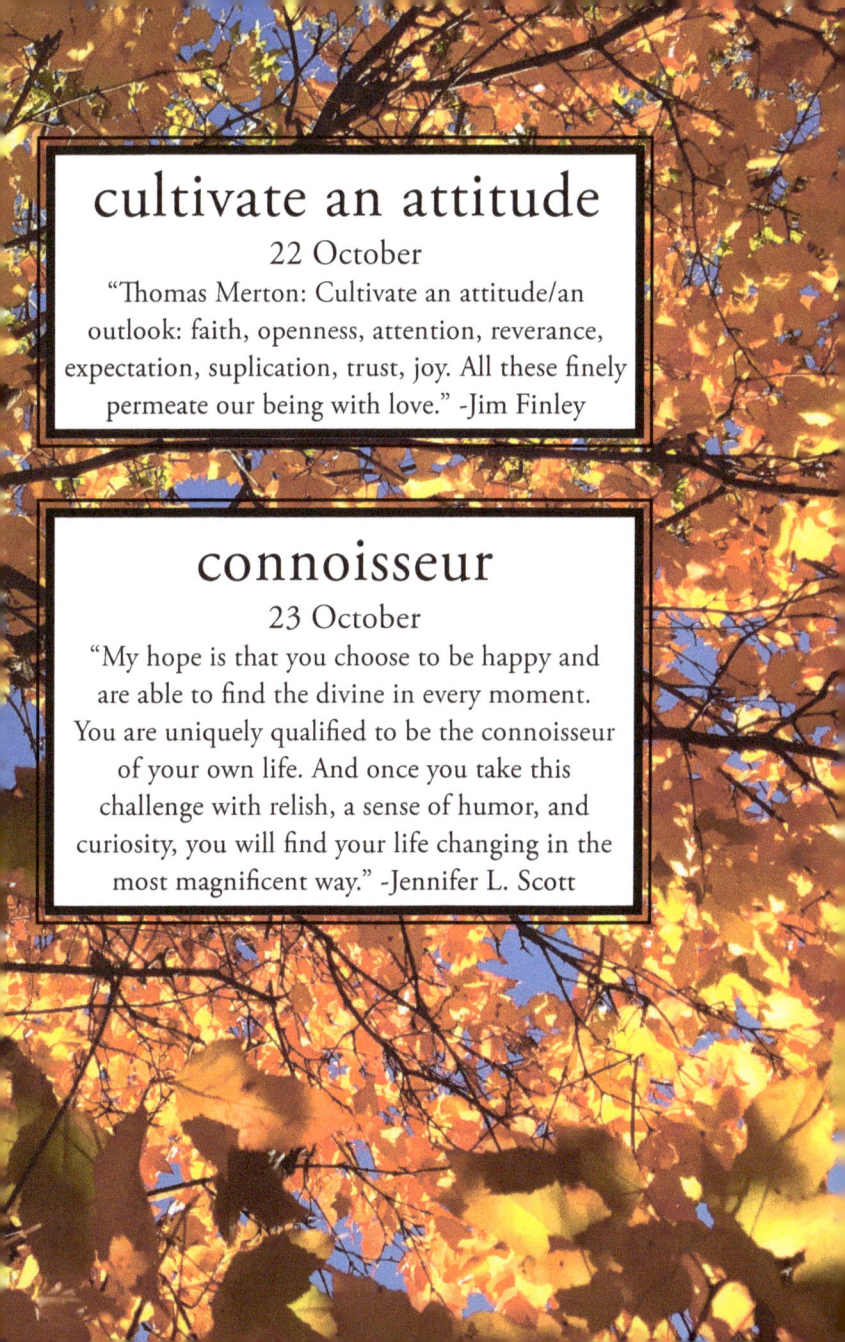

cultivate an attitude
22 October
"Thomas Merton: Cultivate an attitude/an outlook: faith, openness, attention, reverance, expectation, suplication, trust, joy. All these finely permeate our being with love." -Jim Finley

connoisseur
23 October
"My hope is that you choose to be happy and are able to find the divine in every moment. You are uniquely qualified to be the connoisseur of your own life. And once you take this challenge with relish, a sense of humor, and curiosity, you will find your life changing in the most magnificent way." -Jennifer L. Scott

here & now

24 October

"In Vietnamese, 'mindfulness' is *chanh niem*, which means to be truly present in the moment. When you eat, you know that you are eating. When you walk, you know that you are walking. The opposite of mindfulness is forgetfulness. You eat but you don't know that you are eating, because your mind is elsewhere. When you bring your mind back to what is happening in the here and now, that is mindfulness, and mindfulness can bring you a lot of life, pleasure, and joy."
-Thich Nhat Hanh

brighten
25 October

"When you've finished putting your house in order, your life will change dramatically. Once you have experienced what it's like to have a truly ordered house, you'll feel your whole world brighten." -Marie Kondo

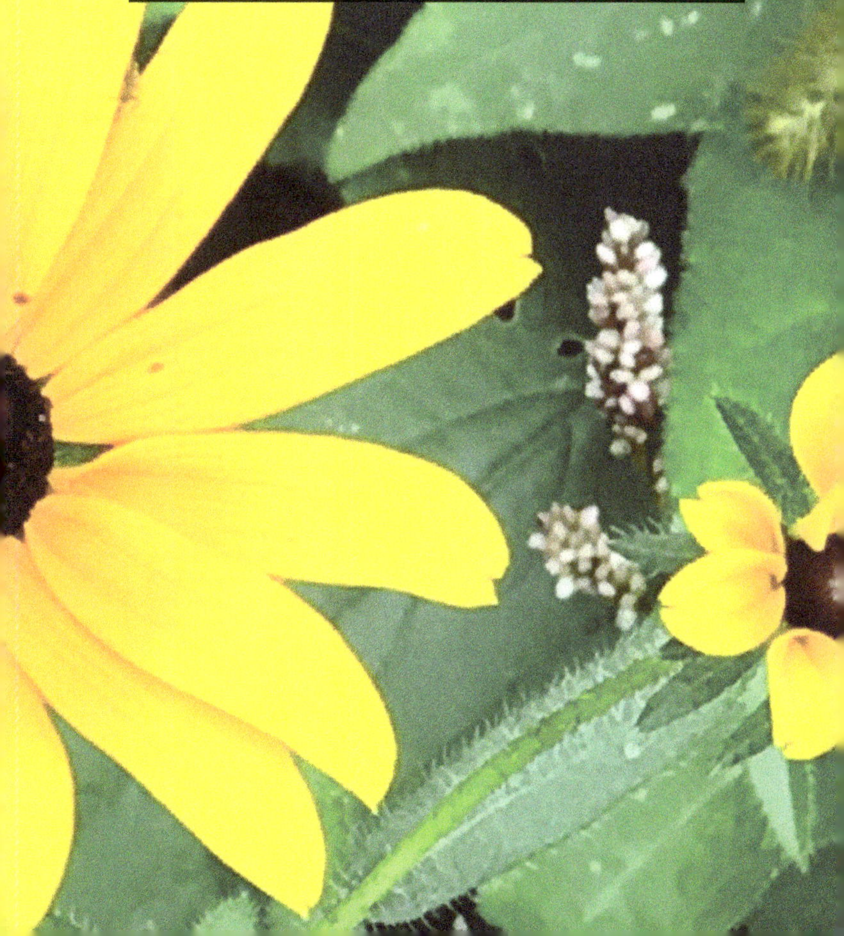

peace
26 October

"As you relax, your parasympathetic nervous system gets more active, which calms down the fight-or-flight sympathetic nervous system. Tension drains out of your body, your heart rate and breathing slow down, and digestion eases - all of which turns down the dial on internal signals of threat, helping you relax even further...when you take advantage of the 'all is well' signals coming up into your brain from your body by deliberately focusing on the fact that you are actually all right, almost every single moment of your life offers a wonderful opportunity to step out of fear and anger and into peace." -Rick Hanson PhD

opportunities
27 October

"Subtracting unneeded stuff multiplies opportunities to pursue things you care about. The result is exponential growth in personal satisfaction. Maybe the life you've always wanted is buried under everything you own!"
-Joshua Becker

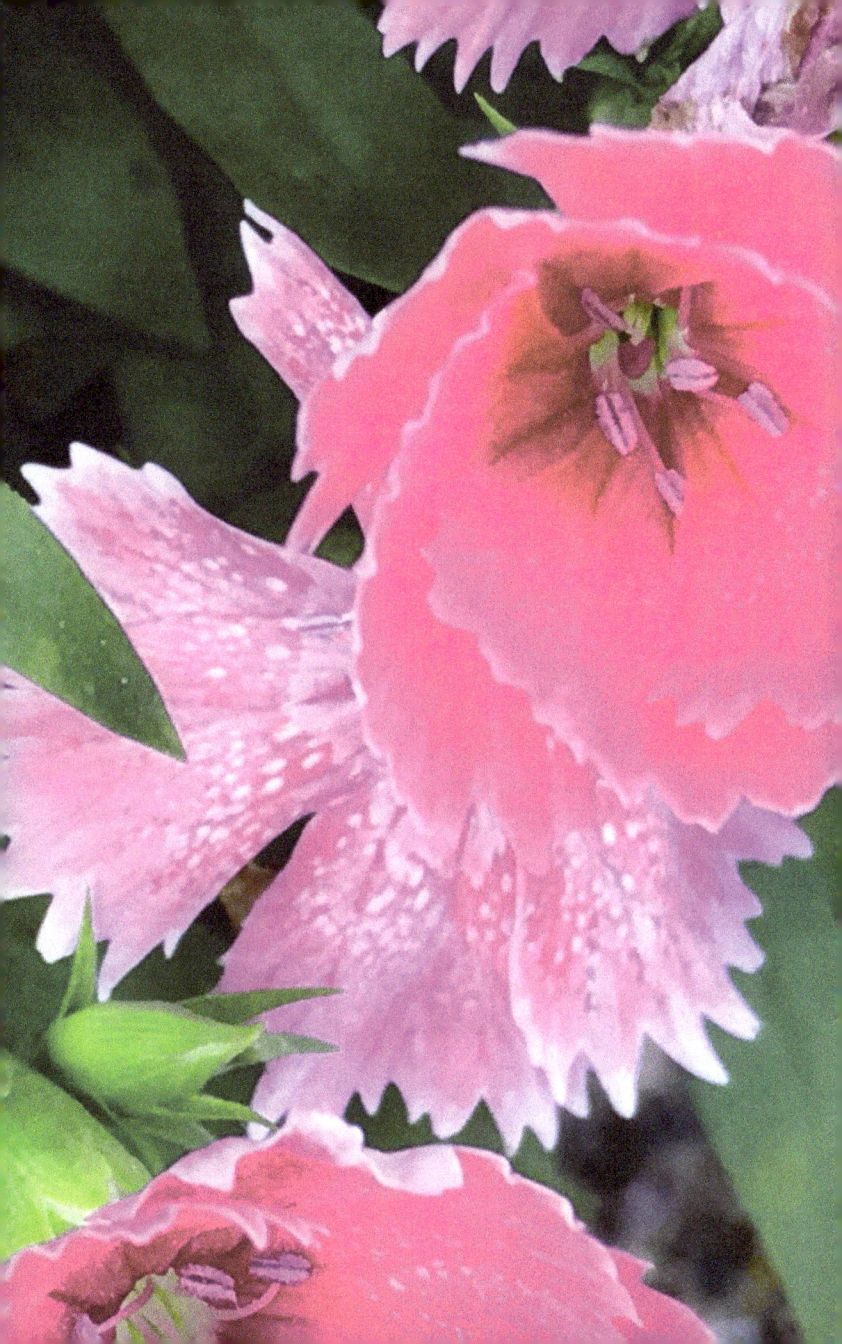

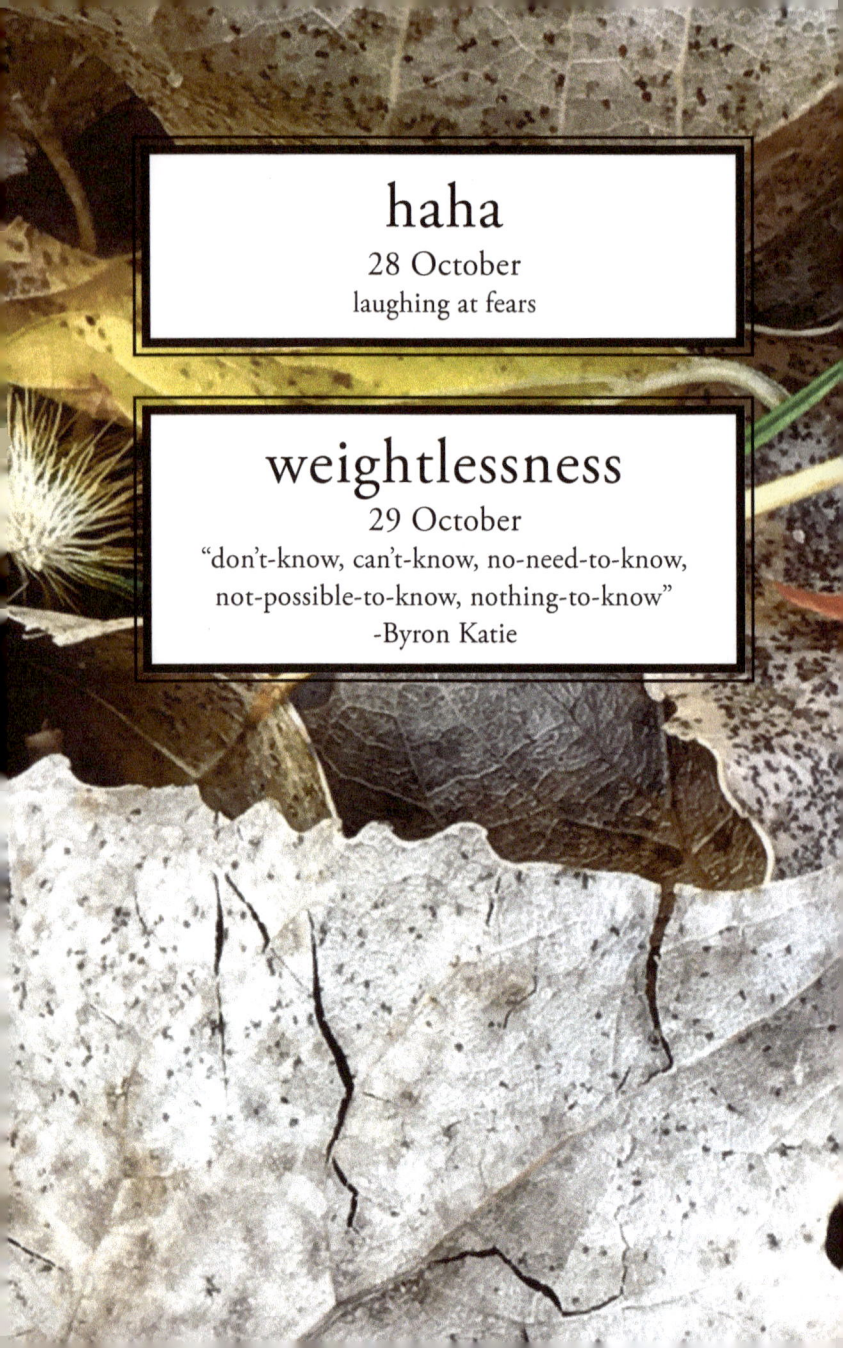

haha
28 October
laughing at fears

weightlessness
29 October
"don't-know, can't-know, no-need-to-know,
not-possible-to-know, nothing-to-know"
-Byron Katie

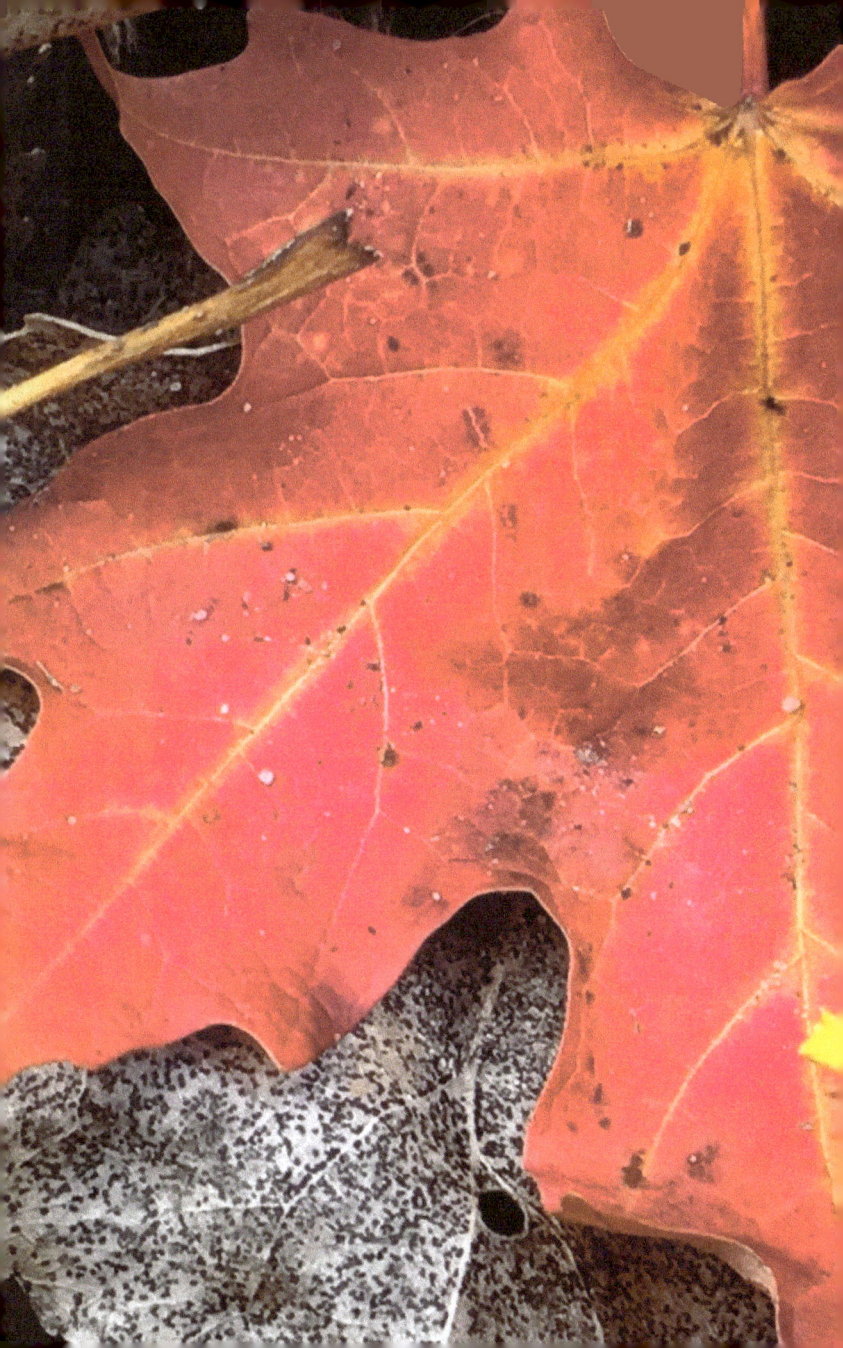

holy thoughts
30 October
"The sedentary life is the very sin against the Holy Spirit. Only thoughts reached by walking have value." -Friedrich Nietzsche (John Durant)

standing desks
31 October
"Many great writers and thinkers throughout history have discovered that standing, pacing, and walking spur creativity...[some who wrote/worked standing]: Victor Hugo, Nathaniel Hawthorne, Henry Wadsworth Longfellow, Charles Dickens, Virginia Woolf, Ernest Hemingway, Vladimir Nabokov, August Wilson, Thomas Jefferson, Benjamin Franklin, Winston Churchill, Johannes Brahms, Richard Wagner, E.B. White, Philip Roth, Lewis Carroll..."
-John Durant

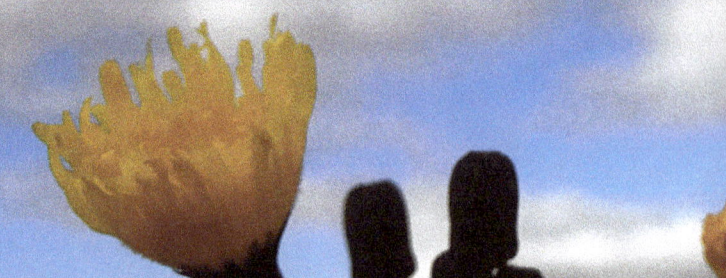

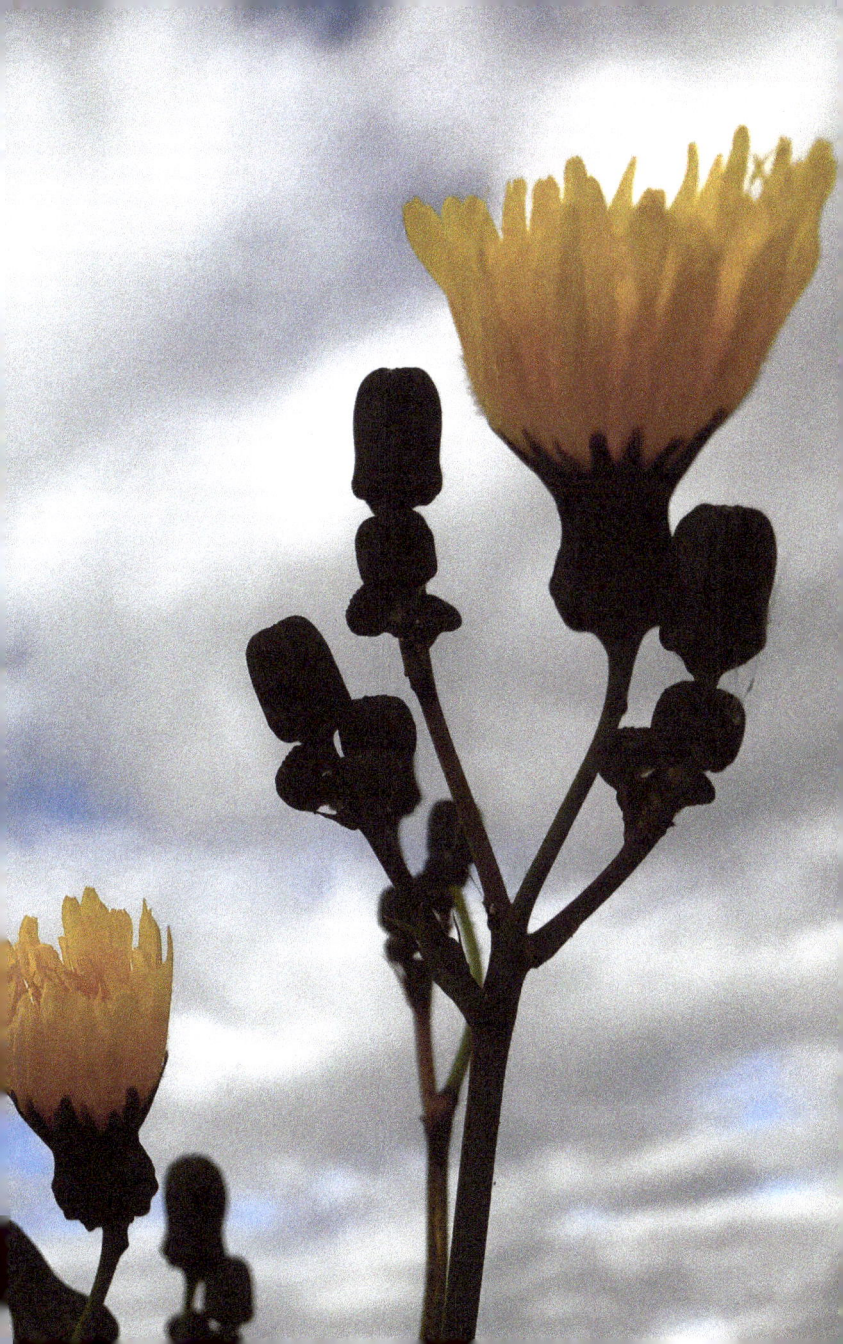

center of health

1 November

"Our nation is in the grip of a hidden epidemic. We've been taking our digestive system for granted for far too long, starving it of actual nutrition while overfeeding it with toxic levels of processed foods and sugar and overtaxing it with environmental chemicals, stress, and excessive antimicrobials...the gut is not simply a food-processing center - the gut is the center of health itself." -Dr Josh Axe

work

2 November

"In some way or other you have to work for the fulfillment of your desires. Put in energy and wait for the results." -Sri Nisargadatta Maharaj

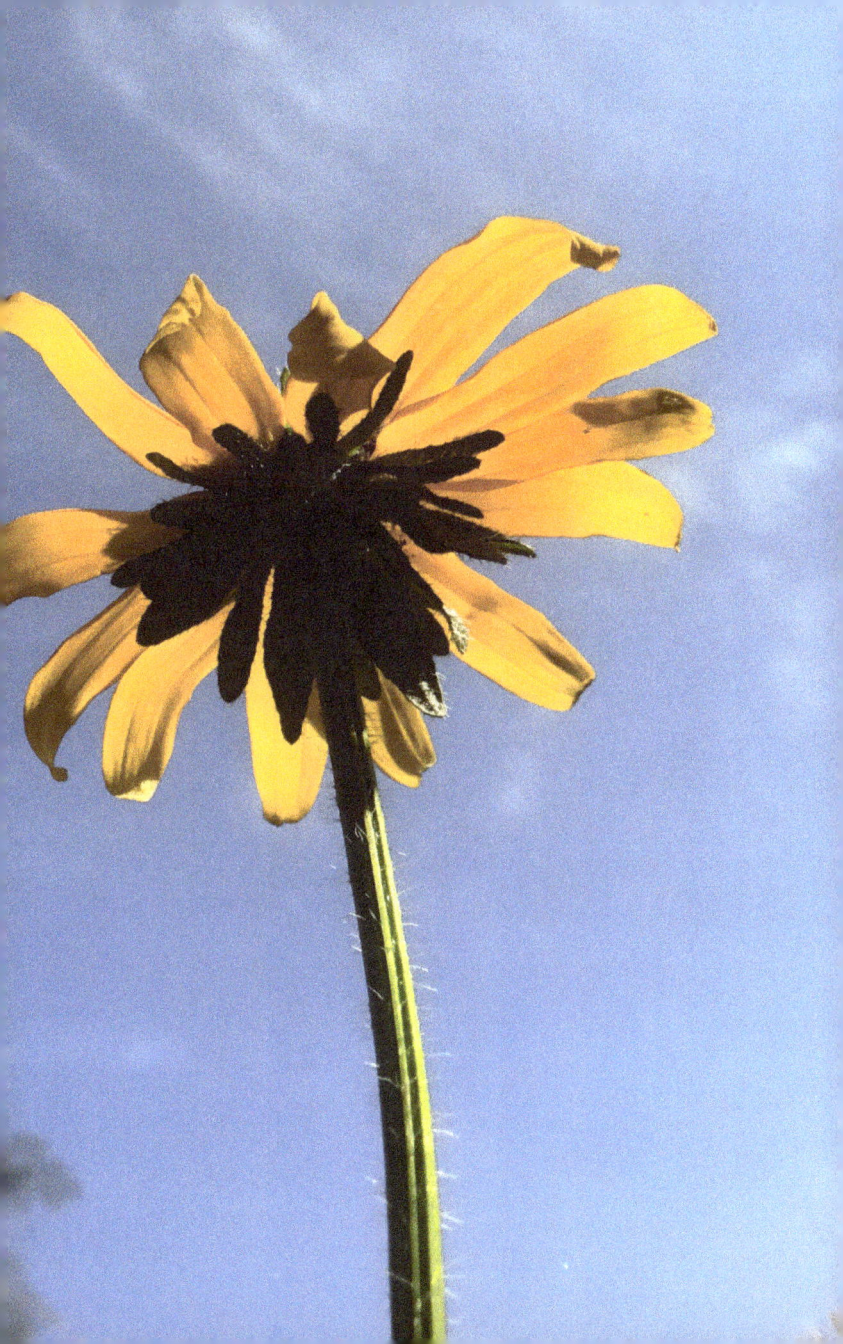

humanity's desire
3 November
"When you desire the common good, the whole world desires with you. Make humanity's desire your own and work for it. There you cannot fail."
-Sri Nisargadatta Maharaj

meditation
4 November
"Meditation will help you to find your bonds, loosen them, untie them and cast off your moorings. When you are no longer attached to anything, you have done your share. The rest will be done for you." -Sri Nisargadatta Maharaj

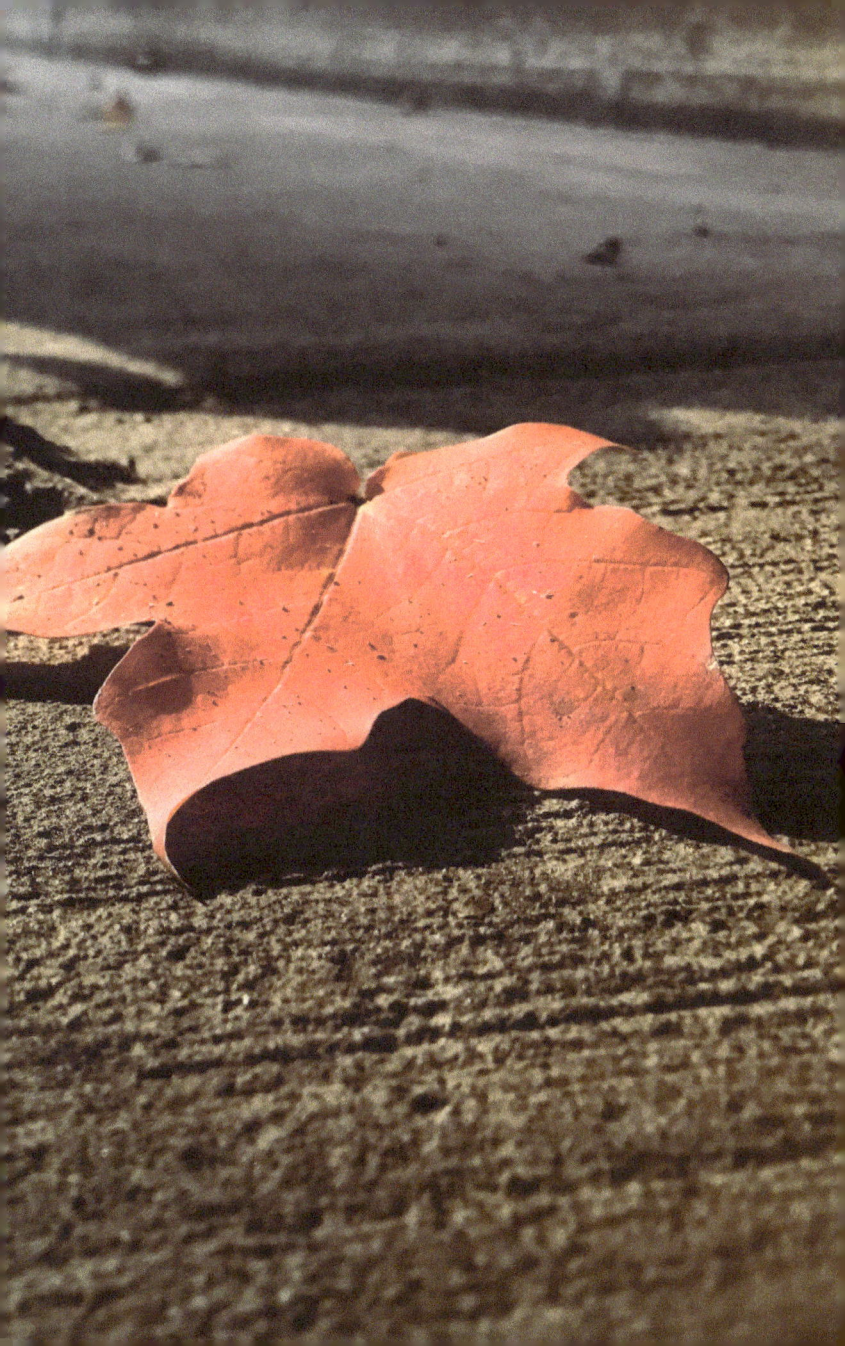

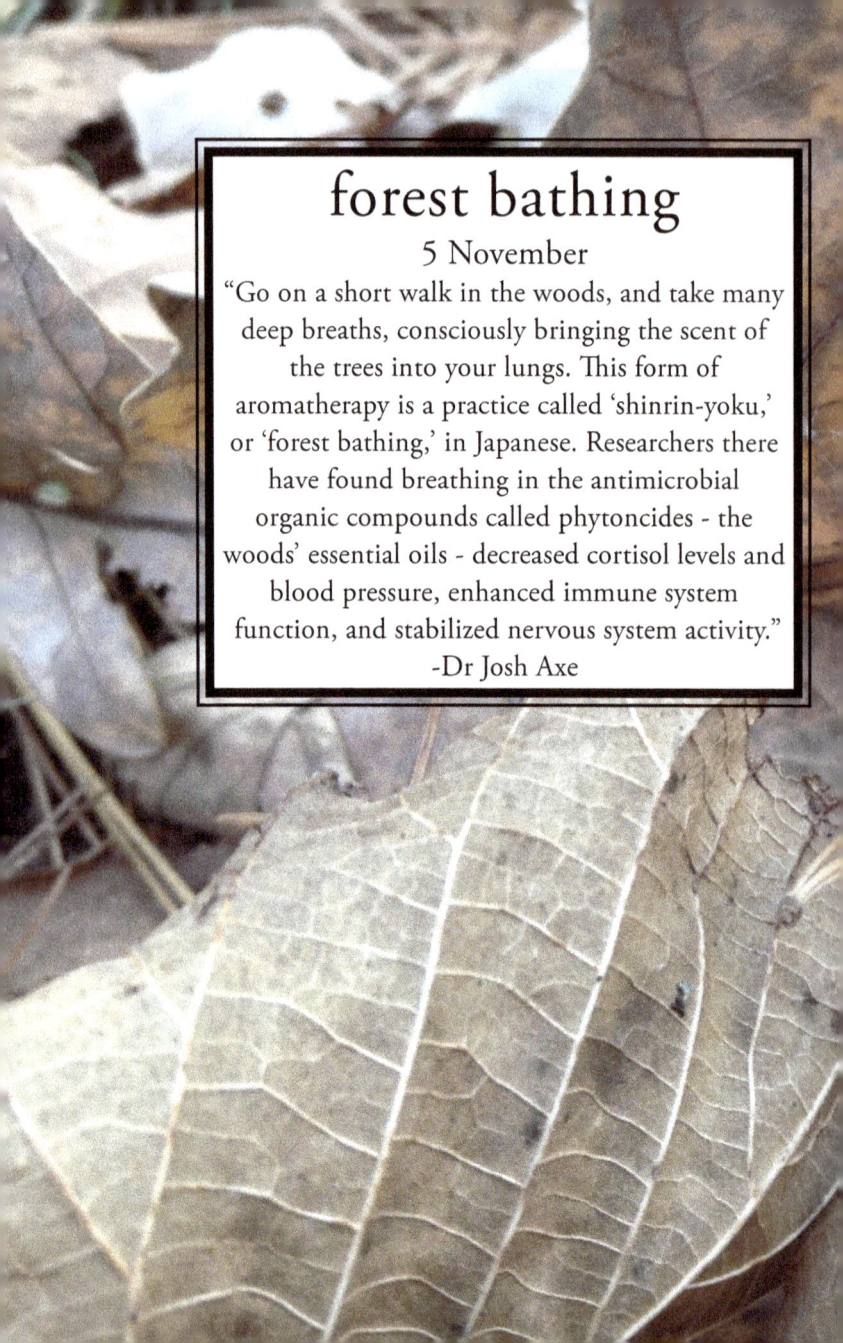

forest bathing
5 November

"Go on a short walk in the woods, and take many deep breaths, consciously bringing the scent of the trees into your lungs. This form of aromatherapy is a practice called 'shinrin-yoku,' or 'forest bathing,' in Japanese. Researchers there have found breathing in the antimicrobial organic compounds called phytoncides - the woods' essential oils - decreased cortisol levels and blood pressure, enhanced immune system function, and stabilized nervous system activity."

-Dr Josh Axe

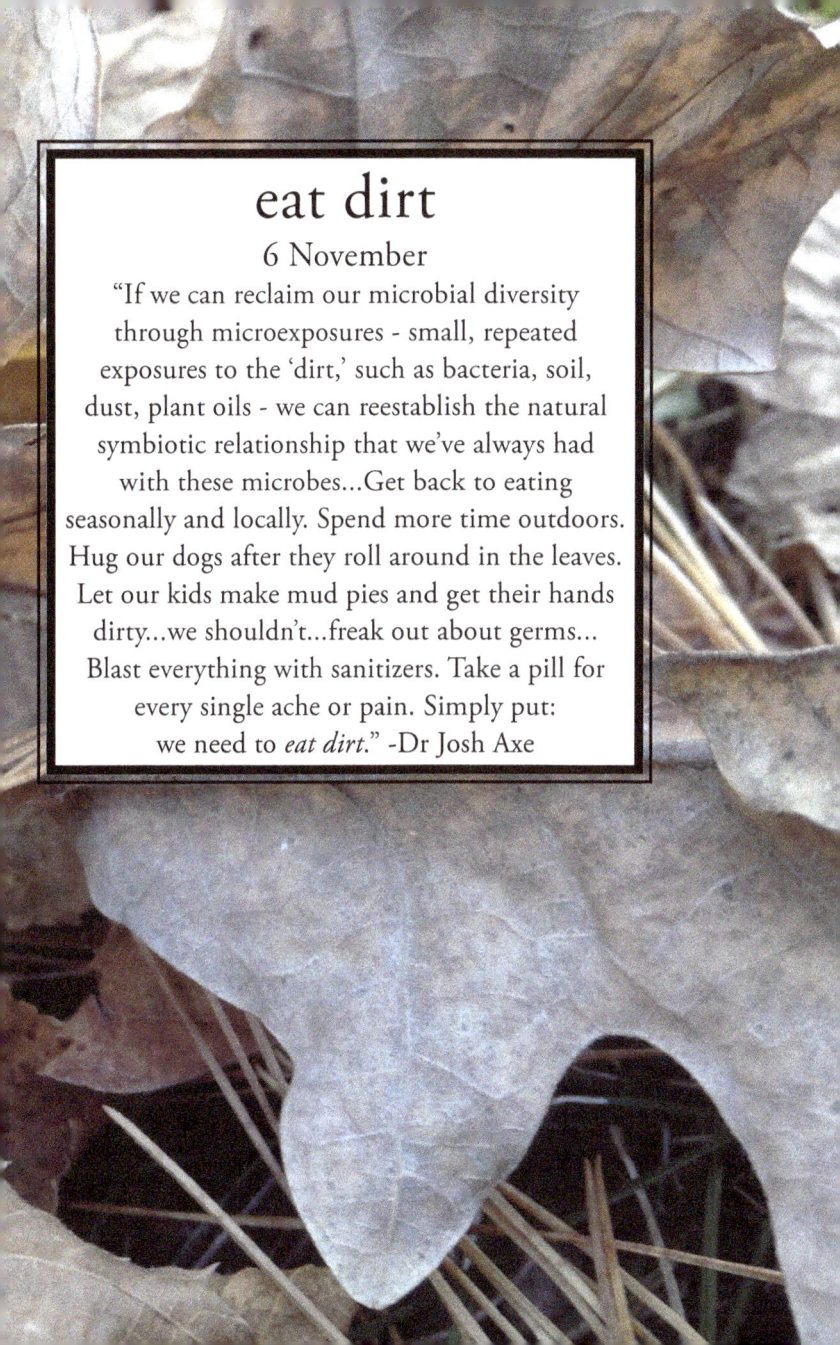

eat dirt

6 November

"If we can reclaim our microbial diversity through microexposures - small, repeated exposures to the 'dirt,' such as bacteria, soil, dust, plant oils - we can reestablish the natural symbiotic relationship that we've always had with these microbes...Get back to eating seasonally and locally. Spend more time outdoors. Hug our dogs after they roll around in the leaves. Let our kids make mud pies and get their hands dirty...we shouldn't...freak out about germs... Blast everything with sanitizers. Take a pill for every single ache or pain. Simply put: we need to *eat dirt*." -Dr Josh Axe

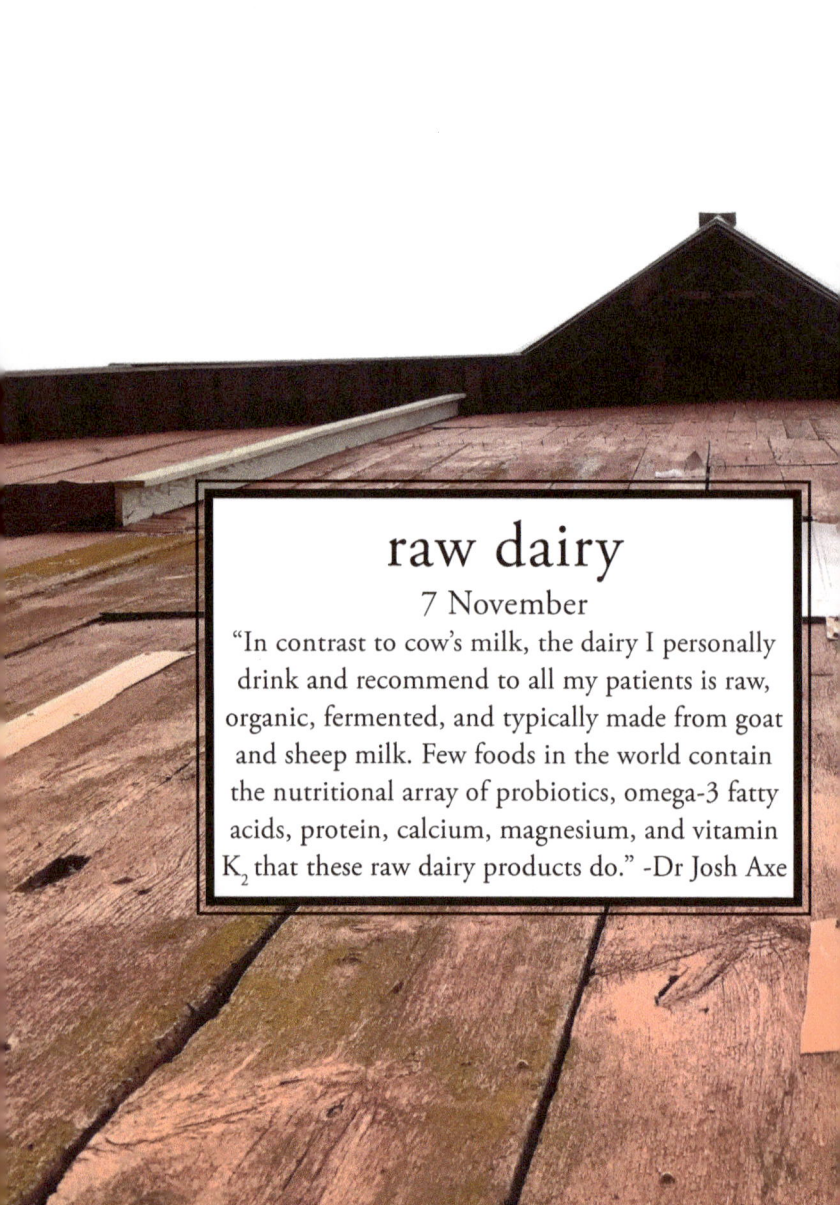

raw dairy
7 November

"In contrast to cow's milk, the dairy I personally drink and recommend to all my patients is raw, organic, fermented, and typically made from goat and sheep milk. Few foods in the world contain the nutritional array of probiotics, omega-3 fatty acids, protein, calcium, magnesium, and vitamin K_2 that these raw dairy products do." -Dr Josh Axe

milk

8 November

"The health of the animal and the processing methods of milk can categorize dairy as either one of the healthier foods in the world or one of the worst...According to a study published in the *Journal of Agricultural and Food Chemisty*, a single glass of pasteurized milk can contain up to twenty different chemicals...I rarely consume cow's milk because even organic versions in this country tend to contain a protein called A1 beta-casein. The result of a relatively recent genetic mutation, this protein is more common among the Holstein cows of American and some European industrial diaries, and can be more inflammatory to the body than gluten...I recommend choosing **raw cow's milk dairy products from only Jersey or Guernsey cows**, when you can find them." -Dr Josh Axe

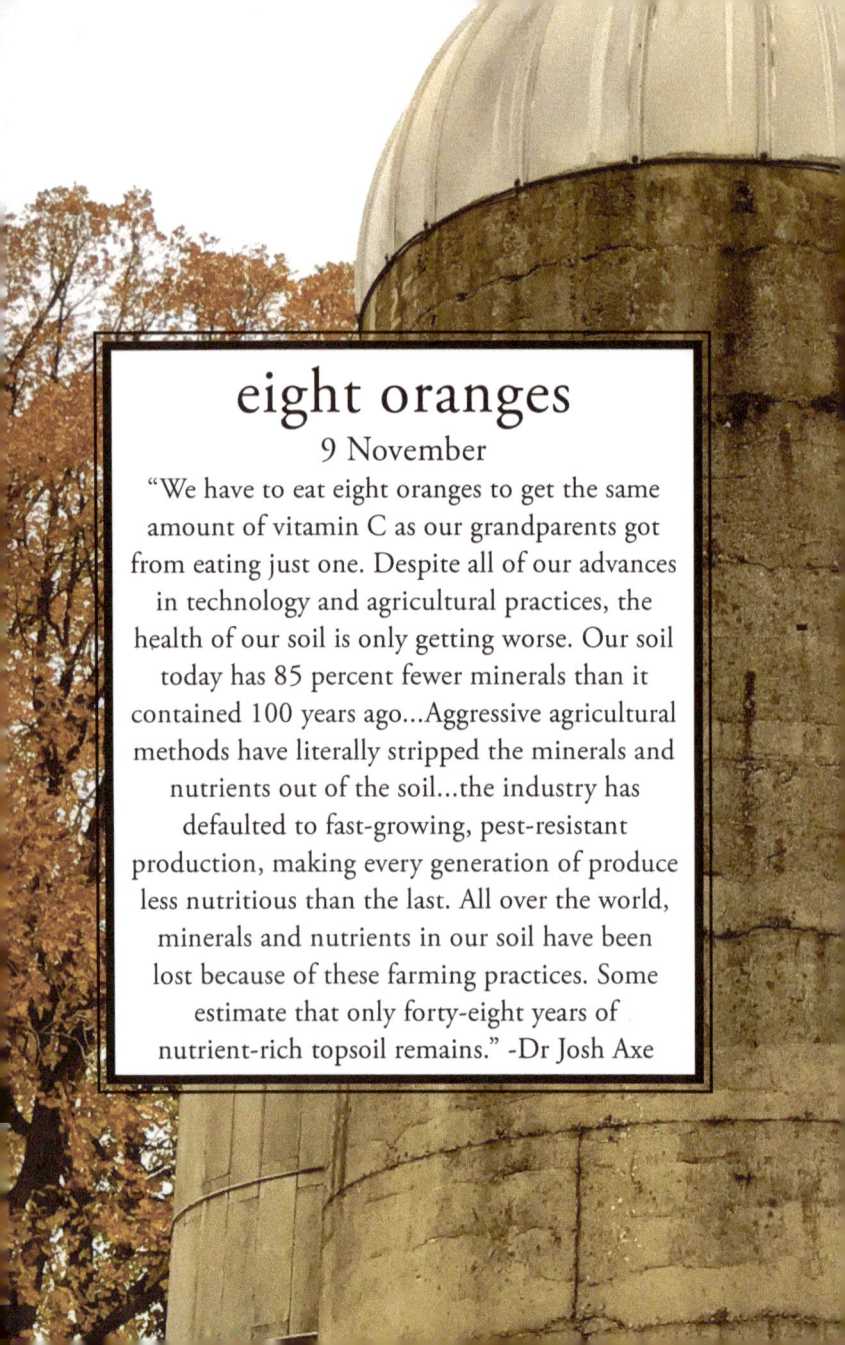

eight oranges
9 November

"We have to eat eight oranges to get the same amount of vitamin C as our grandparents got from eating just one. Despite all of our advances in technology and agricultural practices, the health of our soil is only getting worse. Our soil today has 85 percent fewer minerals than it contained 100 years ago...Aggressive agricultural methods have literally stripped the minerals and nutrients out of the soil...the industry has defaulted to fast-growing, pest-resistant production, making every generation of produce less nutritious than the last. All over the world, minerals and nutrients in our soil have been lost because of these farming practices. Some estimate that only forty-eight years of nutrient-rich topsoil remains." -Dr Josh Axe

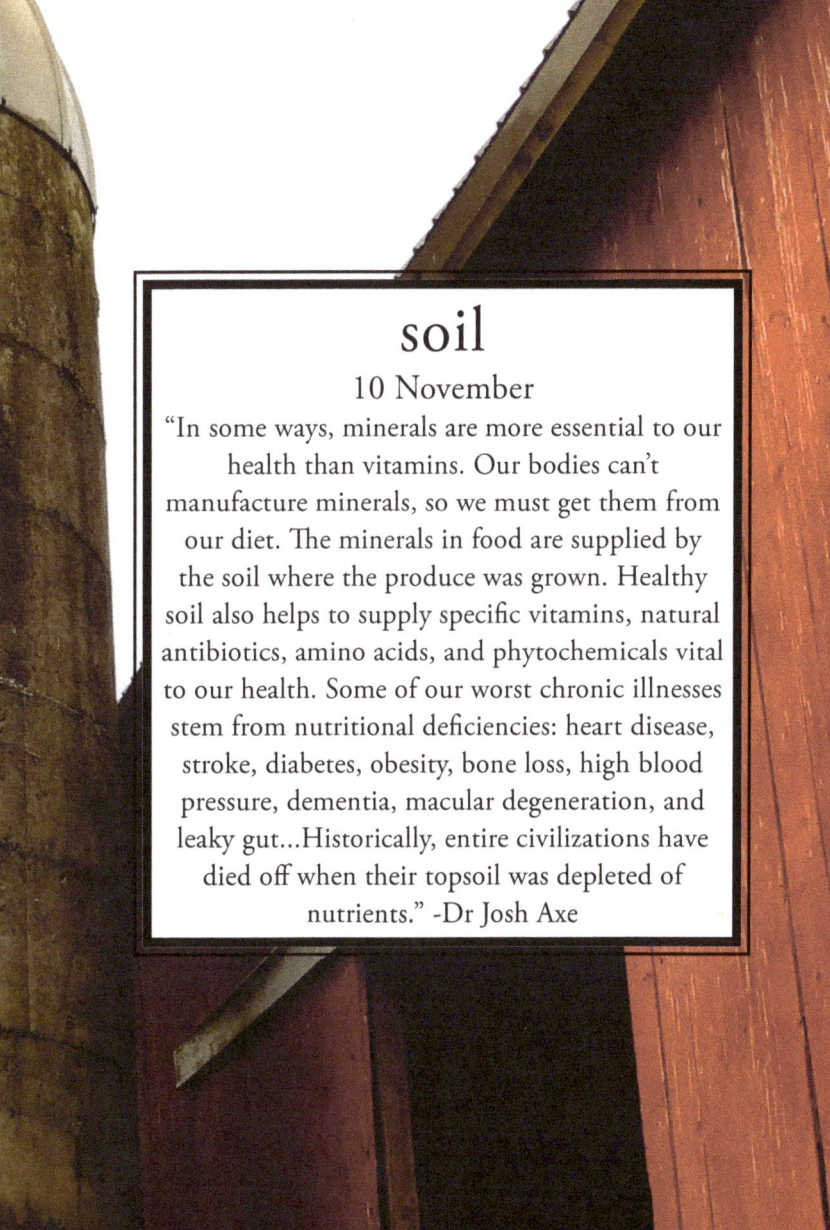

soil

10 November

"In some ways, minerals are more essential to our health than vitamins. Our bodies can't manufacture minerals, so we must get them from our diet. The minerals in food are supplied by the soil where the produce was grown. Healthy soil also helps to supply specific vitamins, natural antibiotics, amino acids, and phytochemicals vital to our health. Some of our worst chronic illnesses stem from nutritional deficiencies: heart disease, stroke, diabetes, obesity, bone loss, high blood pressure, dementia, macular degeneration, and leaky gut...Historically, entire civilizations have died off when their topsoil was depleted of nutrients." -Dr Josh Axe

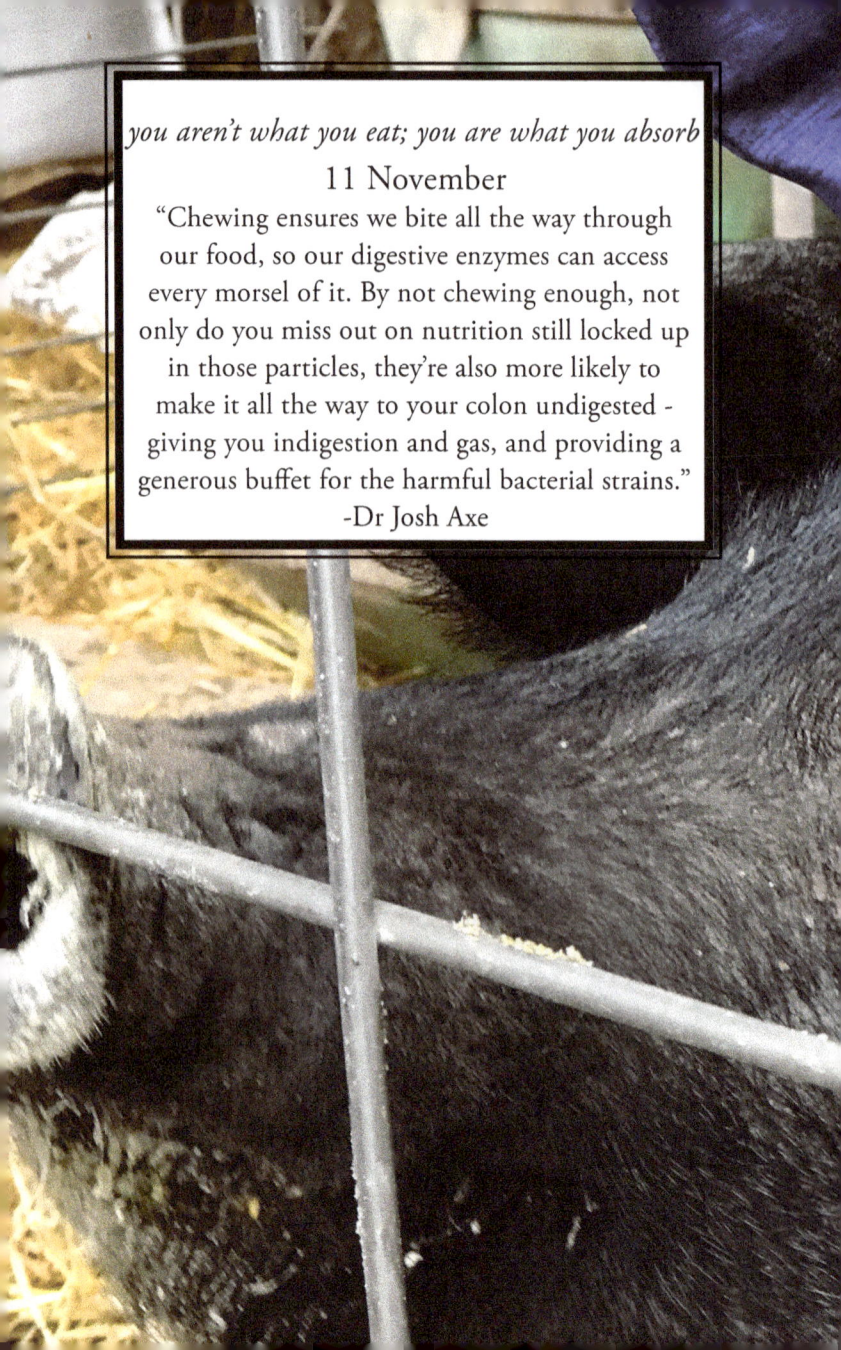

you aren't what you eat; you are what you absorb

11 November

"Chewing ensures we bite all the way through our food, so our digestive enzymes can access every morsel of it. By not chewing enough, not only do you miss out on nutrition still locked up in those particles, they're also more likely to make it all the way to your colon undigested - giving you indigestion and gas, and providing a generous buffet for the harmful bacterial strains."

-Dr Josh Axe

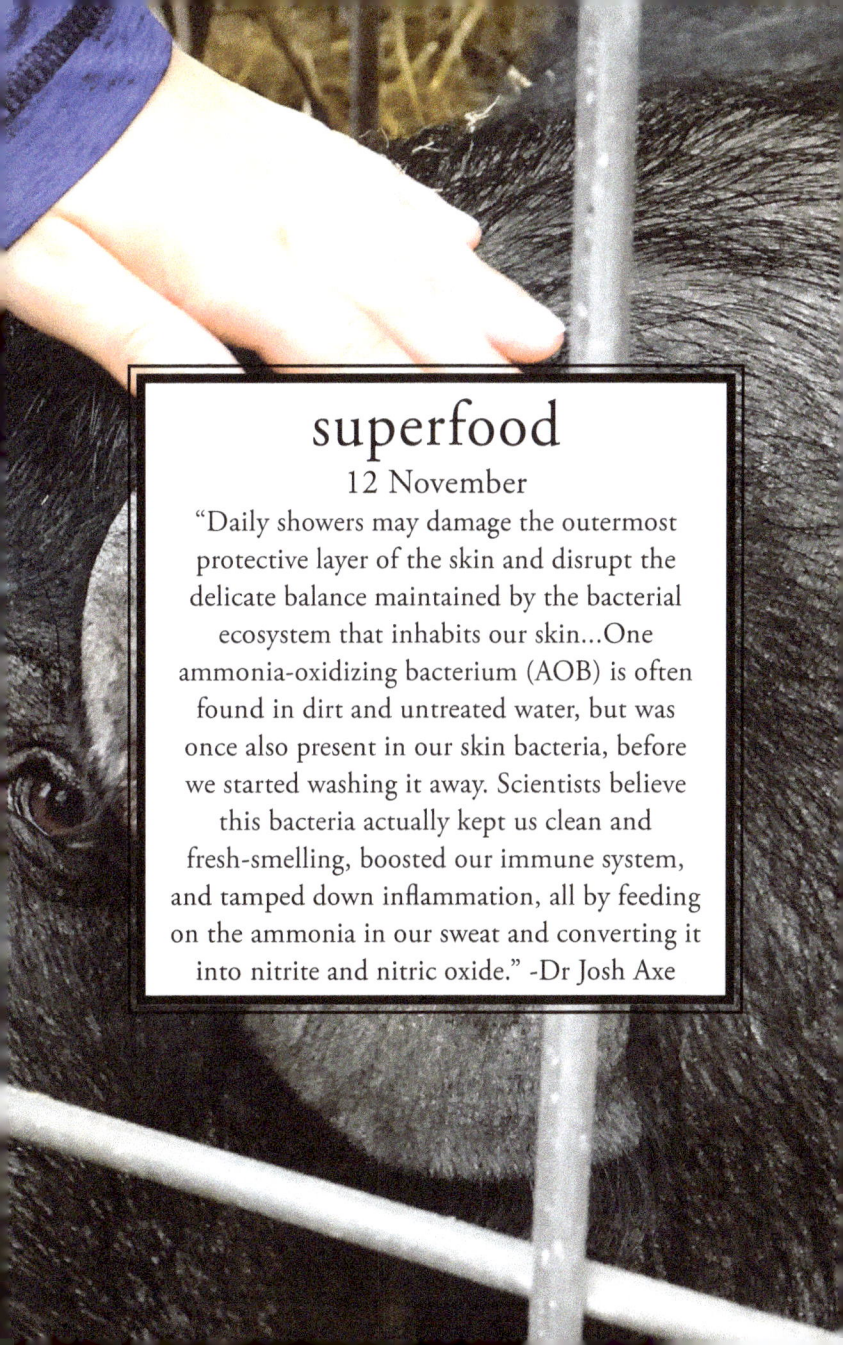

superfood
12 November

"Daily showers may damage the outermost protective layer of the skin and disrupt the delicate balance maintained by the bacterial ecosystem that inhabits our skin...One ammonia-oxidizing bacterium (AOB) is often found in dirt and untreated water, but was once also present in our skin bacteria, before we started washing it away. Scientists believe this bacteria actually kept us clean and fresh-smelling, boosted our immune system, and tamped down inflammation, all by feeding on the ammonia in our sweat and converting it into nitrite and nitric oxide." -Dr Josh Axe

empty

13 November

"Empty snack foods (empty calories - in the form of refined sweeteners, white flour and rancid and hydrogenated vegetable oils - that make up the vast majority of comercially produced snack foods), consumed in great quantities by our youth, have resulted in a generation of teenagers imbued with the vague feeling that they have been cheated - as indeed they have." -Sally Fallon

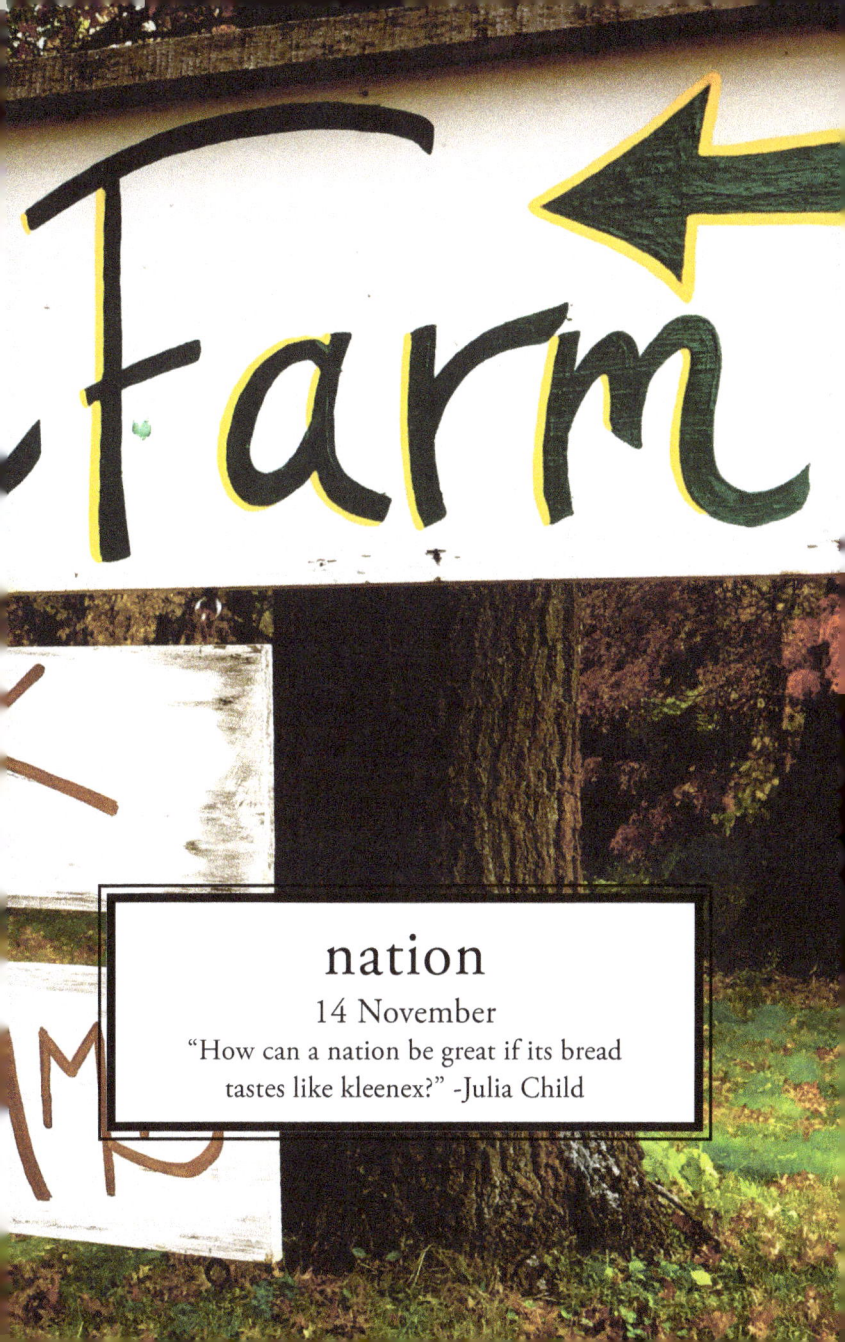

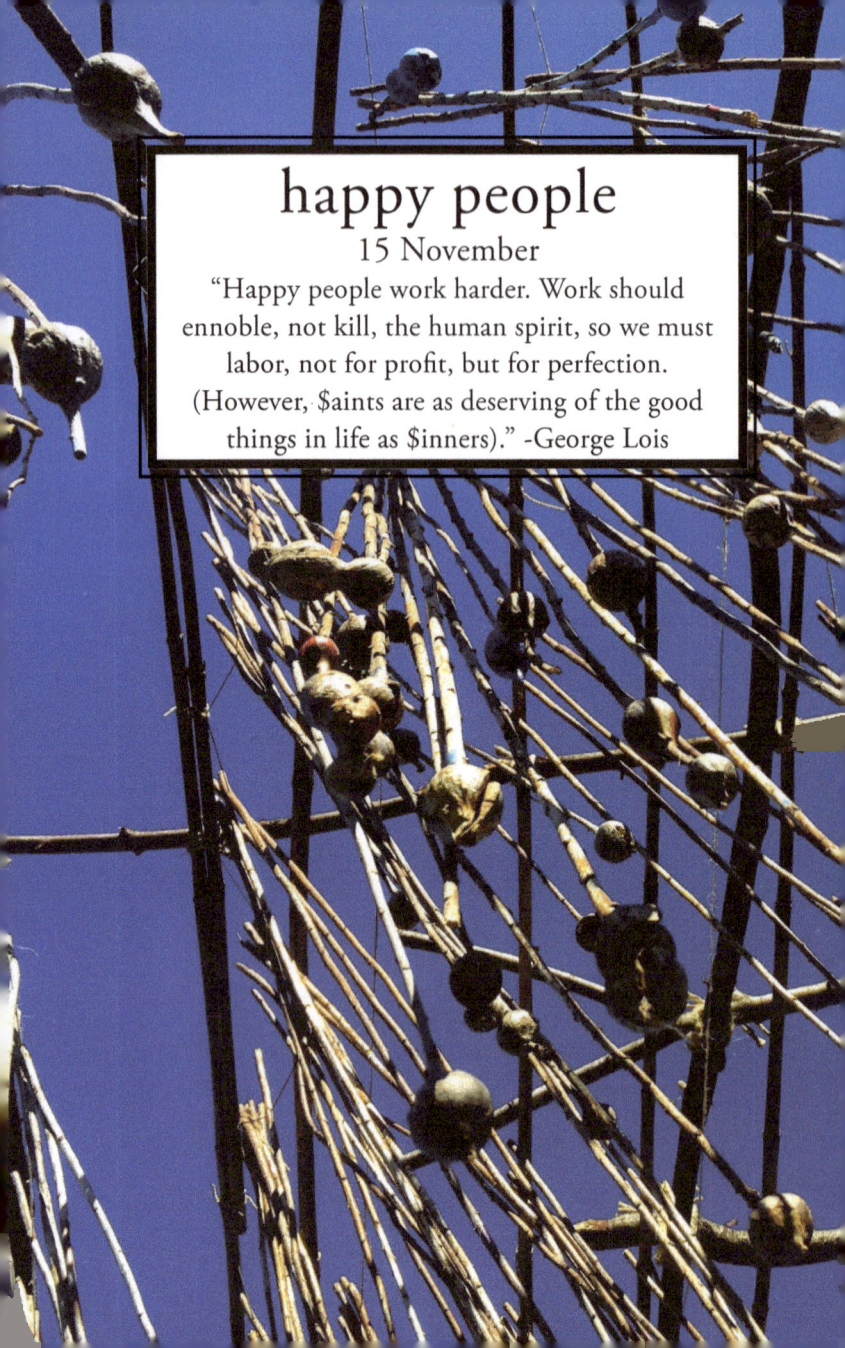

happy people
15 November

"Happy people work harder. Work should ennoble, not kill, the human spirit, so we must labor, not for profit, but for perfection. (However, $aints are as deserving of the good things in life as $inners)." -George Lois

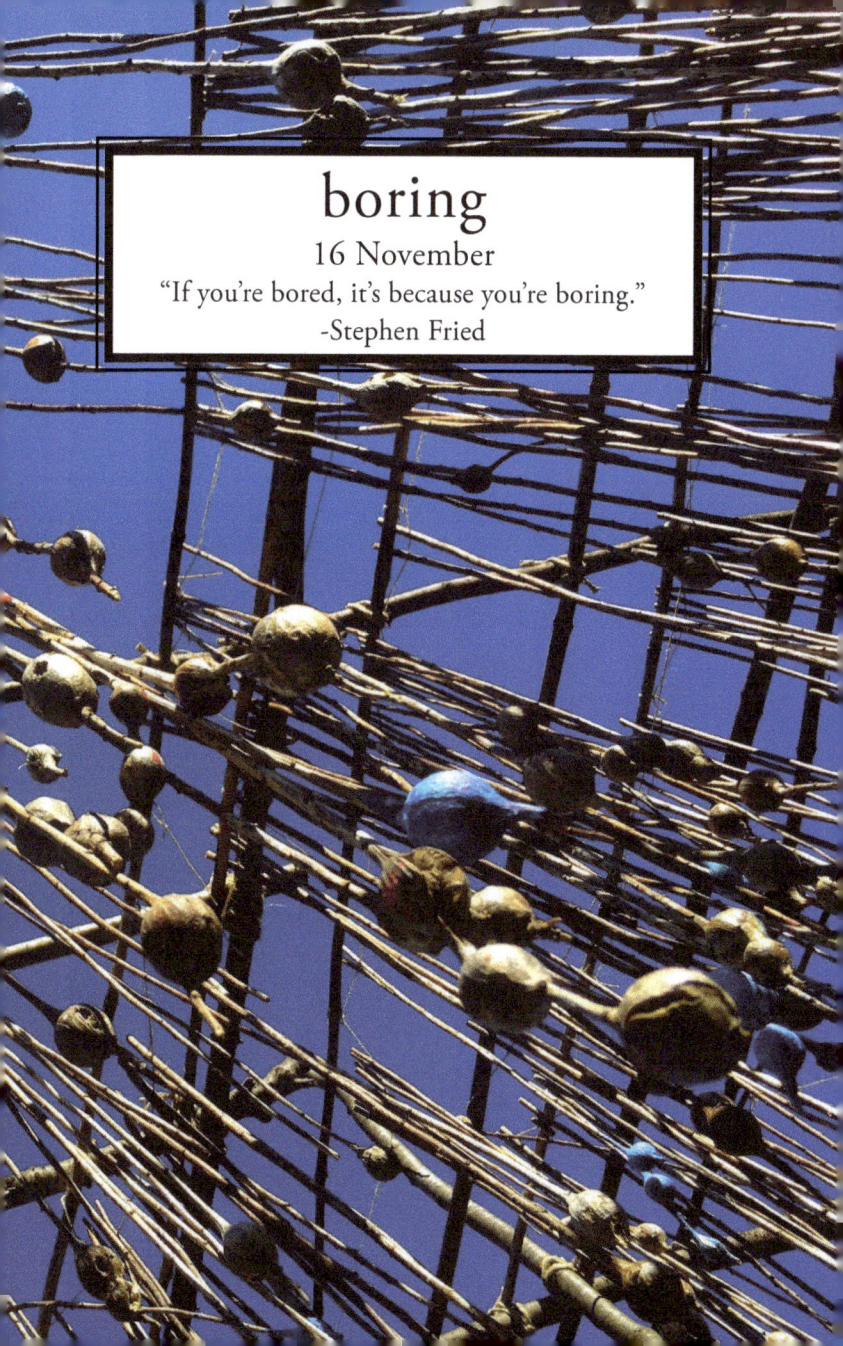

boring
16 November
"If you're bored, it's because you're boring."
-Stephen Fried

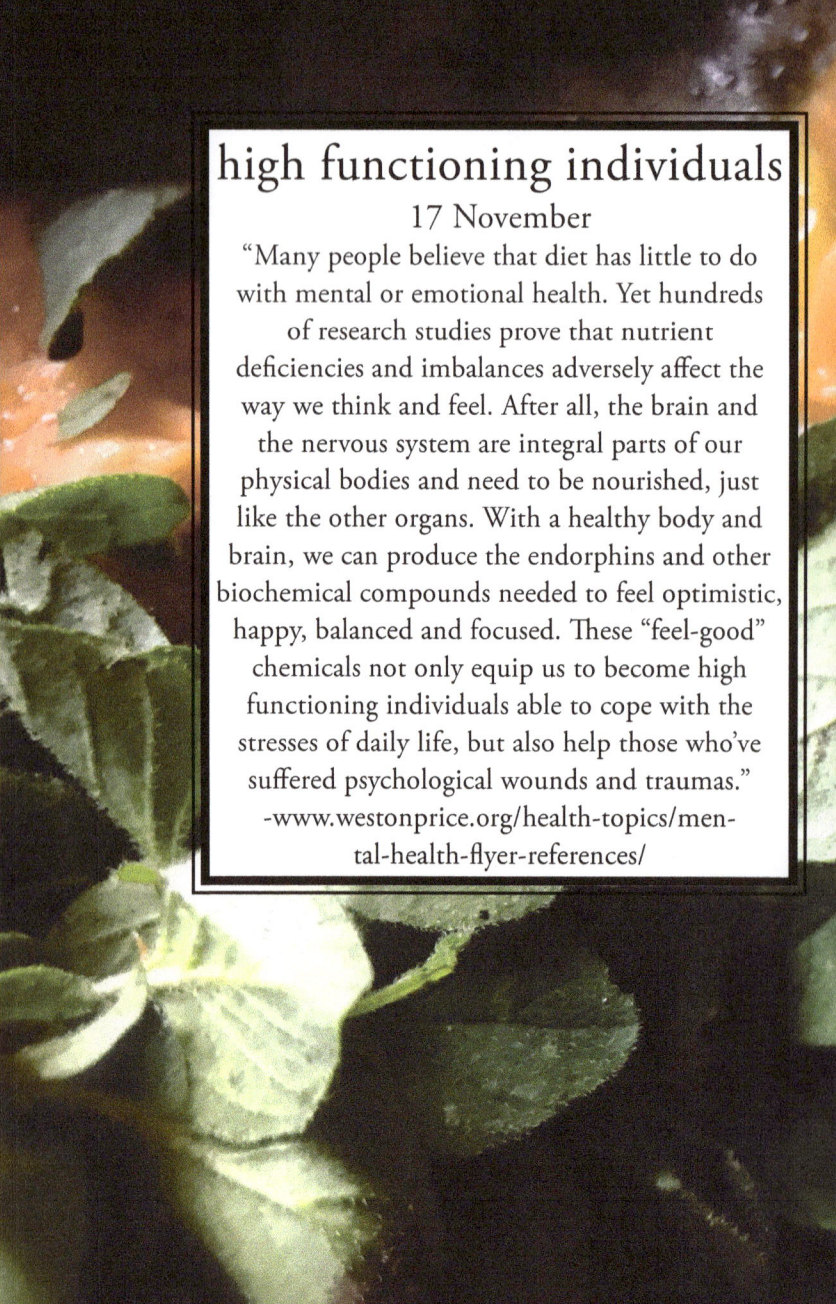

high functioning individuals
17 November

"Many people believe that diet has little to do with mental or emotional health. Yet hundreds of research studies prove that nutrient deficiencies and imbalances adversely affect the way we think and feel. After all, the brain and the nervous system are integral parts of our physical bodies and need to be nourished, just like the other organs. With a healthy body and brain, we can produce the endorphins and other biochemical compounds needed to feel optimistic, happy, balanced and focused. These "feel-good" chemicals not only equip us to become high functioning individuals able to cope with the stresses of daily life, but also help those who've suffered psychological wounds and traumas."
-www.westonprice.org/health-topics/mental-health-flyer-references/

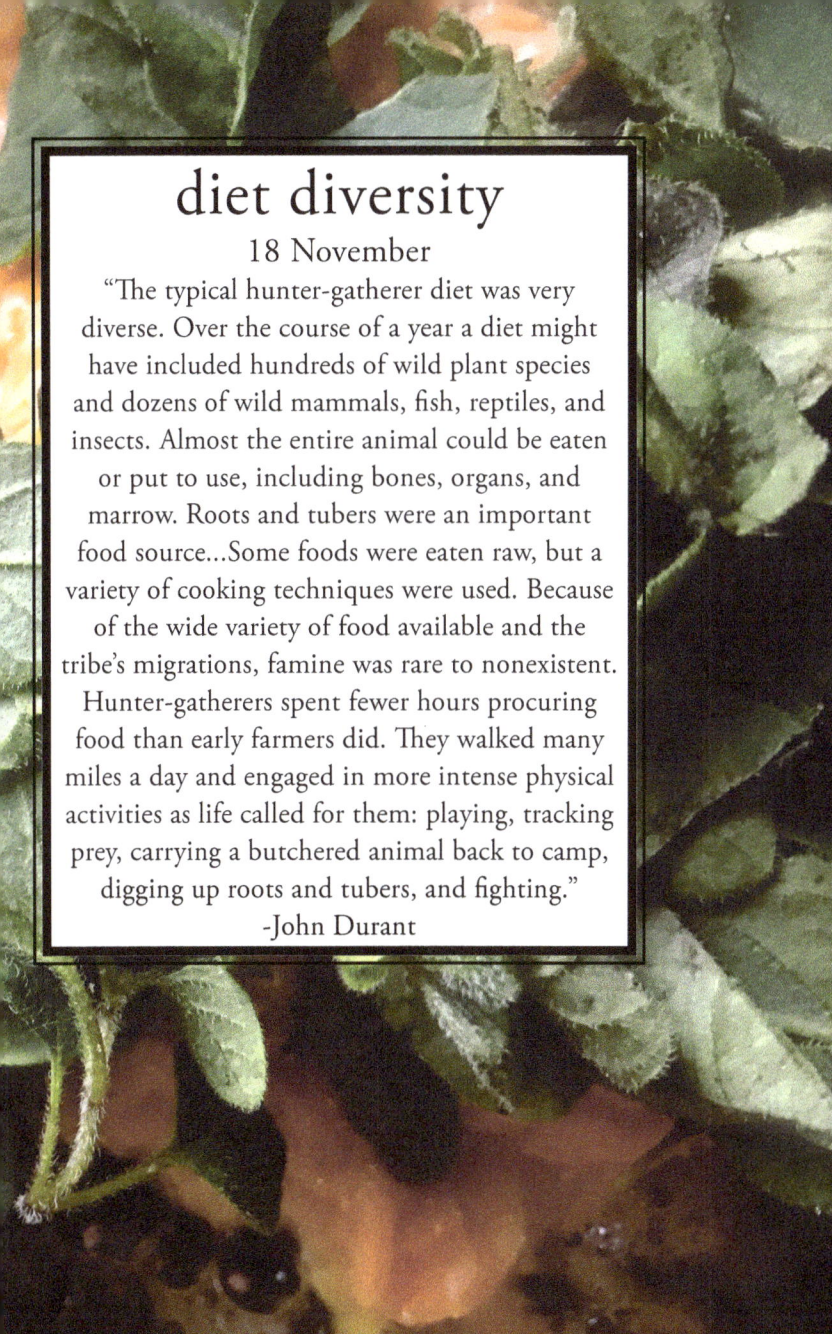

diet diversity
18 November

"The typical hunter-gatherer diet was very diverse. Over the course of a year a diet might have included hundreds of wild plant species and dozens of wild mammals, fish, reptiles, and insects. Almost the entire animal could be eaten or put to use, including bones, organs, and marrow. Roots and tubers were an important food source...Some foods were eaten raw, but a variety of cooking techniques were used. Because of the wide variety of food available and the tribe's migrations, famine was rare to nonexistent. Hunter-gatherers spent fewer hours procuring food than early farmers did. They walked many miles a day and engaged in more intense physical activities as life called for them: playing, tracking prey, carrying a butchered animal back to camp, digging up roots and tubers, and fighting."
-John Durant

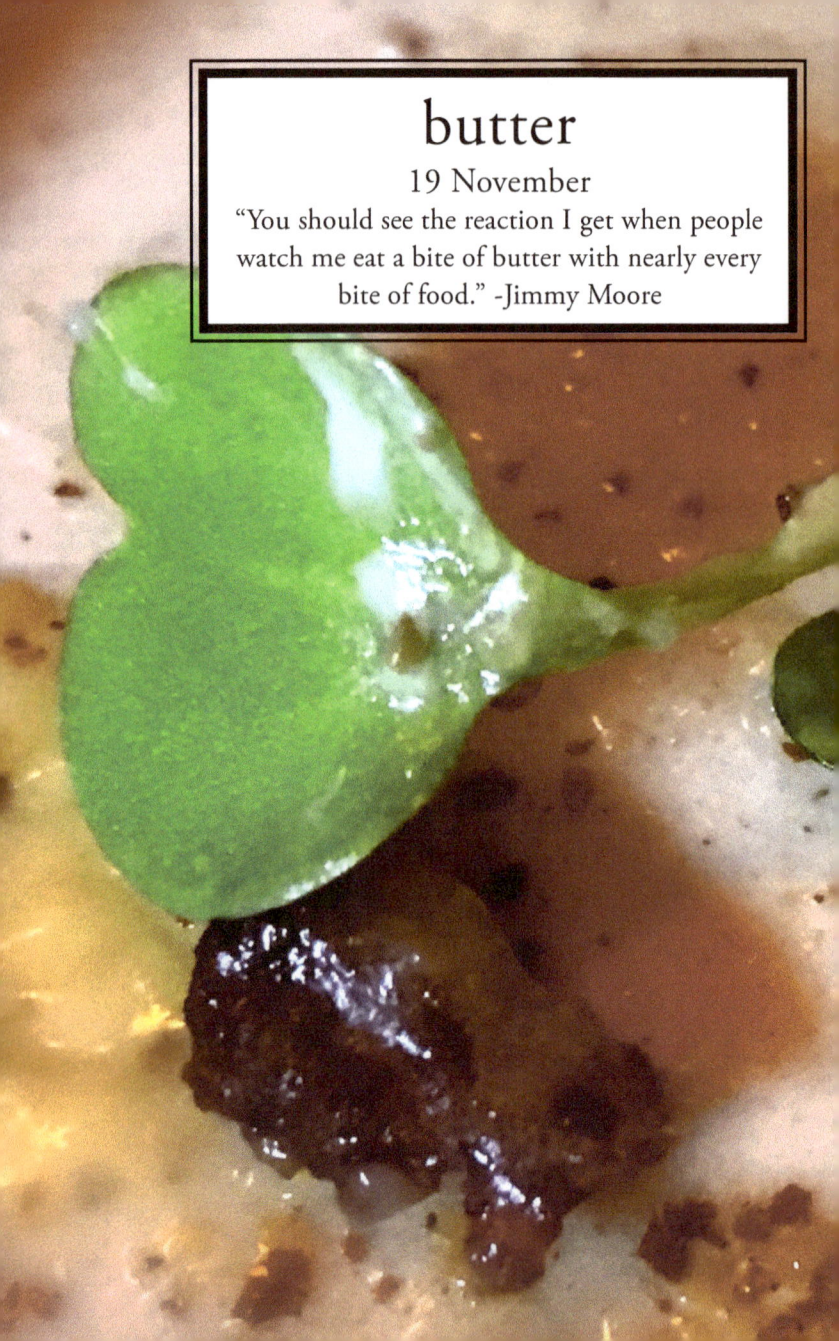

butter

19 November
"You should see the reaction I get when people watch me eat a bite of butter with nearly every bite of food." -Jimmy Moore

'the happy diet'
20 November

"A meal should be pretty substantial, especially if it ends up being your only meal of the day. Maybe that breakfast of two eggs and two slices of bacon should become four eggs cooked in butter and topped with cheddar cheese and sour cream, three slices of bacon, and an avocado. The former meal will likely have you looking for more food in a few hours, whereas the latter meal might take your mind off of food for the rest of the day. What freedom you can experience by making IF [intermittant fasting] a part of your life!"

-Jimmy Moore

Rosita Real Foods™

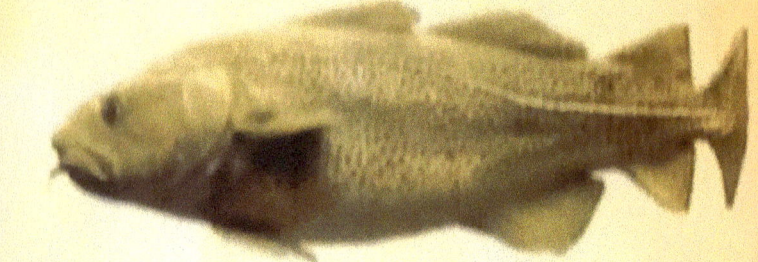

EXTRA-VIRGIN COD LIVER OIL

Morrhuae Oleum

- Wild & Raw
- No Heat or Chemicals Used
- Ancient Extraction Method

Sustainably Harvested & Produced in Norway
5 FL. OZ (150 ml) Dietary Supplement

everyone
21 November

"Nearly everyone can achieve a healthy weight and a long, healthy life by eating as they were meant to eat." -Paul Jaminet PhD & Shou-Ching Jaminet PhD

power of sour
22 November

"It's essential to include more probiotic-rich foods in our diets. As a culture, we have gotten away from eating probiotic foods because they often have a tart, sometimes bitter taste. Instead, our taste buds have been trained to crave sweet and salty foods. It's time to embrace the power of sour and the benefits of bitter foods because these flavors are indicative of probiotics, organic acids, and other compounds that support the growth of microbes in the gut." -Dr Josh Axe

worship

23 November

"Work is worship. Working hard and doing great work is as imperative as breathing. Creating great work warms the heart and enriches the soul. Those of us lucky enough to spend our days doing something we love, something we're good at, are rich. If you do not work passionately (even furiously) at being the best in the world at what you do, you fail your talent, your destiny, and your god." -George Lois

surroundings
24 November
"Surroundings should relate to who you are, what you love, and to what you deem important in life." -George Lois

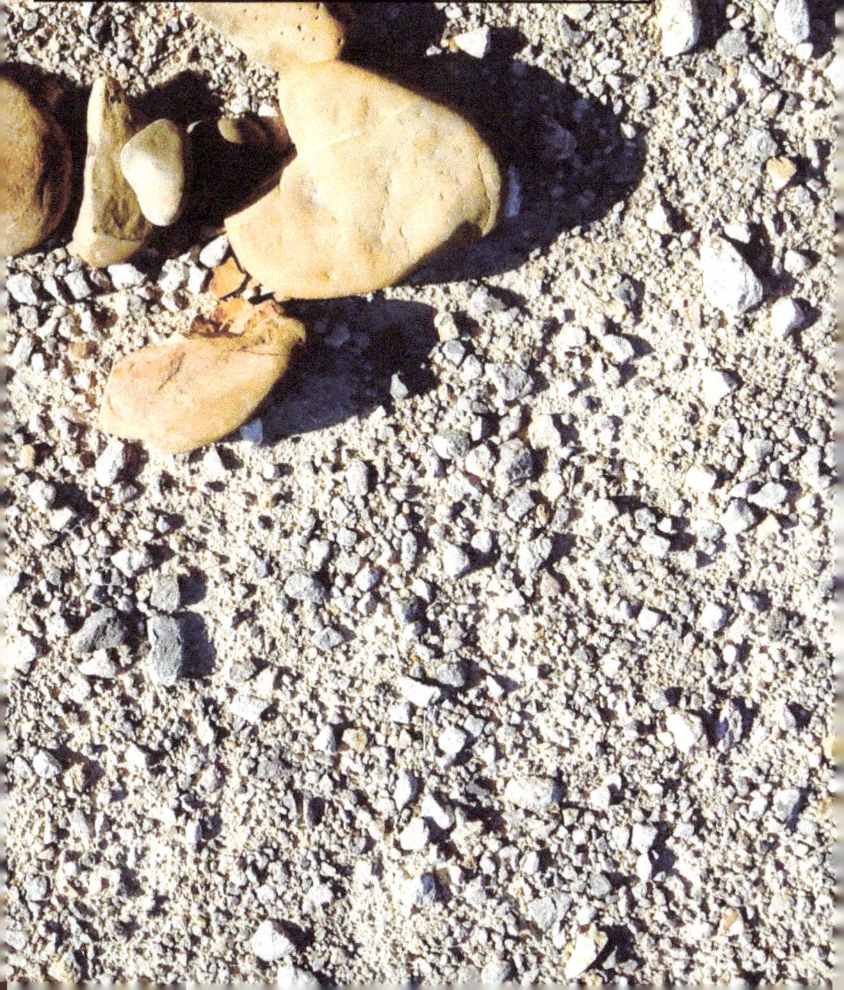

right
25 November

"Desires that lead to sorrow are wrong and those that lead to happiness are right...What helps you to know yourself is right. What prevents it is wrong. To know one's real self is bliss, to forget - is sorrow." -Sri Nisargadatta Maharaj

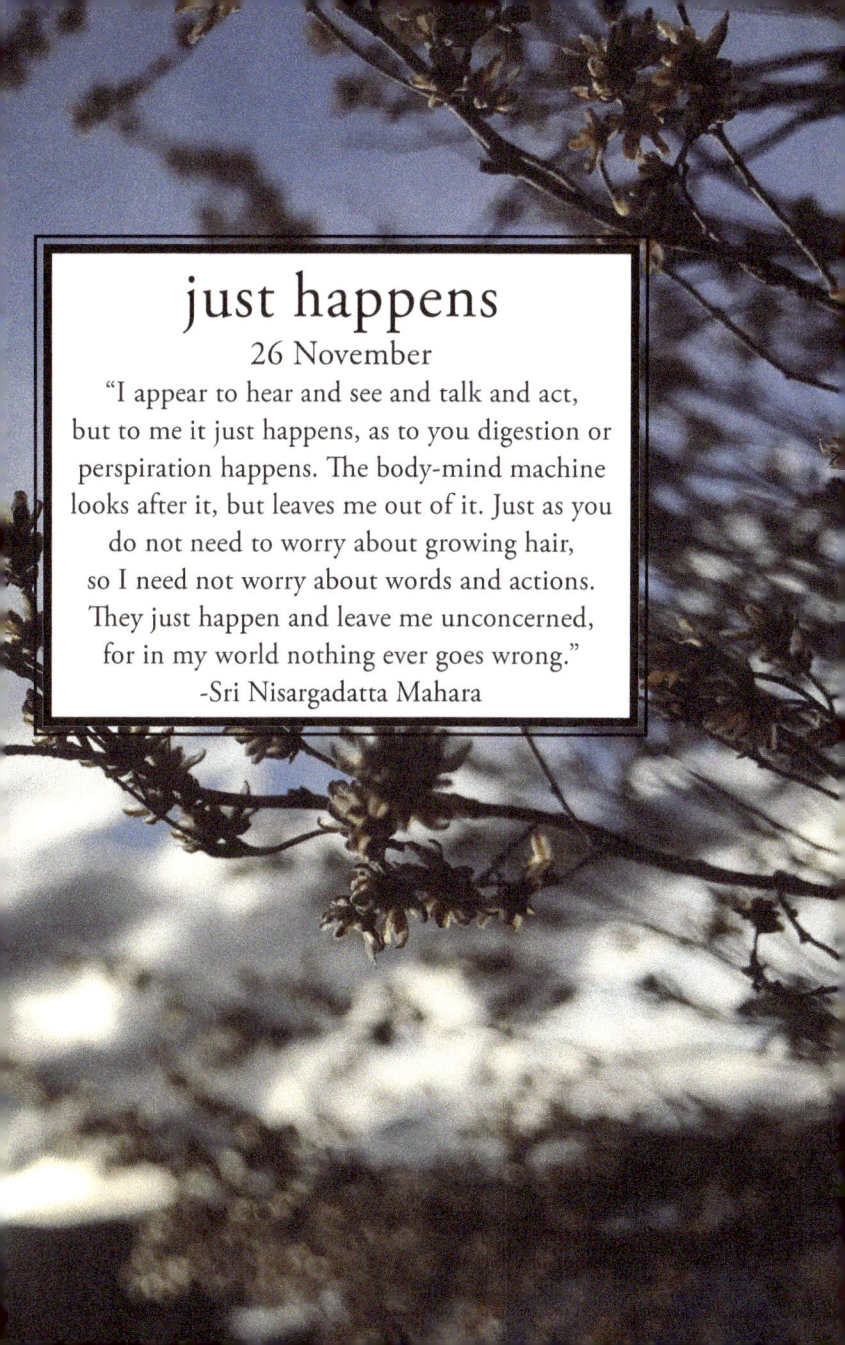

just happens
26 November

"I appear to hear and see and talk and act, but to me it just happens, as to you digestion or perspiration happens. The body-mind machine looks after it, but leaves me out of it. Just as you do not need to worry about growing hair, so I need not worry about words and actions. They just happen and leave me unconcerned, for in my world nothing ever goes wrong."

-Sri Nisargadatta Mahara

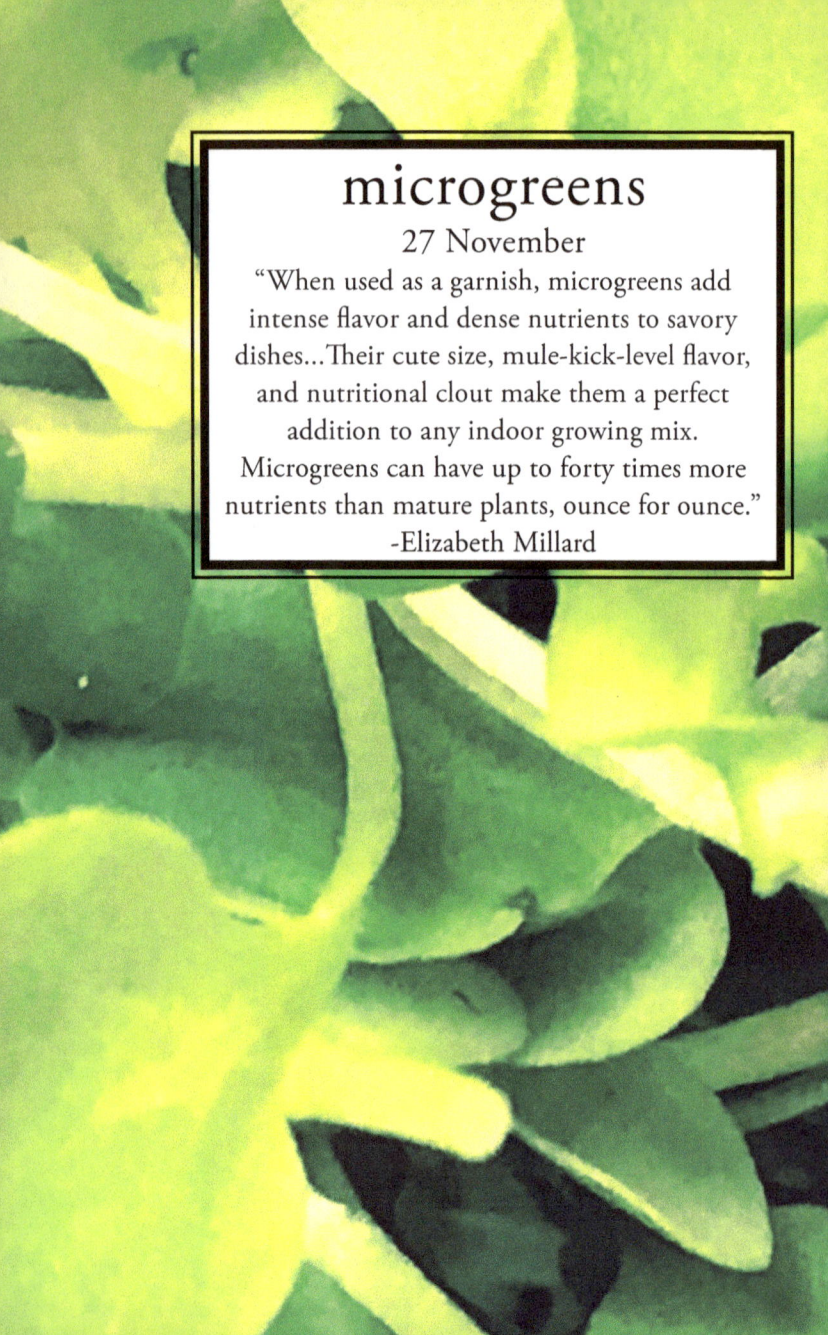

microgreens
27 November

"When used as a garnish, microgreens add intense flavor and dense nutrients to savory dishes…Their cute size, mule-kick-level flavor, and nutritional clout make them a perfect addition to any indoor growing mix. Microgreens can have up to forty times more nutrients than mature plants, ounce for ounce."
-Elizabeth Millard

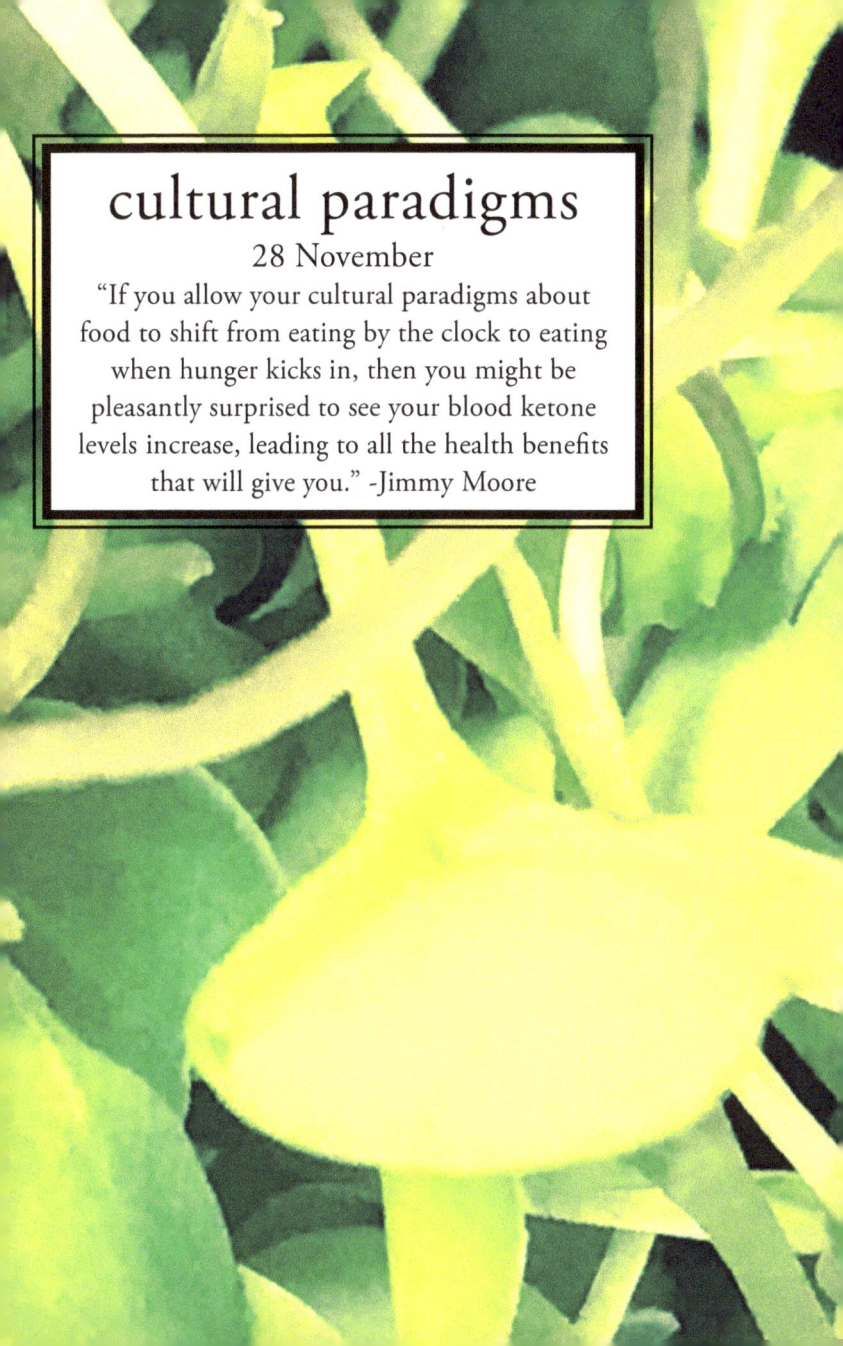

cultural paradigms
28 November

"If you allow your cultural paradigms about food to shift from eating by the clock to eating when hunger kicks in, then you might be pleasantly surprised to see your blood ketone levels increase, leading to all the health benefits that will give you." -Jimmy Moore

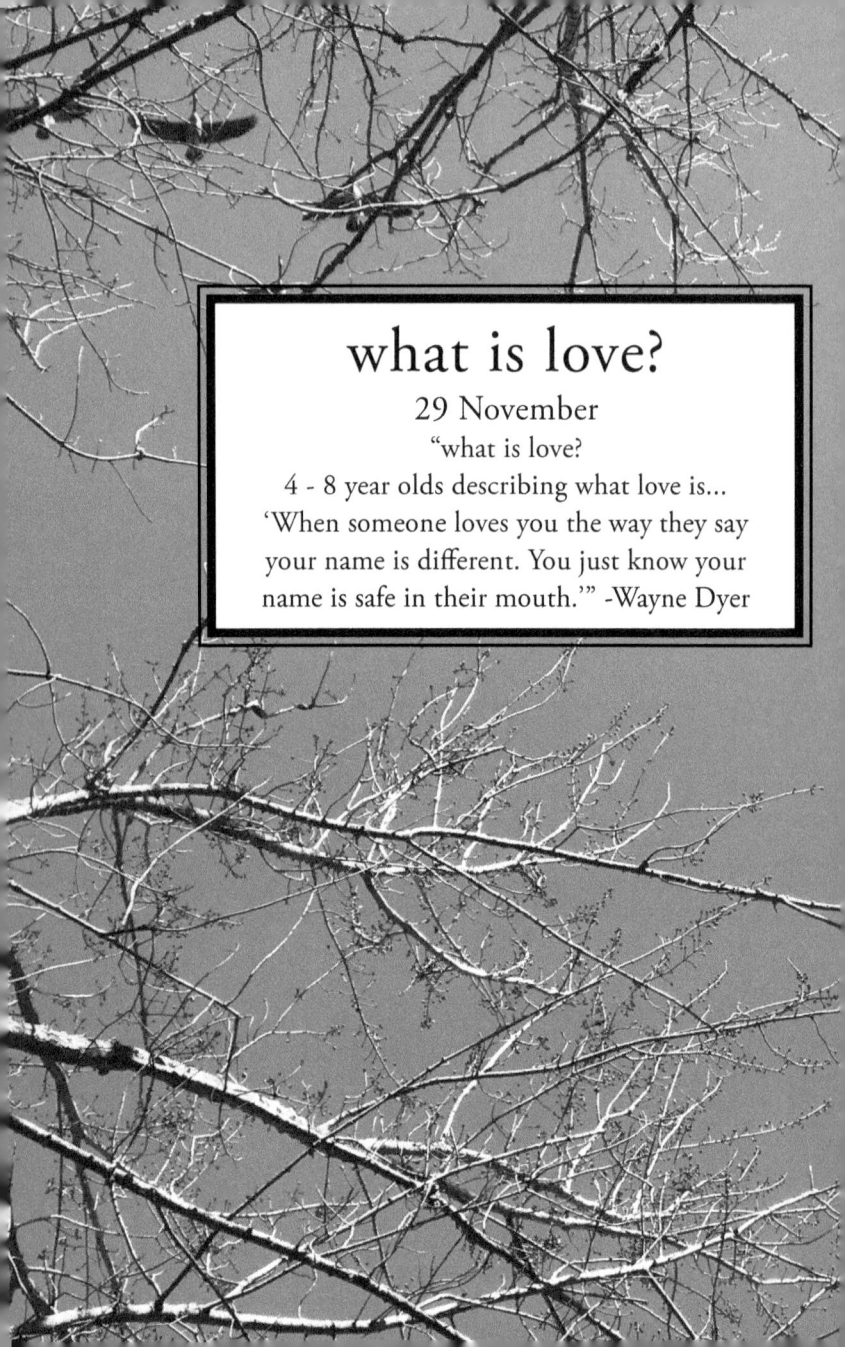

what is love?

29 November

"what is love?
4 - 8 year olds describing what love is...
'When someone loves you the way they say your name is different. You just know your name is safe in their mouth.'" -Wayne Dyer

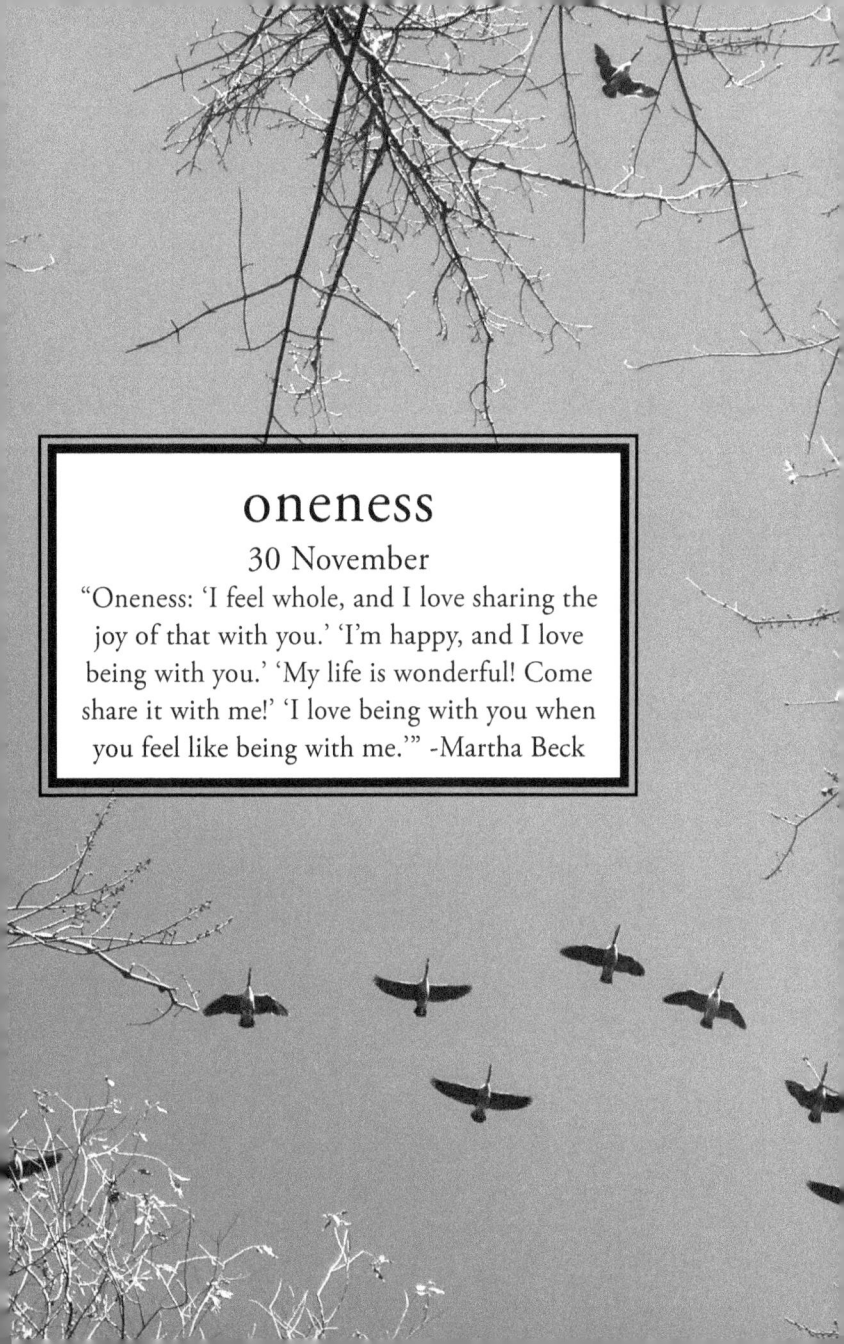

oneness
30 November
"Oneness: 'I feel whole, and I love sharing the joy of that with you.' 'I'm happy, and I love being with you.' 'My life is wonderful! Come share it with me!' 'I love being with you when you feel like being with me.'" -Martha Beck

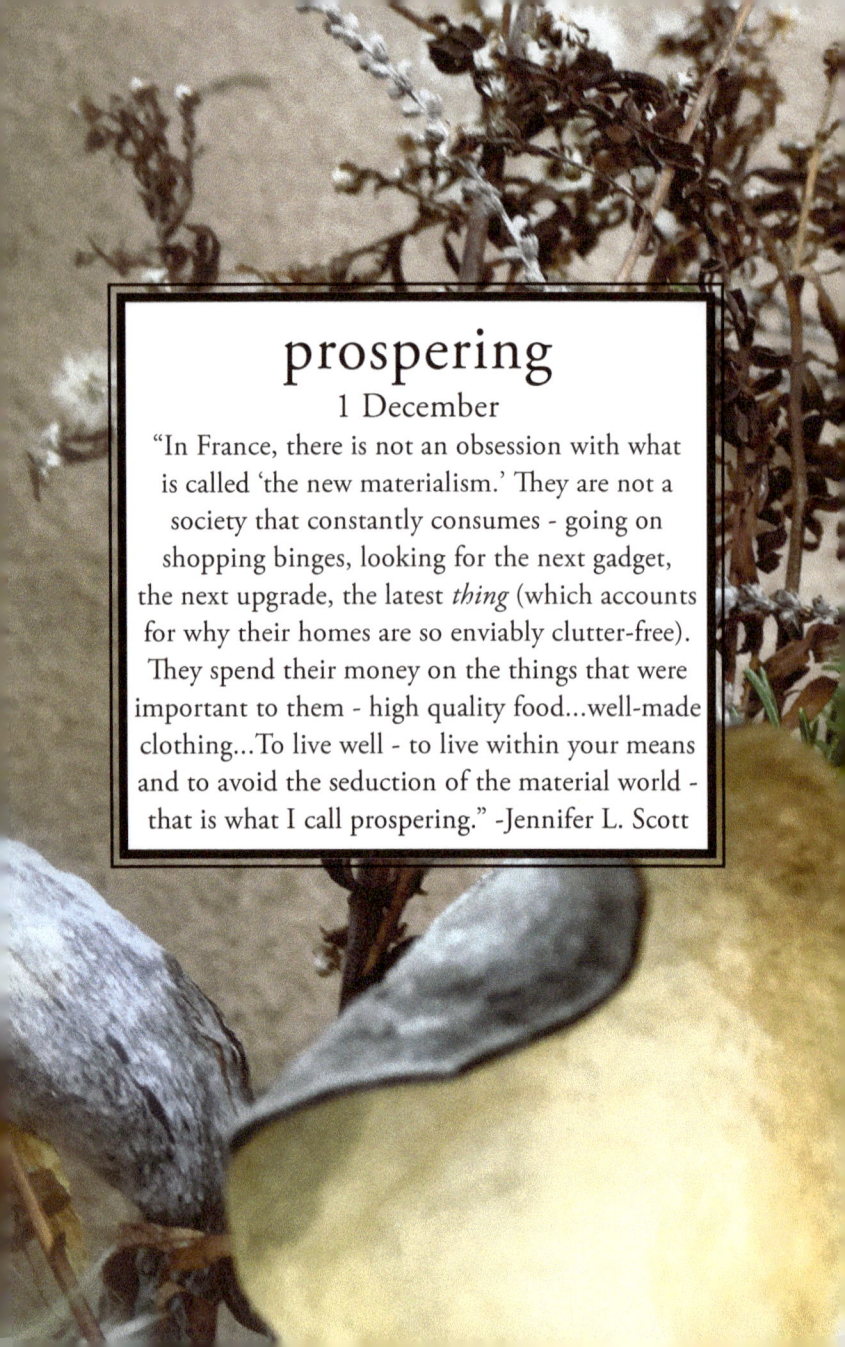

prospering
1 December

"In France, there is not an obsession with what is called 'the new materialism.' They are not a society that constantly consumes - going on shopping binges, looking for the next gadget, the next upgrade, the latest *thing* (which accounts for why their homes are so enviably clutter-free). They spend their money on the things that were important to them - high quality food...well-made clothing...To live well - to live within your means and to avoid the seduction of the material world - that is what I call prospering." -Jennifer L. Scott

3 skirts, 3 pants, 4 tops
2 December

"The benefits of the ten-item wardrobe are vast. Your shopping habits will become healthier. You will waste less money; you will not be a slave to consumerism; you won't be tempted by old pulls that used to draw you in (*final sale! clearance! last chance!*). You will clarify your true style and embrace it. You will be forced to wear your nice clothes on a daily basis by getting rid of the ragged or unflattering ones, and therefore you will look presentable always. When you wake up in the morning, the choice of what to wear will be easy because everything in your wardrobe will go with everything else. Poised people look presentable, assert their style, and are comfortable in their clothing. The ten-item wardrobe will get you there." -Jennifer L. Scott

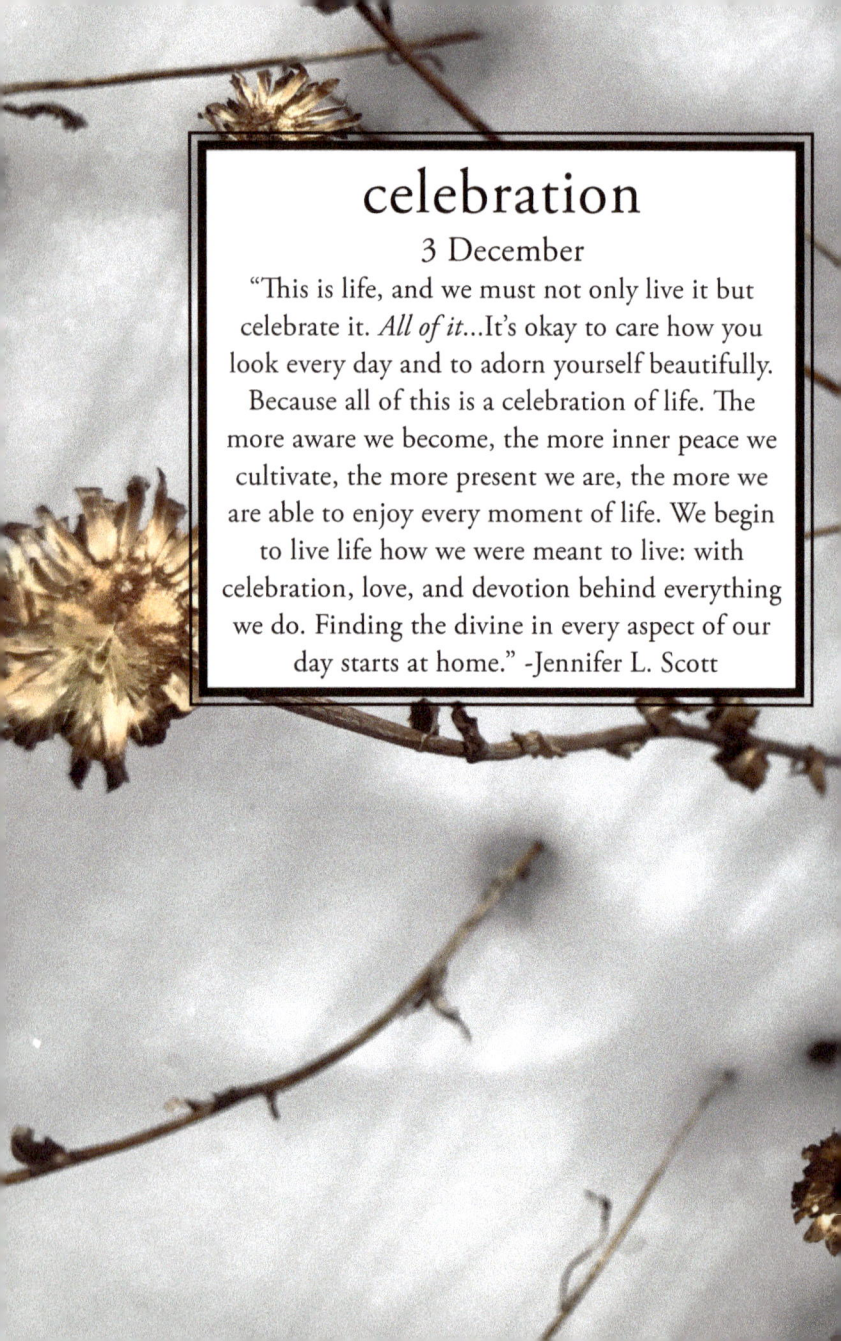

celebration
3 December

"This is life, and we must not only live it but celebrate it. *All of it*...It's okay to care how you look every day and to adorn yourself beautifully. Because all of this is a celebration of life. The more aware we become, the more inner peace we cultivate, the more present we are, the more we are able to enjoy every moment of life. We begin to live life how we were meant to live: with celebration, love, and devotion behind everything we do. Finding the divine in every aspect of our day starts at home." -Jennifer L. Scott

superlife
4 December

"Eat the right foods: meat, seafood, roots and tubers, leafy vegetables, eggs, fruit and nuts. Experiment with full-fat fermented dairy. Aim for a diet where the bulk of calories comes from seafood and animals, but the physical bulk comes from plants. Don't be afraid of fat, eat nose to tail, and eat a variety of plants. Respect ancient culinary wisdom. Follow traditional recipes. Eat fermented foods. Eat raw foods. Make broths and stocks. Cook at low heat, using traditional fats and oils (coconut, beef, butter, ghee, olive). Lead a healthy lifestyle. Sleep as much as possible. Move and exercise regularly. Stay on your feet (stand, walk, run). Get regular, moderate sun. Try some intermittent fasting. Try some hot and cold exposure. Make it meaningful in order to make it an ongoing lifestyle." -John Durant

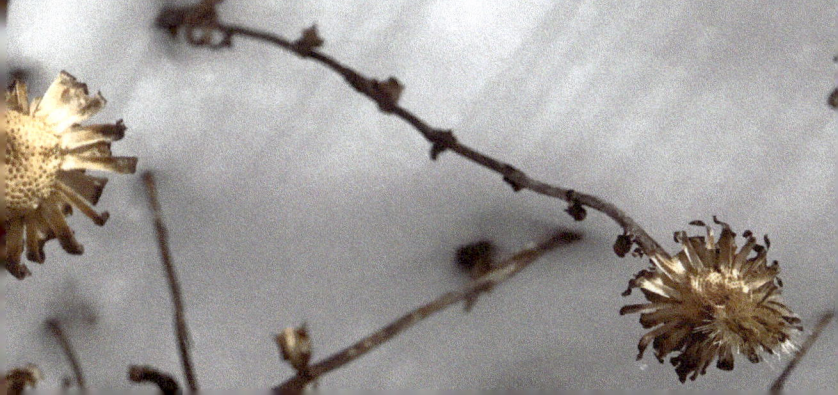

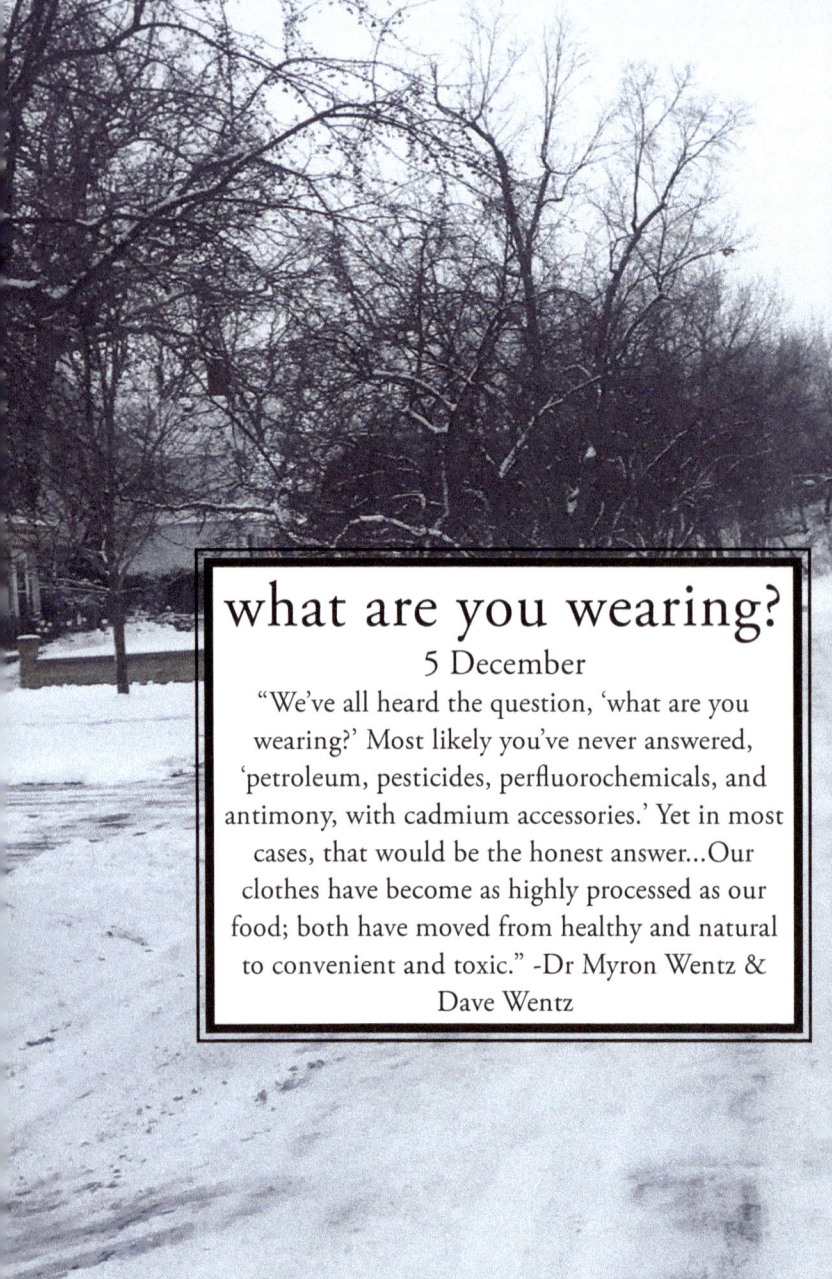

what are you wearing?
5 December

"We've all heard the question, 'what are you wearing?' Most likely you've never answered, 'petroleum, pesticides, perfluorochemicals, and antimony, with cadmium accessories.' Yet in most cases, that would be the honest answer...Our clothes have become as highly processed as our food; both have moved from healthy and natural to convenient and toxic." -Dr Myron Wentz & Dave Wentz

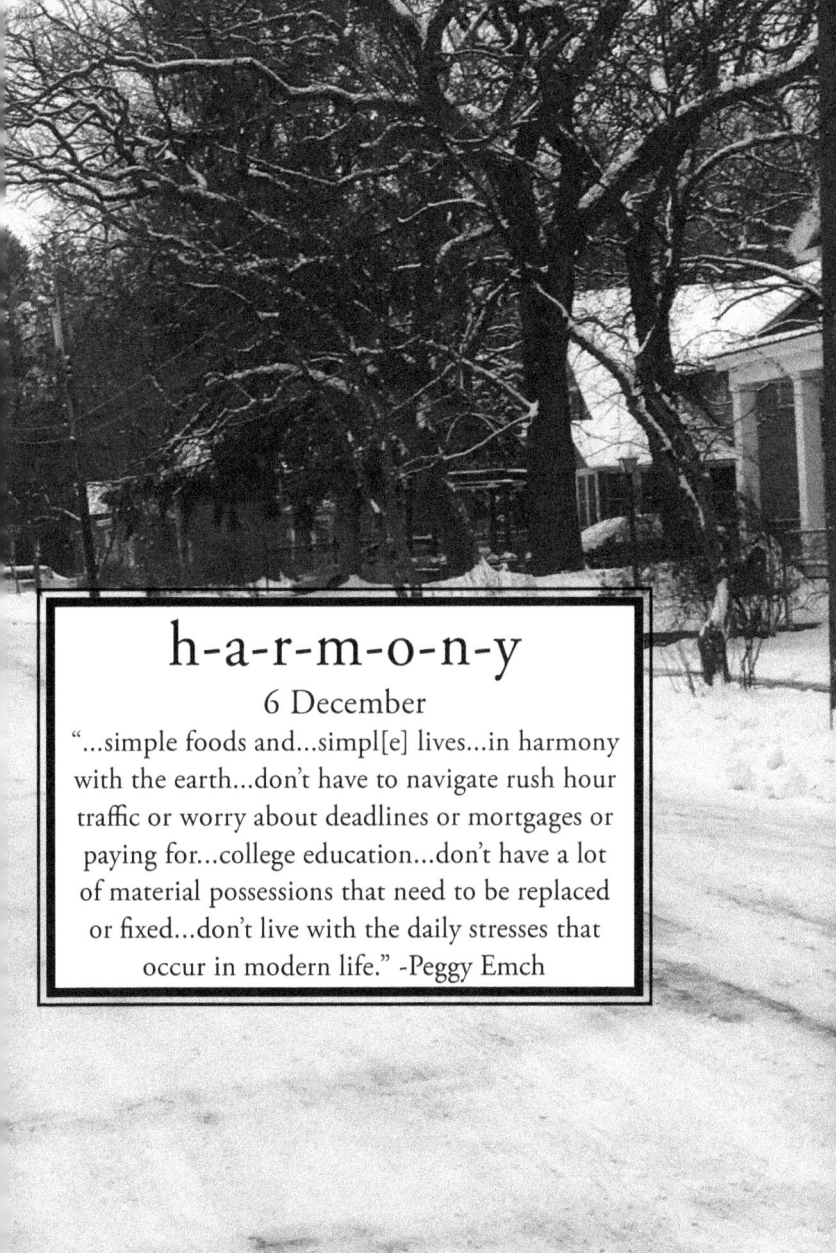

h-a-r-m-o-n-y

6 December

"...simple foods and...simpl[e] lives...in harmony with the earth...don't have to navigate rush hour traffic or worry about deadlines or mortgages or paying for...college education...don't have a lot of material possessions that need to be replaced or fixed...don't live with the daily stresses that occur in modern life." -Peggy Emch

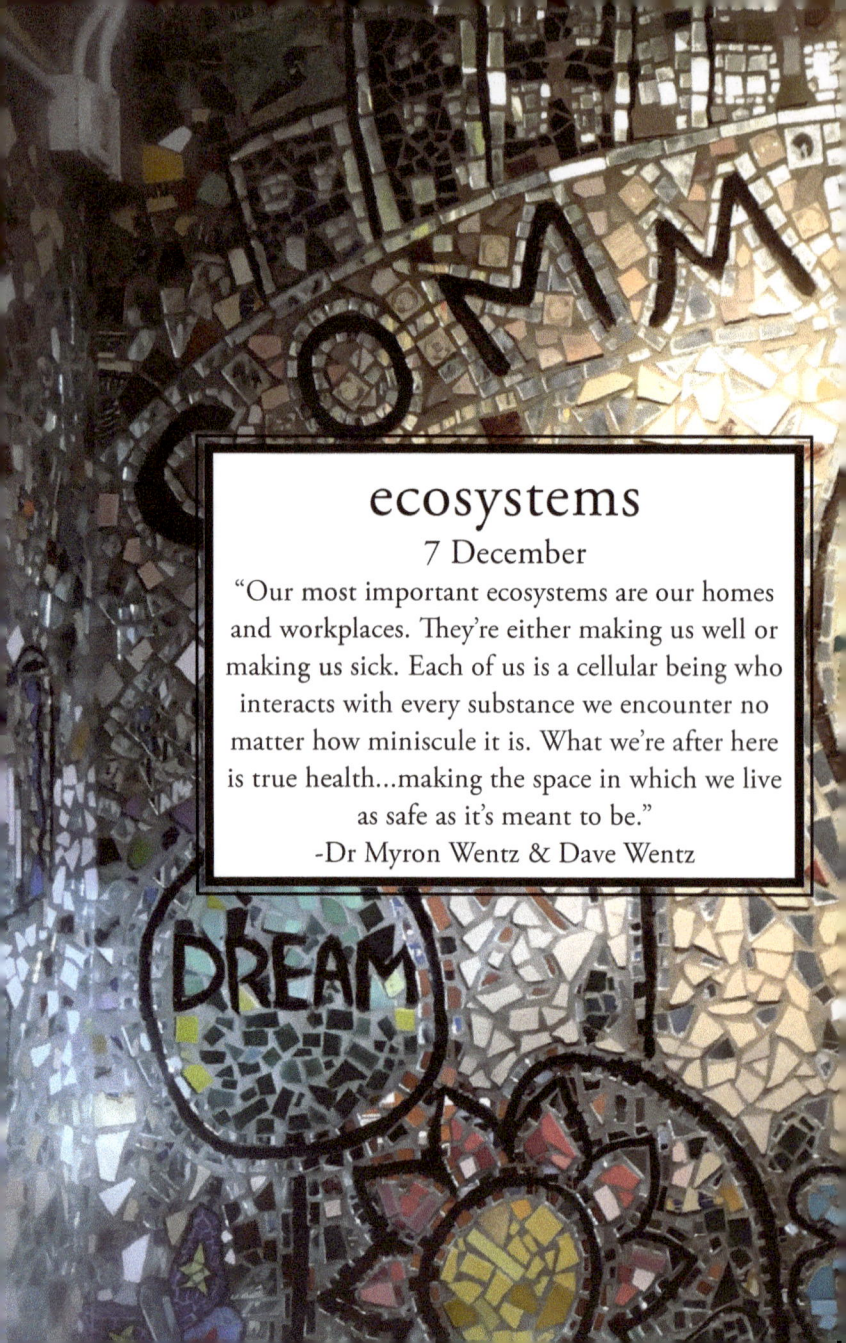

ecosystems
7 December

"Our most important ecosystems are our homes and workplaces. They're either making us well or making us sick. Each of us is a cellular being who interacts with every substance we encounter no matter how miniscule it is. What we're after here is true health...making the space in which we live as safe as it's meant to be."
-Dr Myron Wentz & Dave Wentz

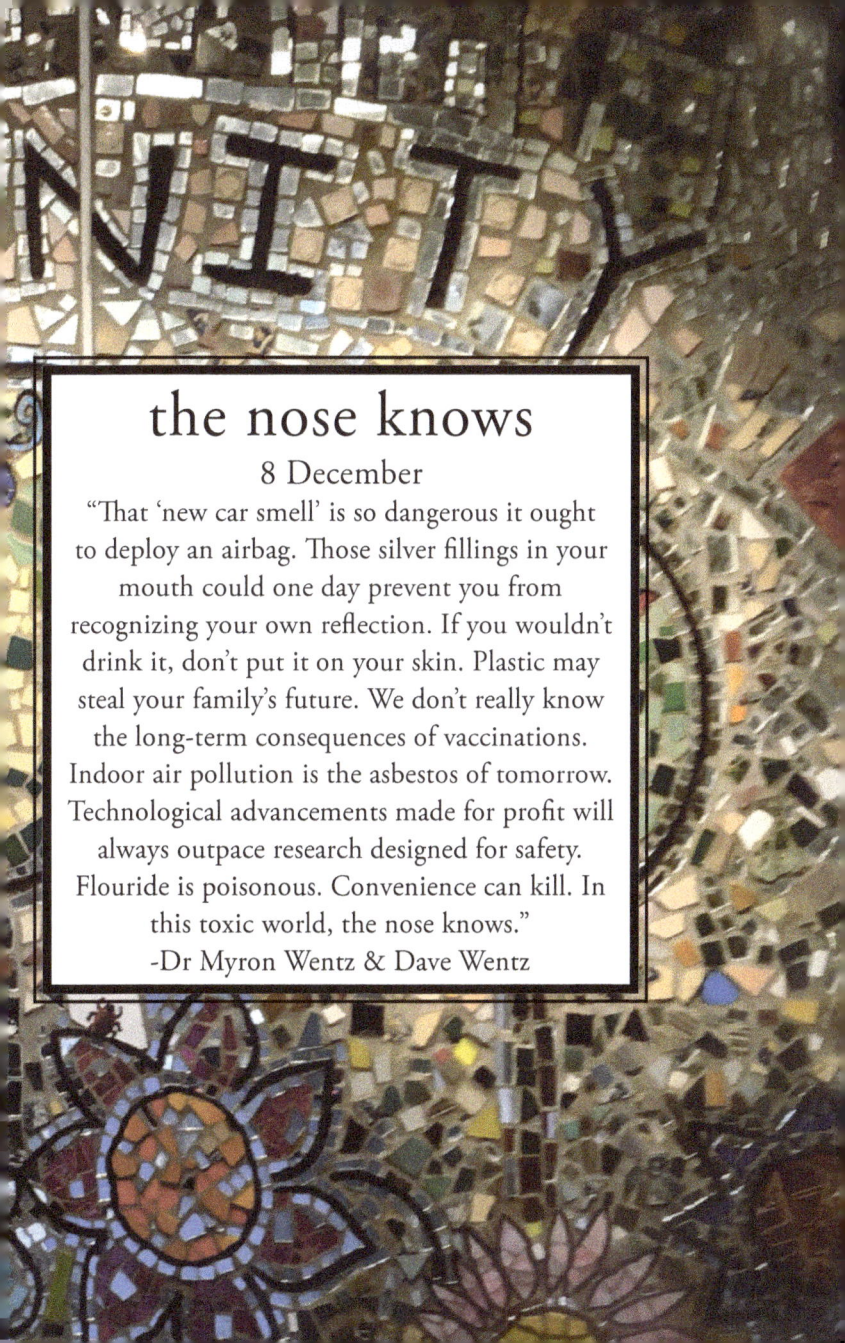

the nose knows
8 December

"That 'new car smell' is so dangerous it ought to deploy an airbag. Those silver fillings in your mouth could one day prevent you from recognizing your own reflection. If you wouldn't drink it, don't put it on your skin. Plastic may steal your family's future. We don't really know the long-term consequences of vaccinations. Indoor air pollution is the asbestos of tomorrow. Technological advancements made for profit will always outpace research designed for safety. Flouride is poisonous. Convenience can kill. In this toxic world, the nose knows."

-Dr Myron Wentz & Dave Wentz

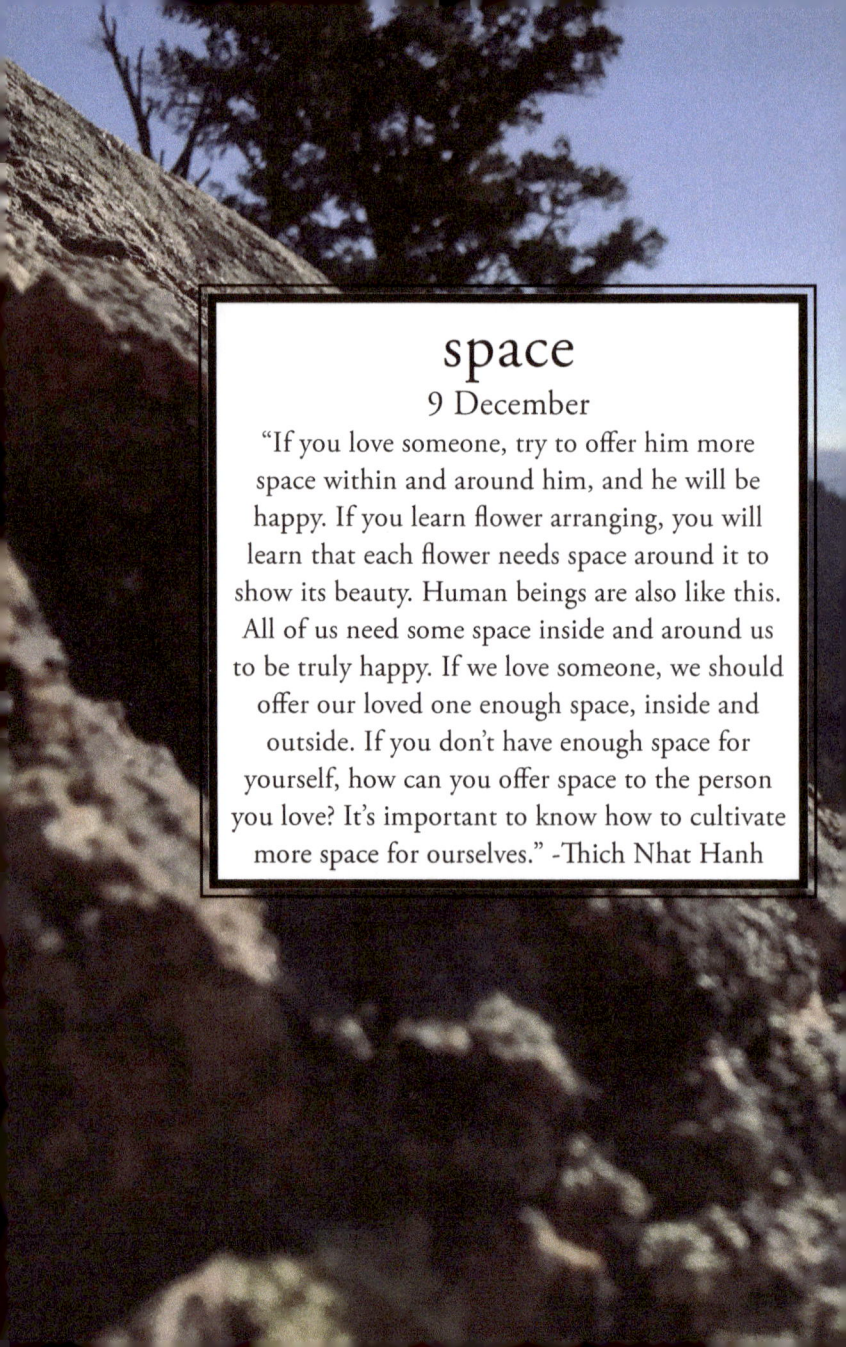

space
9 December

"If you love someone, try to offer him more space within and around him, and he will be happy. If you learn flower arranging, you will learn that each flower needs space around it to show its beauty. Human beings are also like this. All of us need some space inside and around us to be truly happy. If we love someone, we should offer our loved one enough space, inside and outside. If you don't have enough space for yourself, how can you offer space to the person you love? It's important to know how to cultivate more space for ourselves." -Thich Nhat Hanh

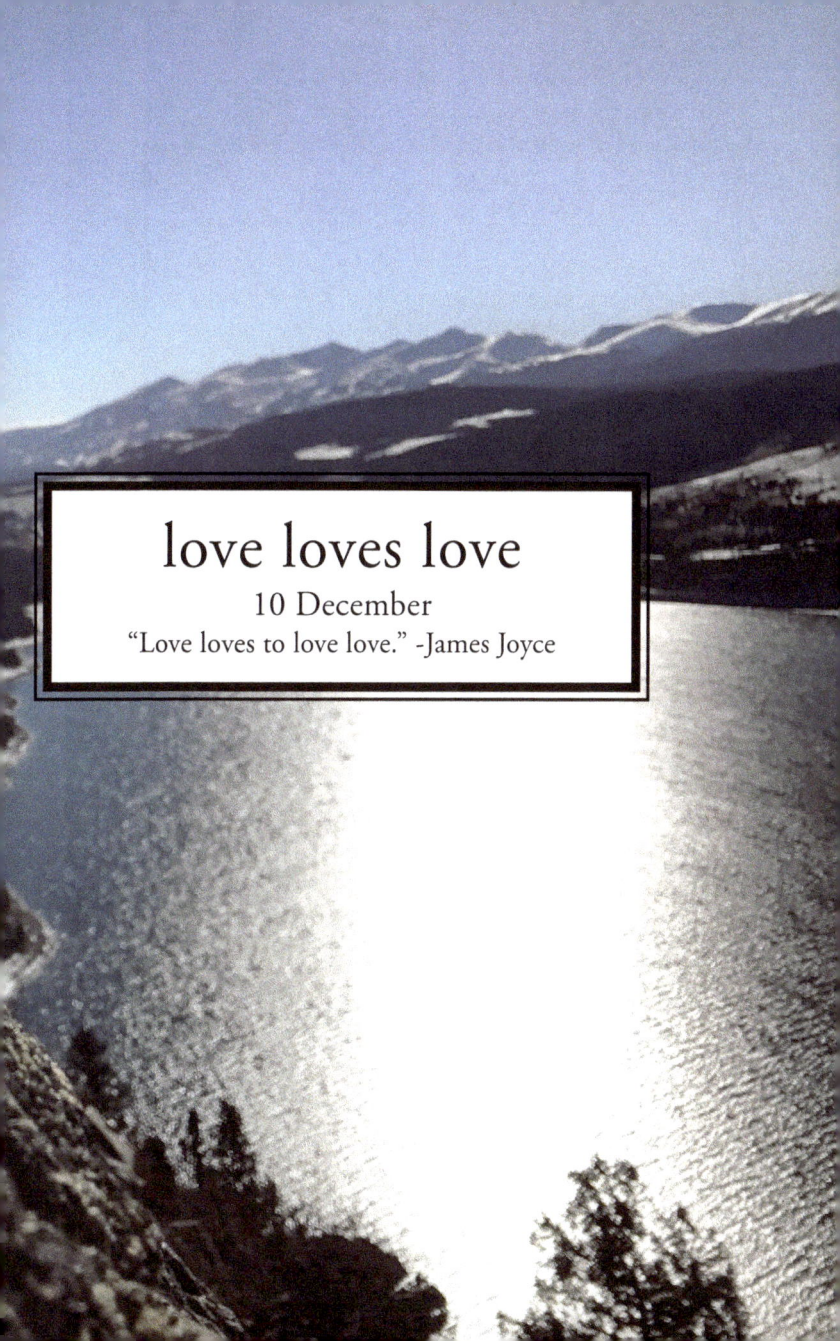

love loves love
10 December
"Love loves to love love." -James Joyce

pouring love
11 December

"What can you expect [from practicing] unconditional love? If you pour love into every single situation and every single person you meet, and beyond that to everyone on the planet and to the infinity of the universe, you will feel yourself becoming a different person: you will sleep more soundly; you will feel at peace virtually all of the time; your relationships will be more deeply spiritual; most significantly, you will begin recognizing the 'coincidences' of your life with greater regularity; your thought forms of unconditional love will begin to produce what you desire without your even being aware of how it is happening; your dreams will be more intense, and the vision of your purpose will become clearer."

-Wayne Dyer

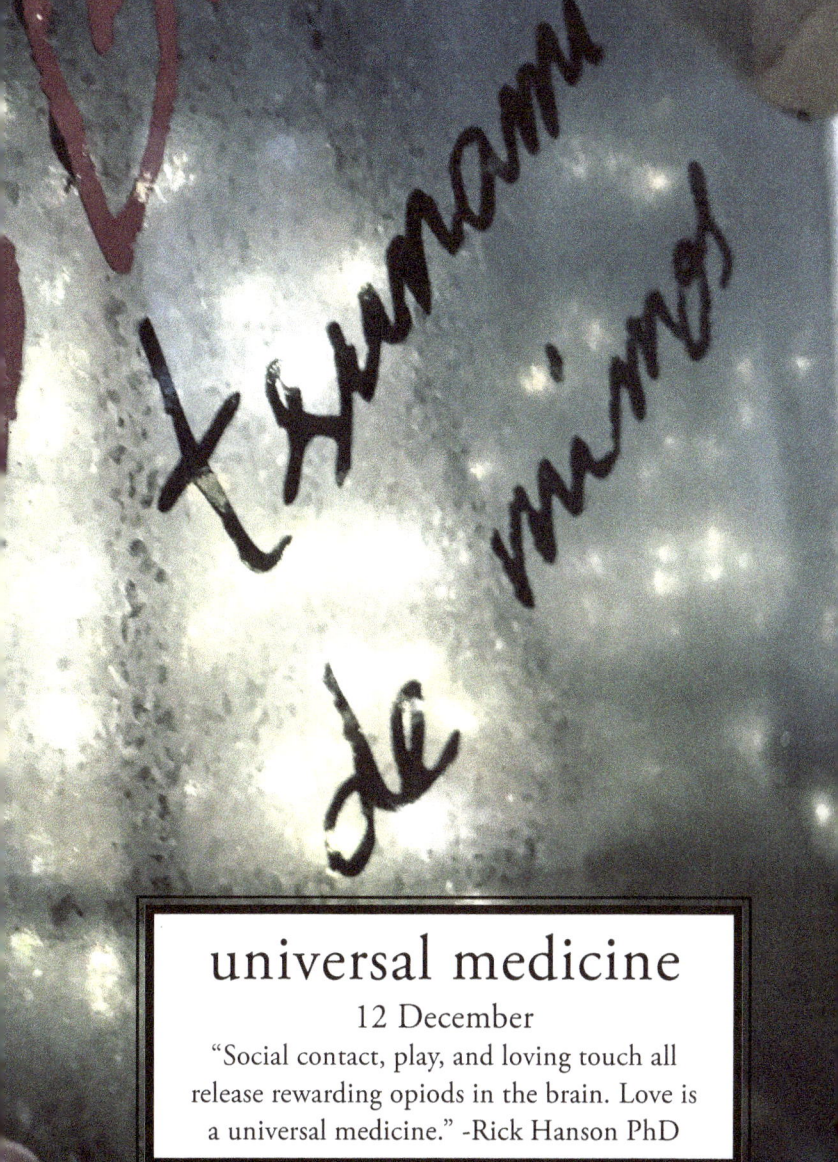

universal medicine
12 December
"Social contact, play, and loving touch all release rewarding opiods in the brain. Love is a universal medicine." -Rick Hanson PhD

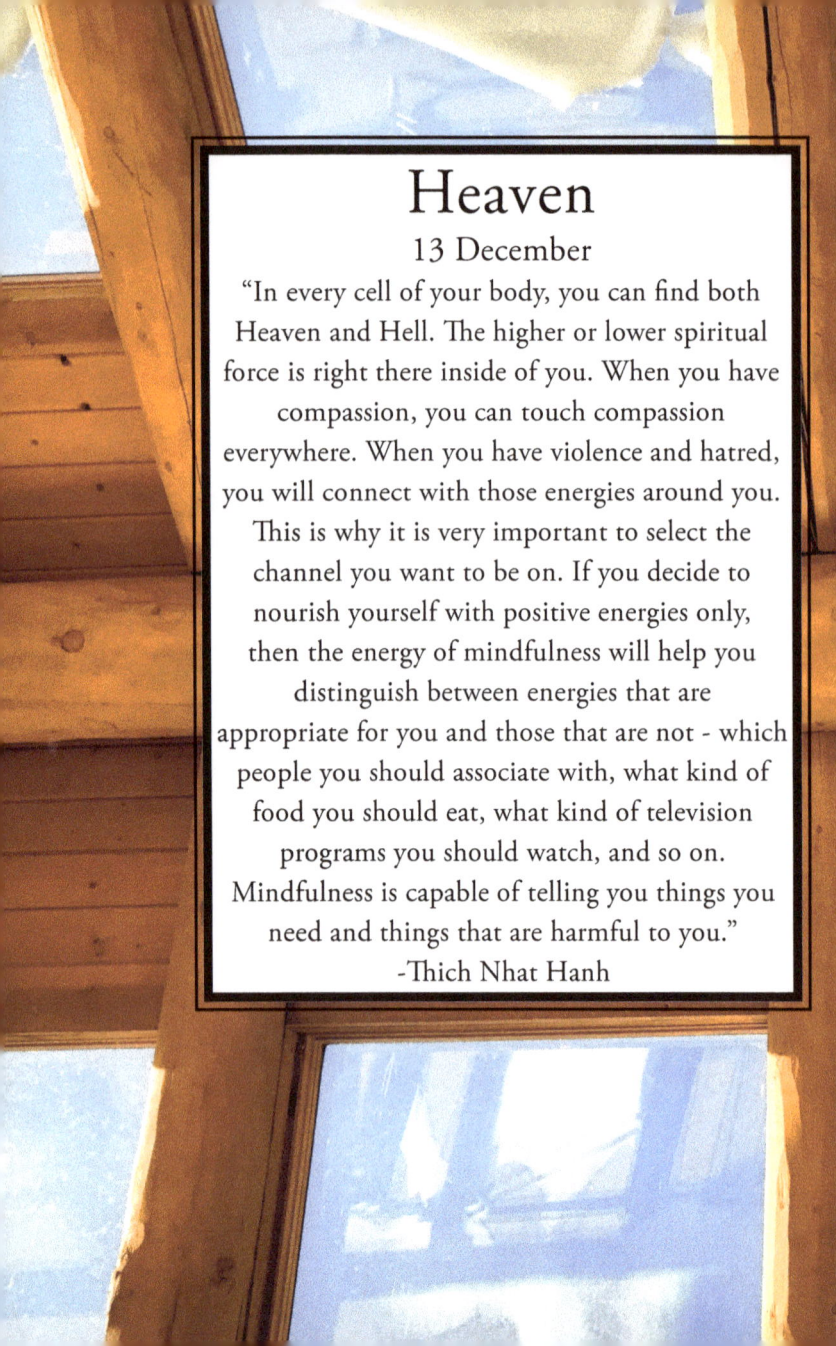

Heaven
13 December

"In every cell of your body, you can find both Heaven and Hell. The higher or lower spiritual force is right there inside of you. When you have compassion, you can touch compassion everywhere. When you have violence and hatred, you will connect with those energies around you. This is why it is very important to select the channel you want to be on. If you decide to nourish yourself with positive energies only, then the energy of mindfulness will help you distinguish between energies that are appropriate for you and those that are not - which people you should associate with, what kind of food you should eat, what kind of television programs you should watch, and so on. Mindfulness is capable of telling you things you need and things that are harmful to you."

-Thich Nhat Hanh

blooming genius
14 December

"Genius thrives in a contemplative environment, where every minute isn't filled with obligations or hoards of people offering advice and insisting on your constant participation in ordinary, mundane endeavors. The genius in you isn't seeking confirmation from others, but quiet space for its ideas to blossom. Genius isn't as much about achieving a big IQ on a standardized test, as it is the exceptionally high level of plain old savvy in any given field of human endeavor...an uncomplicated life with fewer intrusions tolerated, in a simple setting, allows your creative genius to surface and express itself." -Wayne Dyer

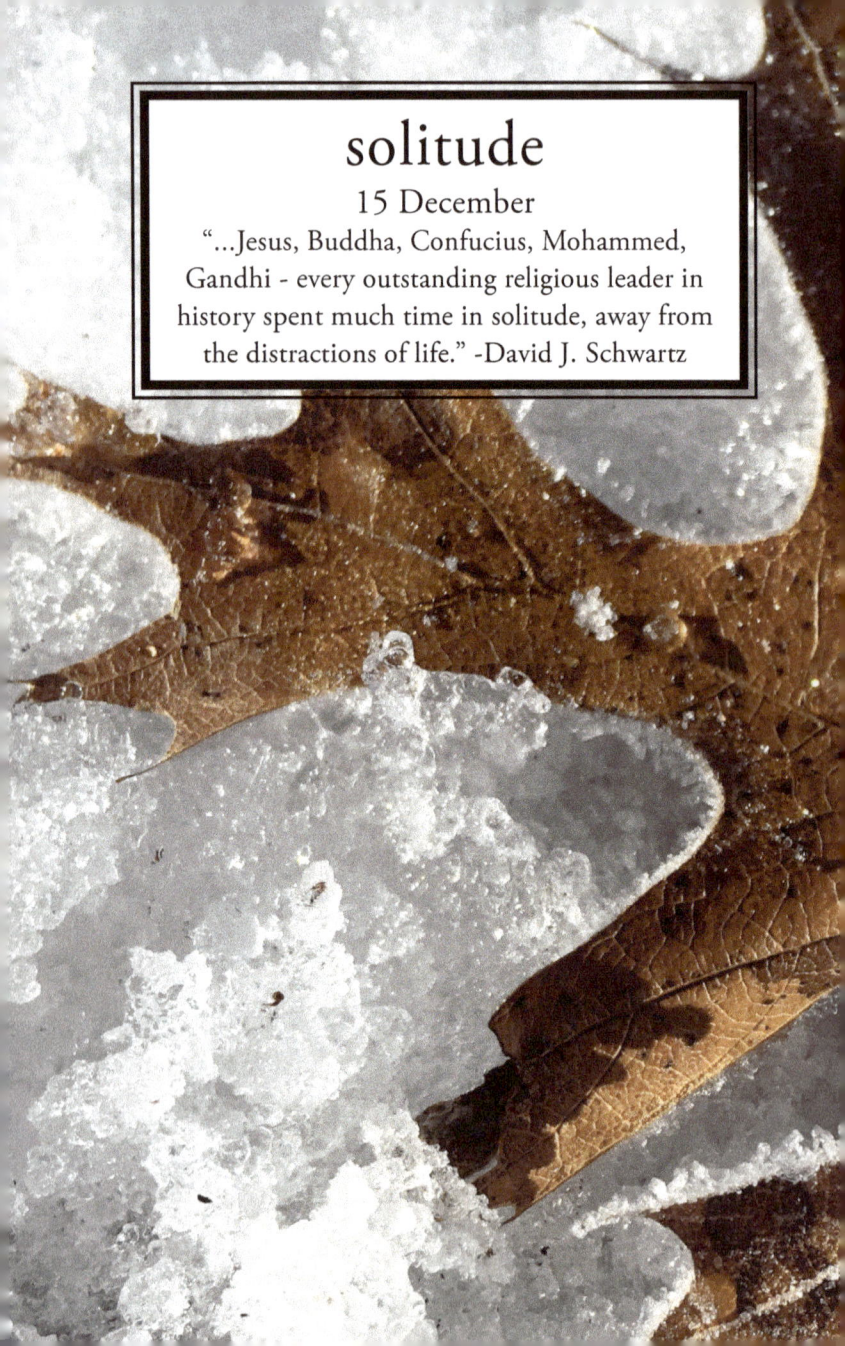

solitude
15 December
"...Jesus, Buddha, Confucius, Mohammed, Gandhi - every outstanding religious leader in history spent much time in solitude, away from the distractions of life." -David J. Schwartz

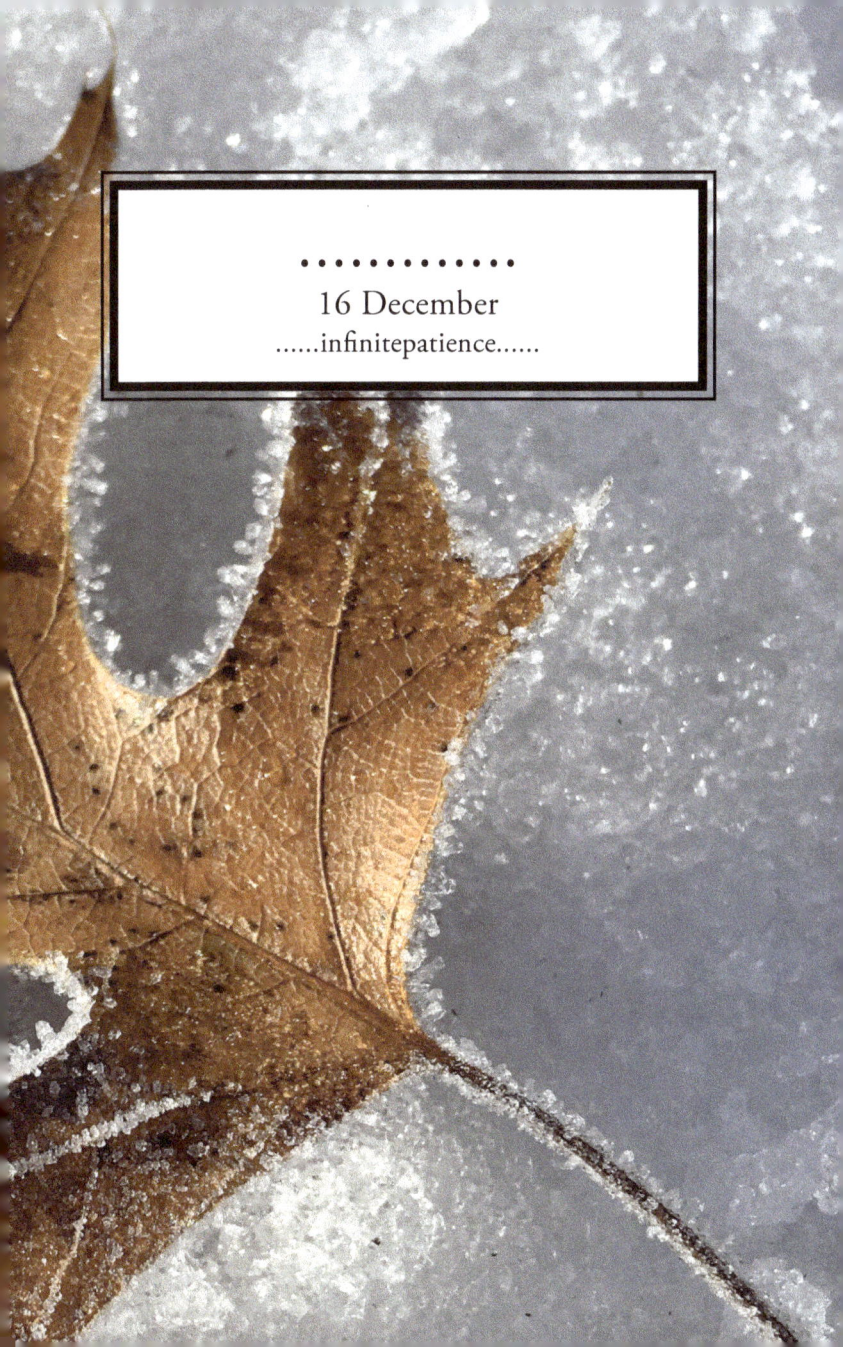

16 December
......infinitepatience......

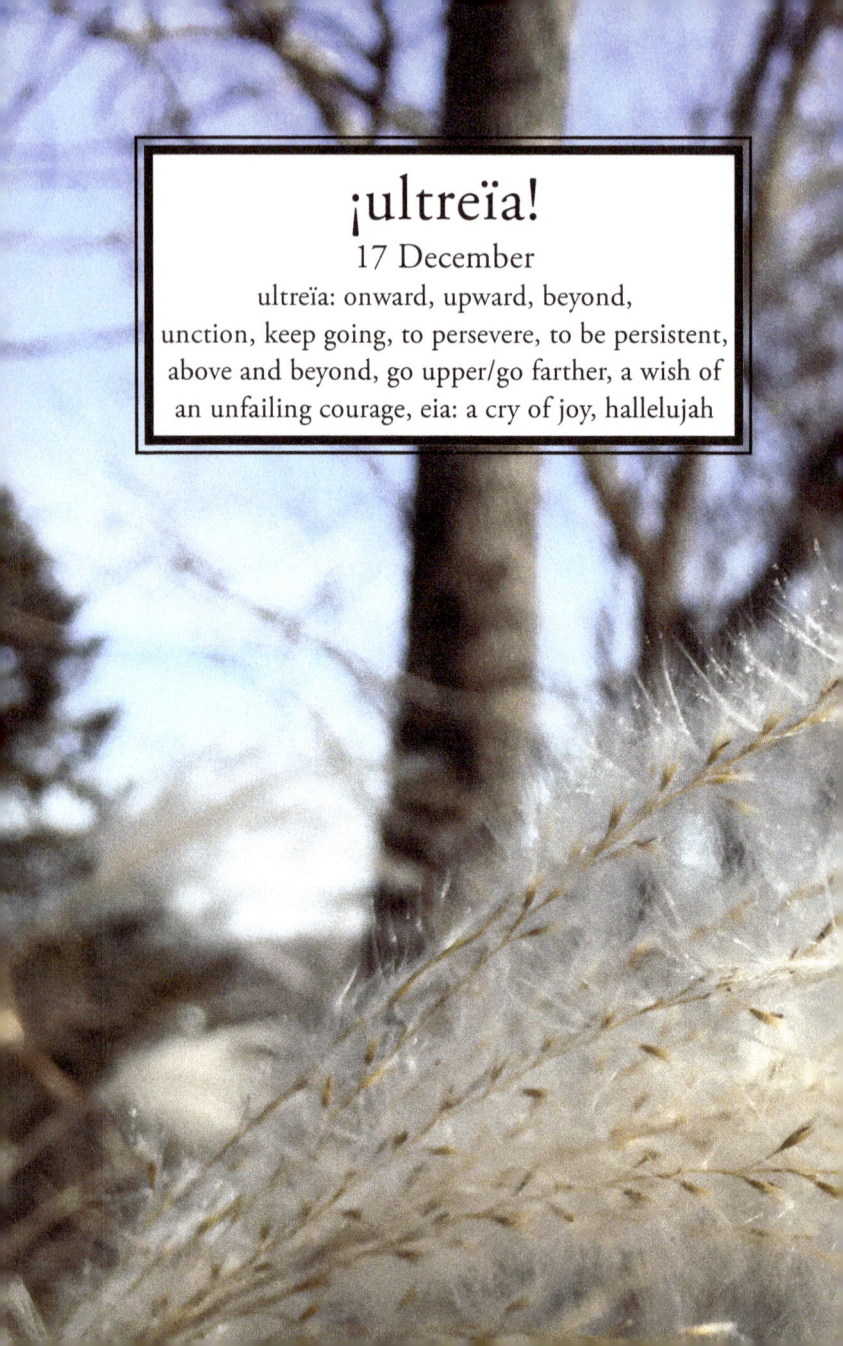

¡ultreïa!
17 December

ultreïa: onward, upward, beyond, unction, keep going, to persevere, to be persistent, above and beyond, go upper/go farther, a wish of an unfailing courage, eia: a cry of joy, hallelujah

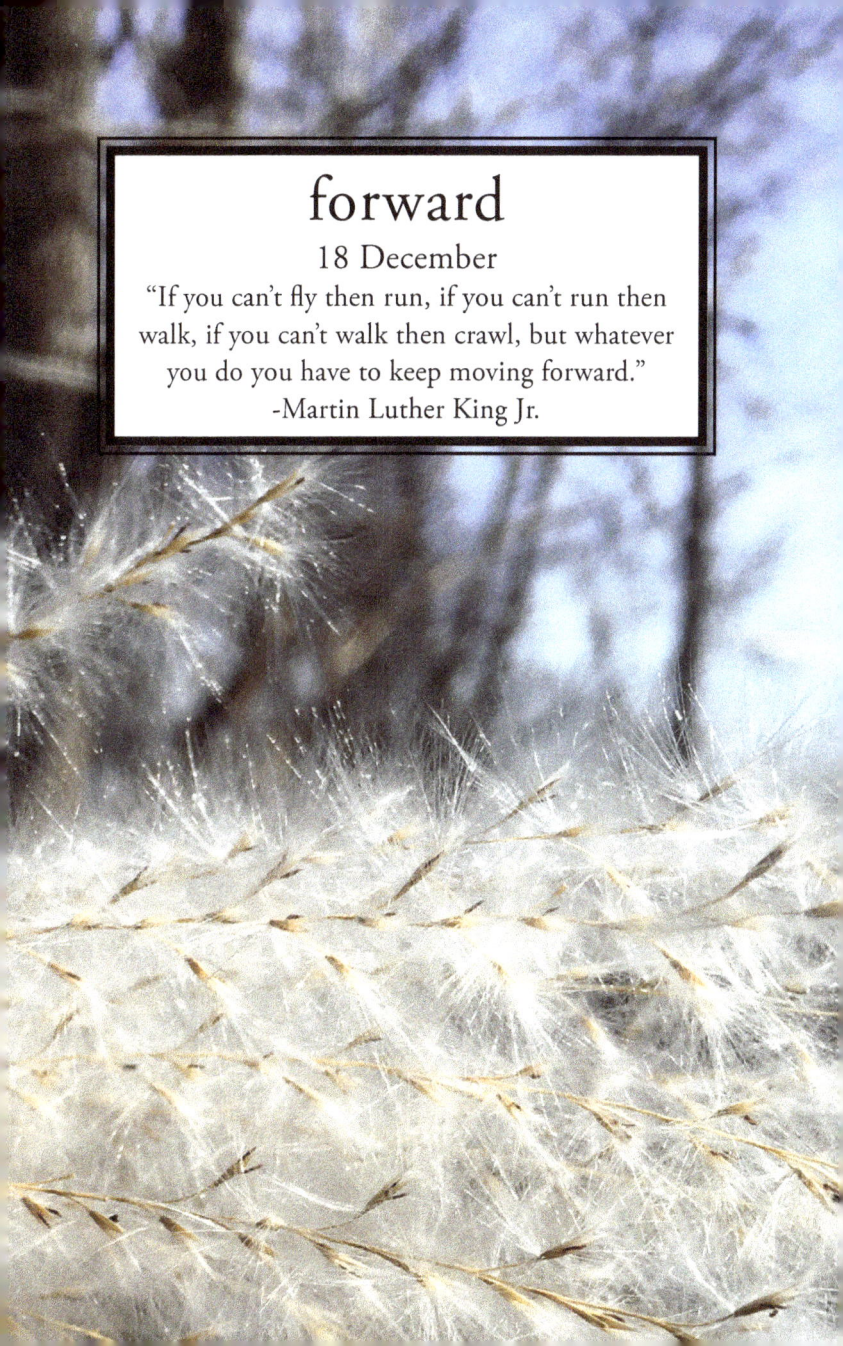

forward

18 December

"If you can't fly then run, if you can't run then walk, if you can't walk then crawl, but whatever you do you have to keep moving forward."
-Martin Luther King Jr.

rejuvenation
19 December

"One of the best-kept secrets for restful, rejuvenating sleep is the quality of your experiences during the day. When you live each moment completely and fully appreciate the world around you, you do not accumulate stress; therefore, dynamic daily activity directly benefits the quality of your sleep." -chopra.com

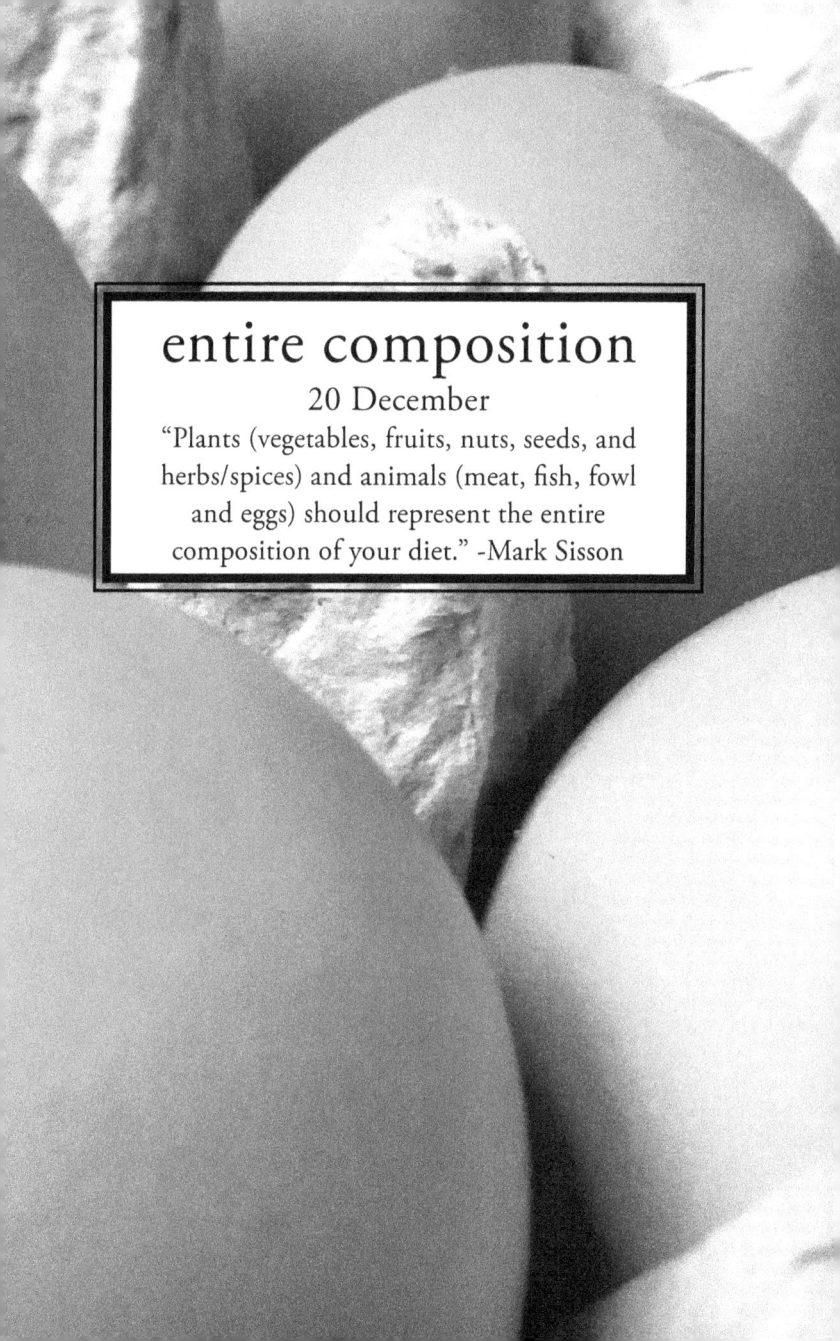

entire composition
20 December
"Plants (vegetables, fruits, nuts, seeds, and herbs/spices) and animals (meat, fish, fowl and eggs) should represent the entire composition of your diet." -Mark Sisson

L-O-V-E

21 December

"Love is composed of a single soul
inhabiting two bodies." -Aristotle

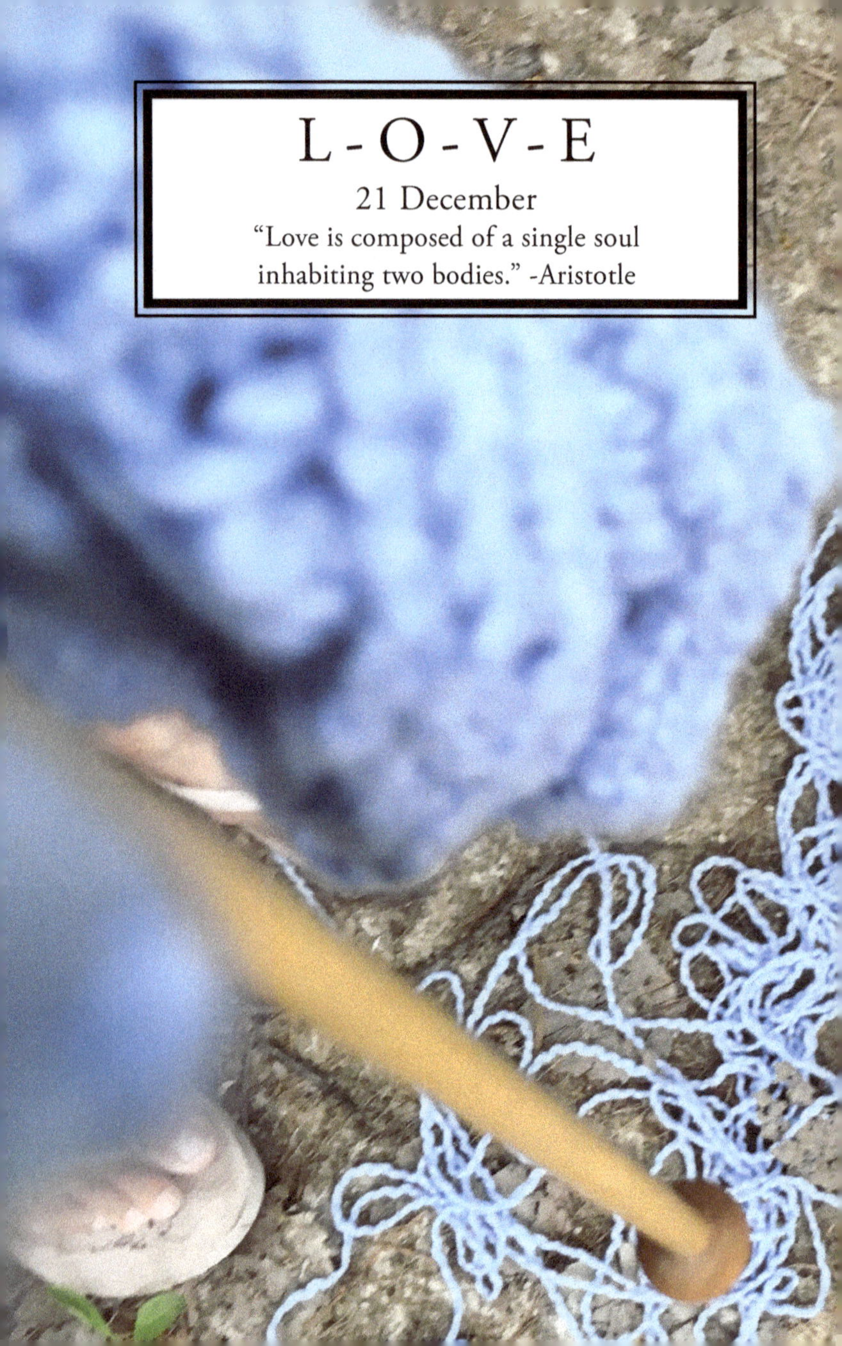

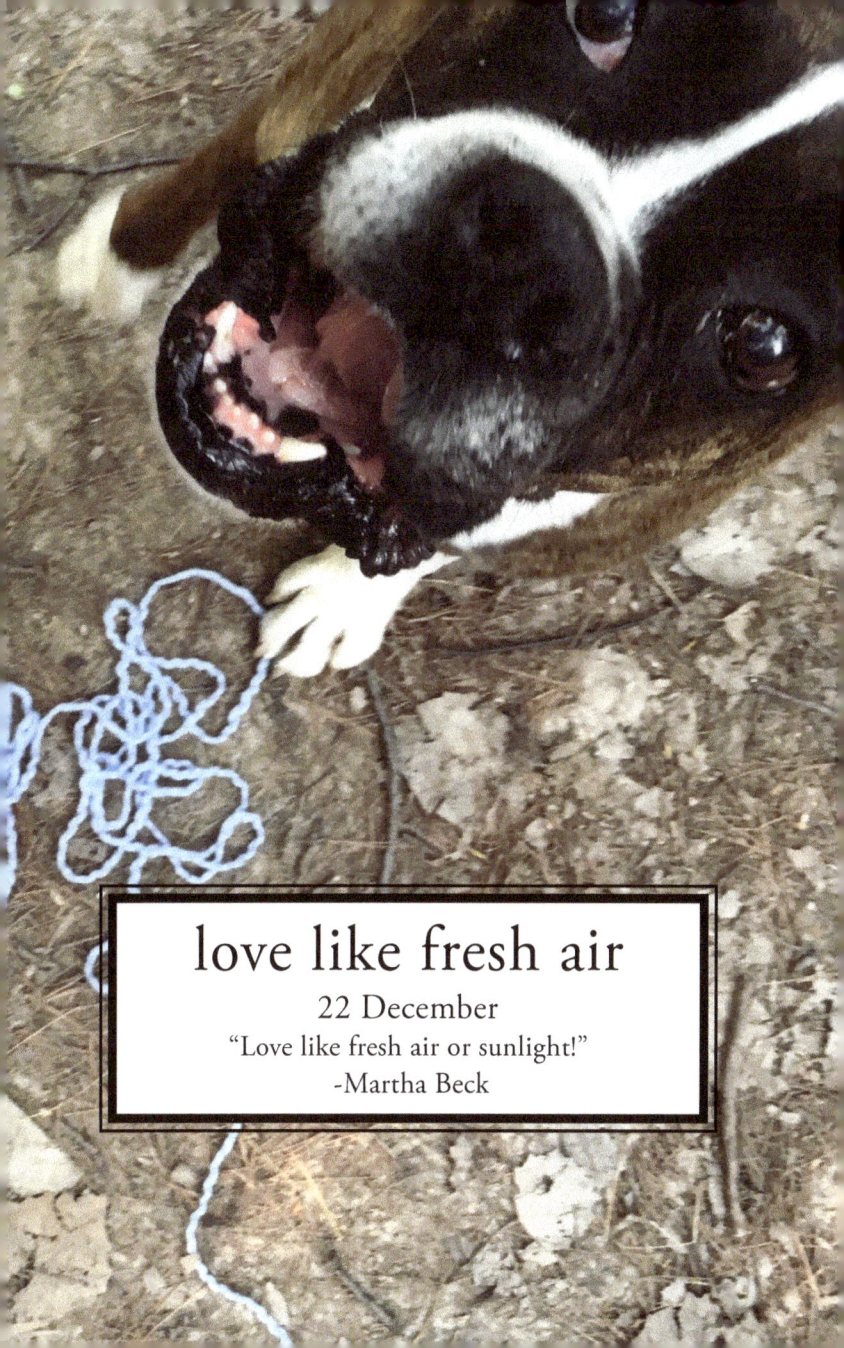

love like fresh air

22 December
"Love like fresh air or sunlight!"
-Martha Beck

doing my best
23 December
"Always do your best."
-Don Miguel Ruiz

ta-daaa
24 December
"self-actualization:
1. needs no approval
2. free of both criticism and flattery
3. feels neither superior to anyone nor inferior to anyone 4. experiences fearless action because detached from the influence of situations, circumstances, events and relationships"
-Deepak Chopra

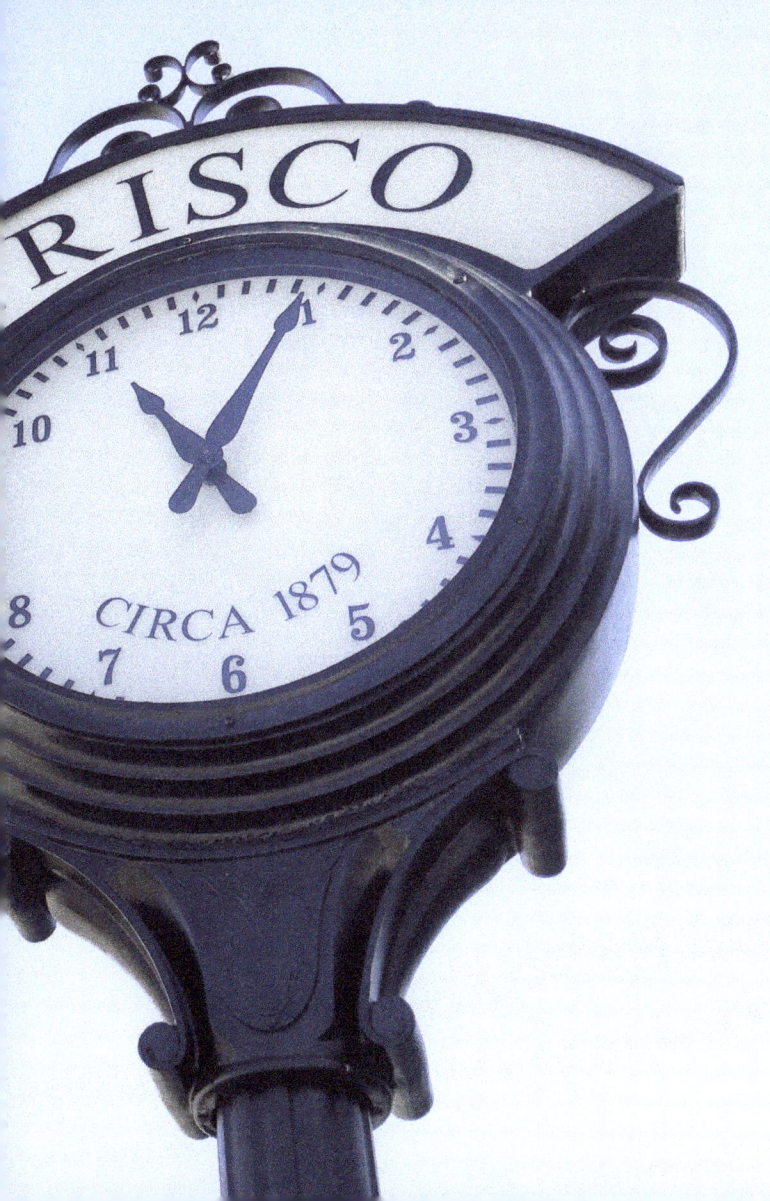

self-compassion

25 December

"Compassion: the wish that
a living being not suffer
kindness: the wish that a being be happy,
usually with feelings of warmth
self-compassion: compassion toward yourself and
a sense that many others have difficulties and
pains like your own (studies show self-compassion
lowers stress and self-criticism while increasing
resilience and self-worth)." -Rick Hanson PhD

LOVE

26 December
"Love is a deep empathy with the other's 'beingness.' You recognize yourself, your essence, in the other...so you can no longer inflict suffering on the other." -Eckhart Tolle

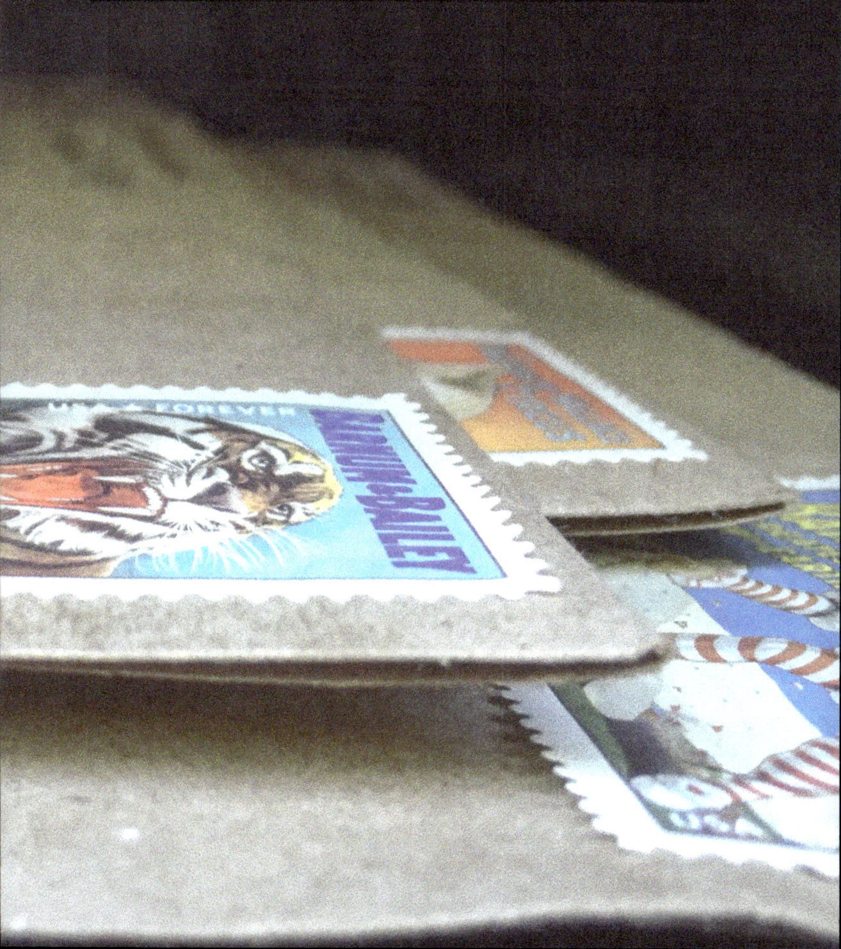

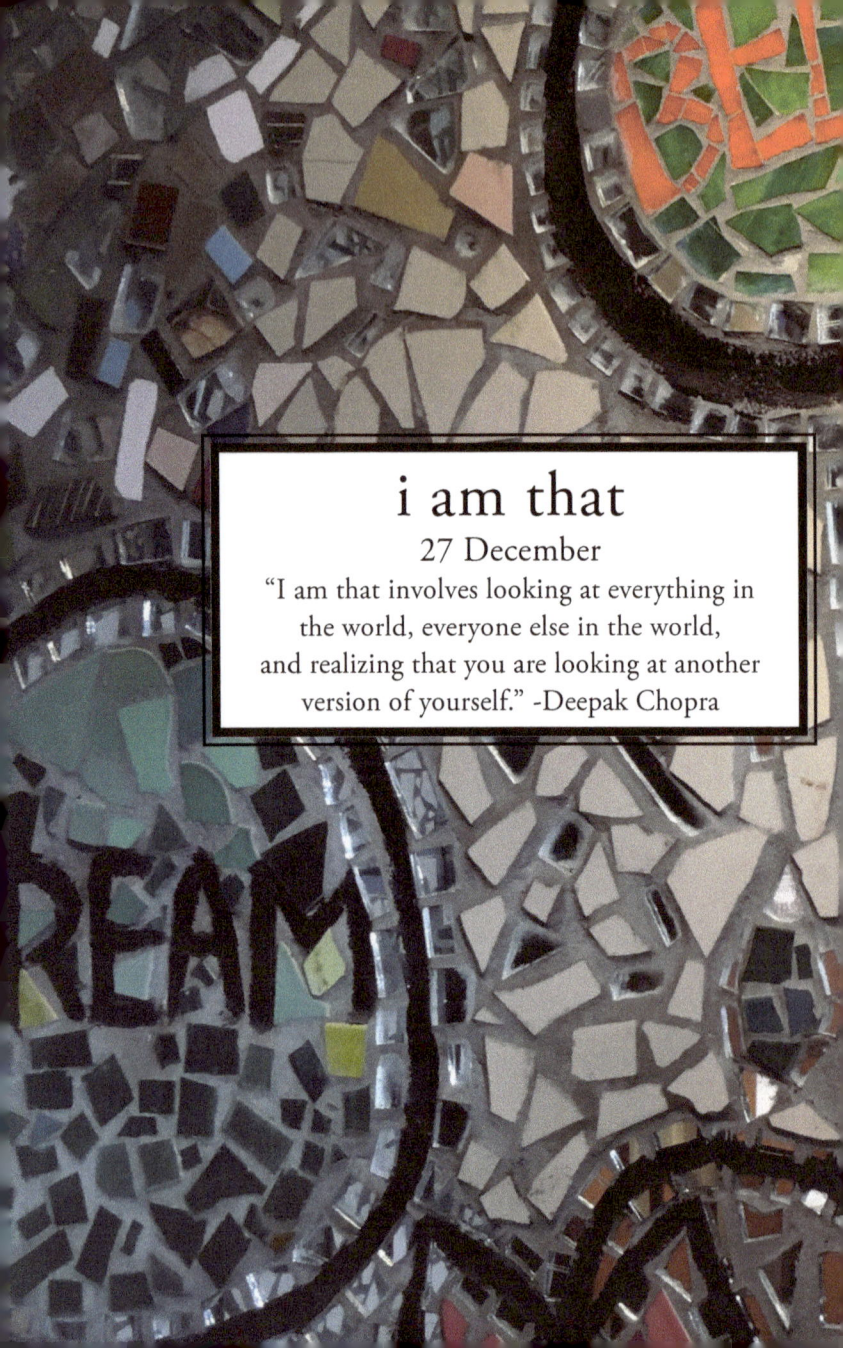

i am that
27 December
"I am that involves looking at everything in the world, everyone else in the world, and realizing that you are looking at another version of yourself." -Deepak Chopra

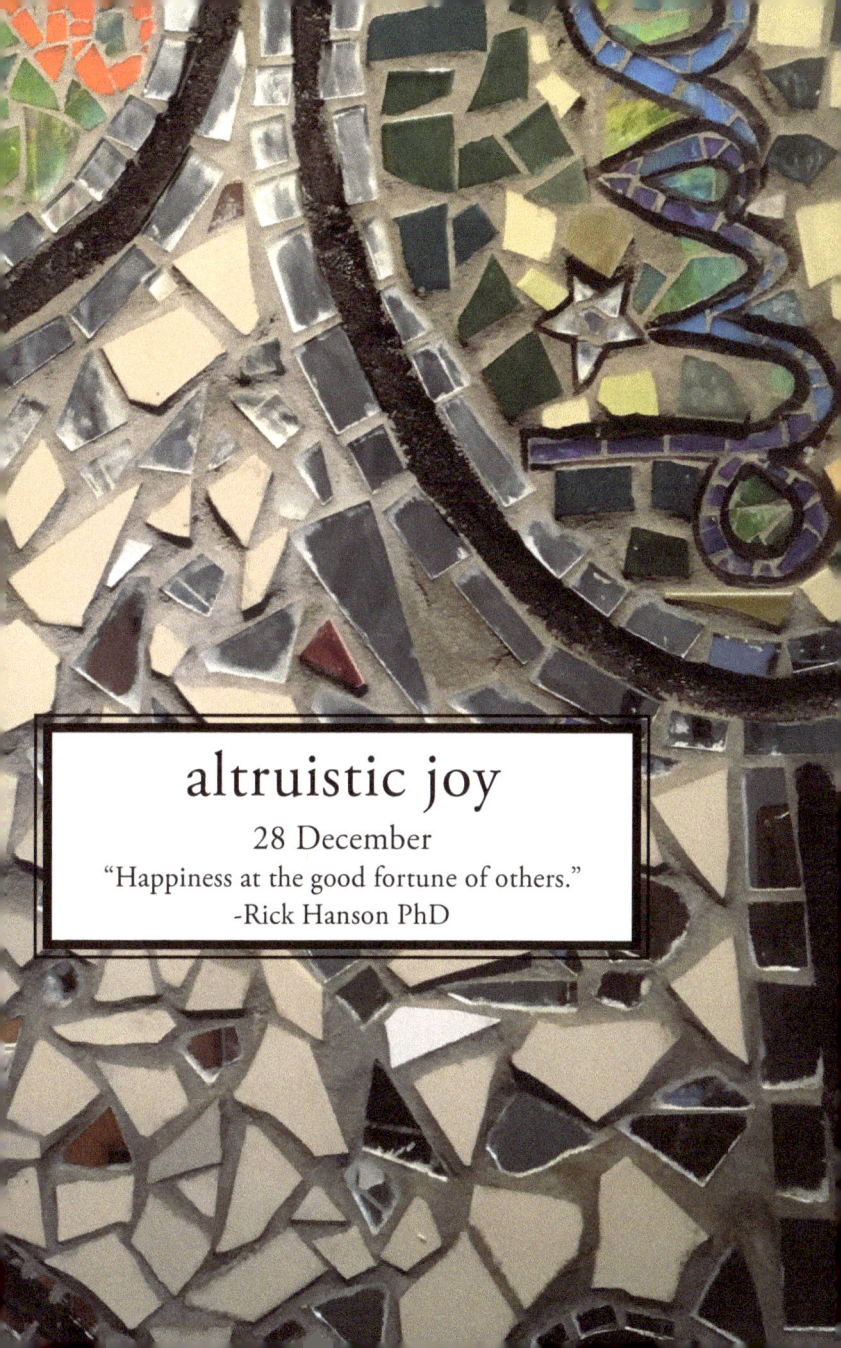

altruistic joy

28 December
"Happiness at the good fortune of others."
-Rick Hanson PhD

advice
29 December
"The quality of any advice anybody has to offer has to be judged against the quality of life they actually lead." -Douglas Adams (Guy Kawasaki)

thank you
30 December
"If the only prayer you said was thank you, that would be enough." -Meister Eckhart

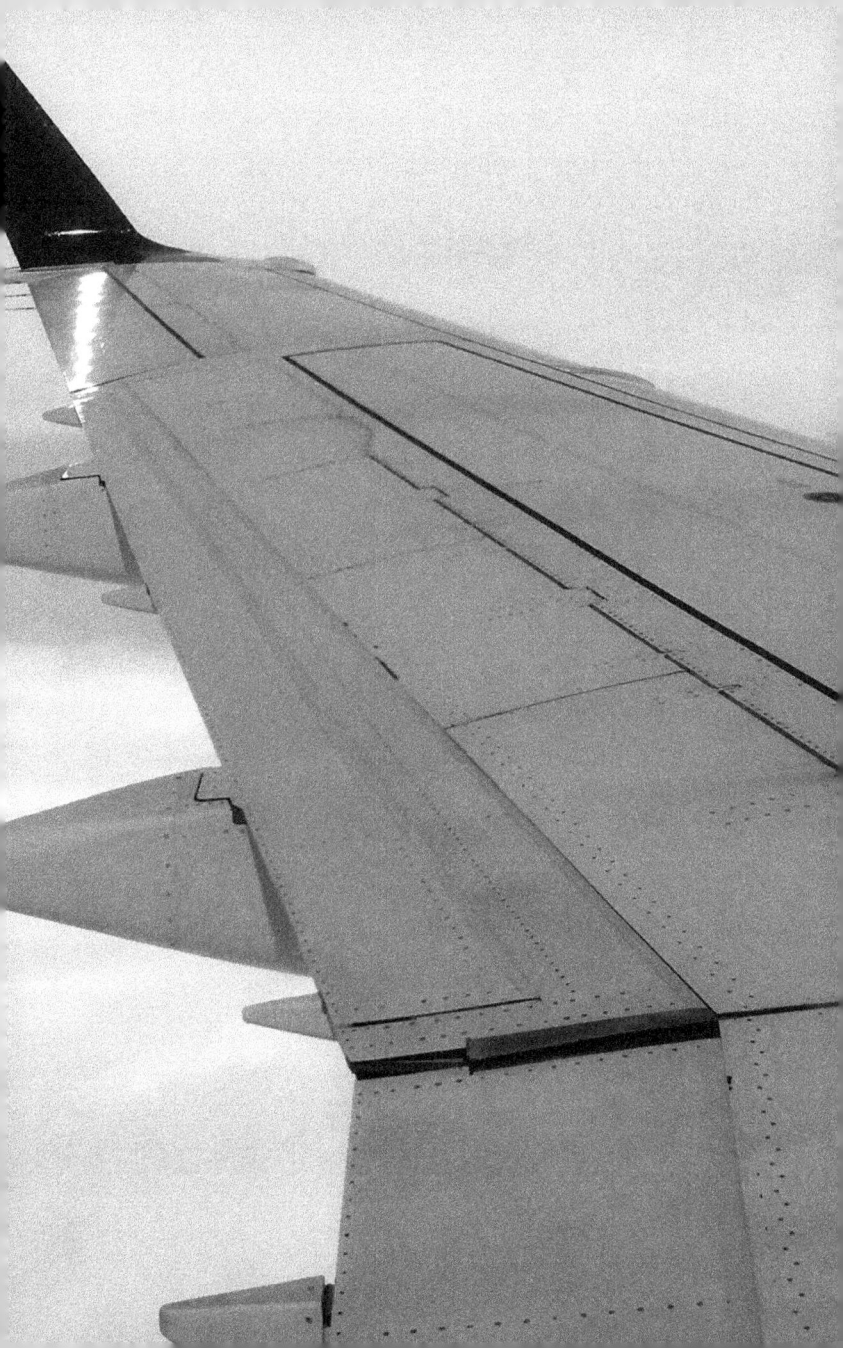

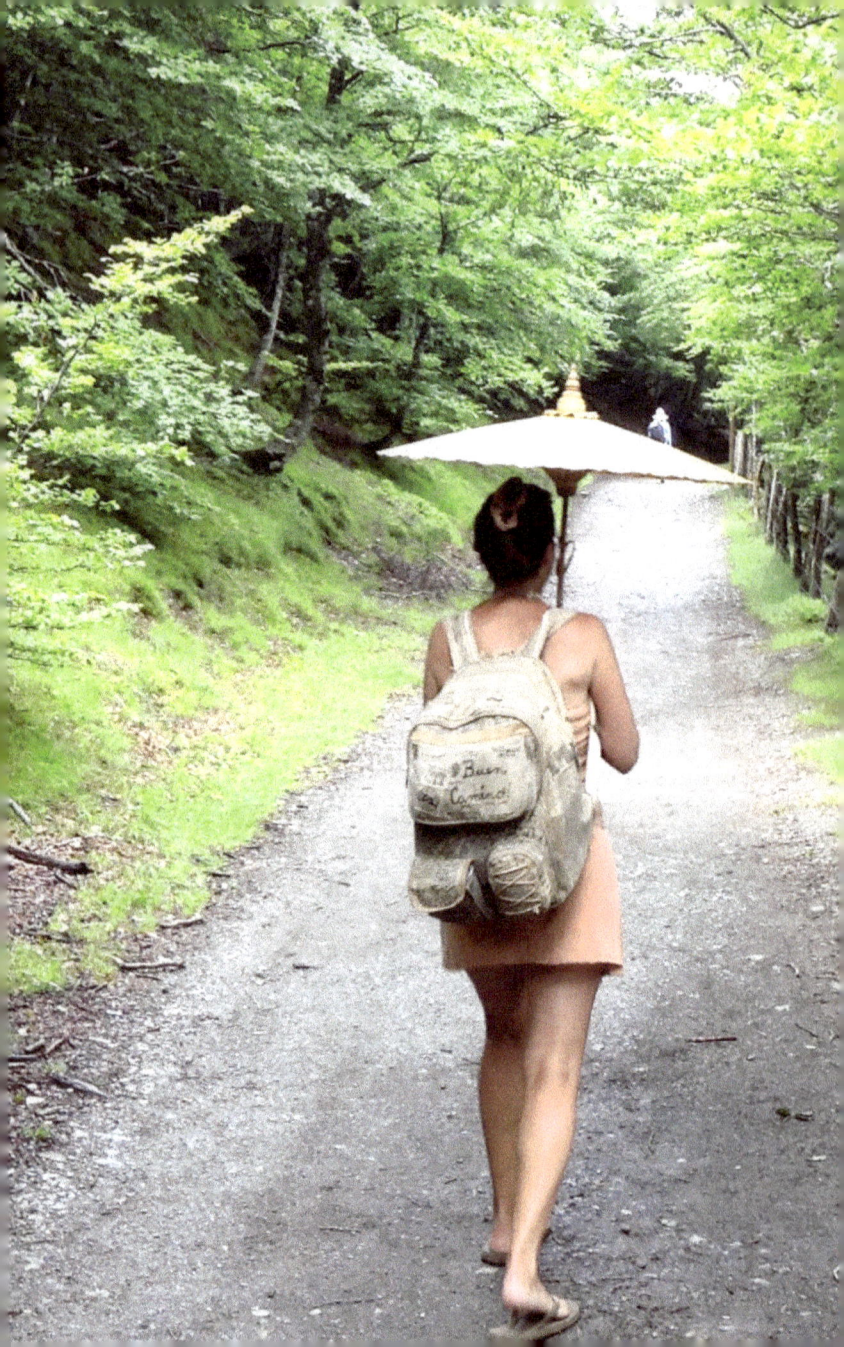

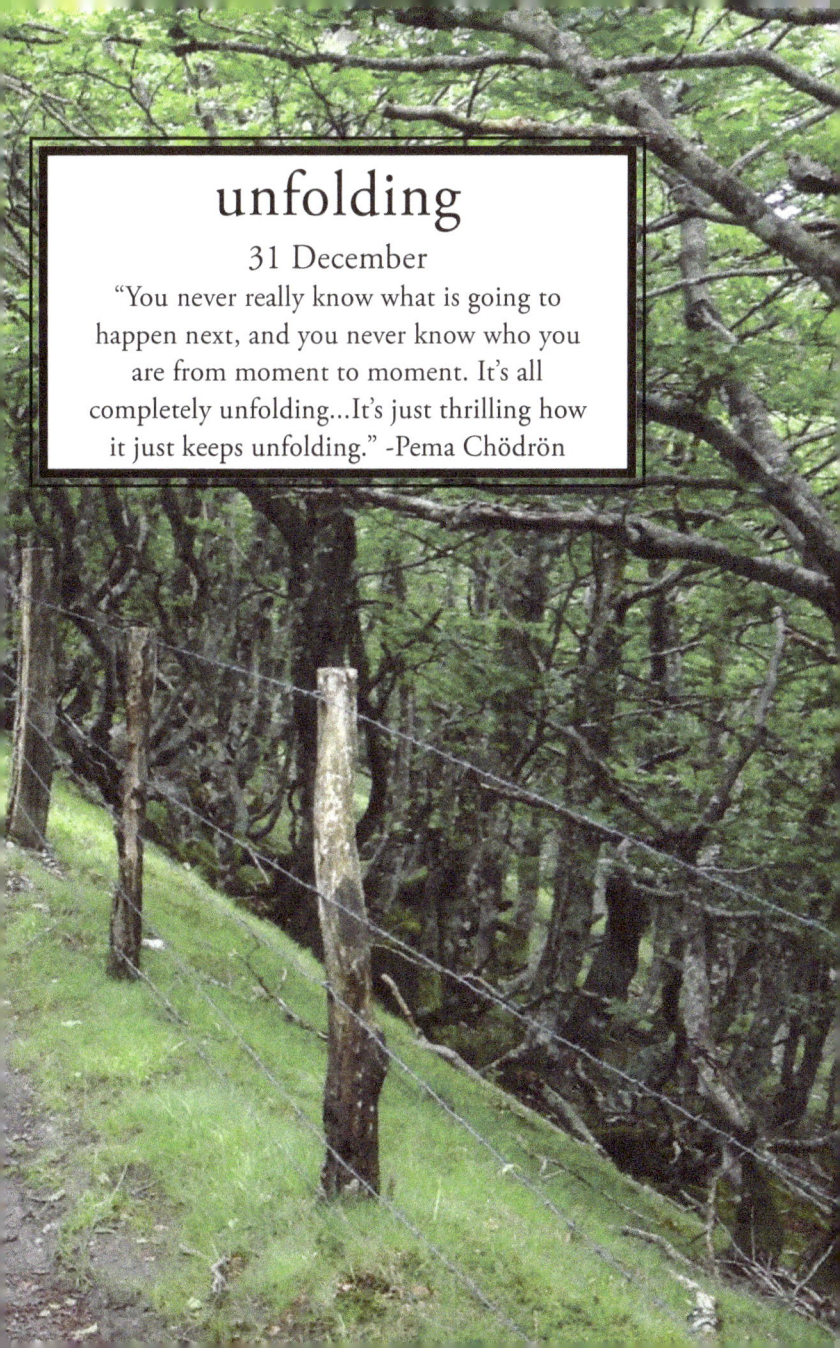

unfolding

31 December

"You never really know what is going to happen next, and you never know who you are from moment to moment. It's all completely unfolding…It's just thrilling how it just keeps unfolding." -Pema Chödrön

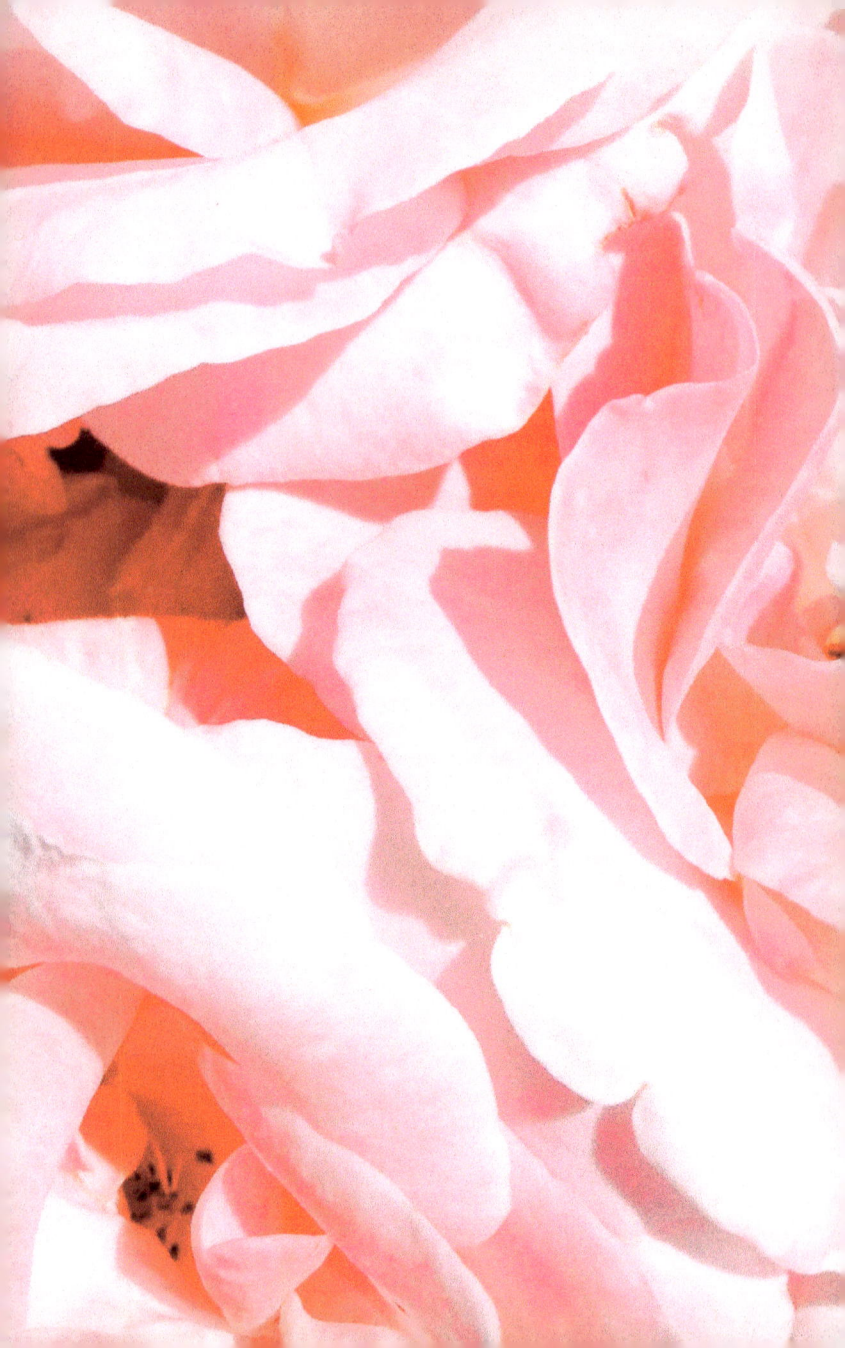

www.ingramcontent.com/pod-product-compliance
Lightning Source LLC
Chambersburg PA
CBHW040327300426
44113CB00020B/2673